Pediatric Cardiology: Diagnosis and Management

Pediatric Cardiology: Diagnosis and Management

Edited by Sara Thornton

AMERICAN
MEDICAL PUBLISHERS
www.americanmedicalpublishers.com

American Medical Publishers,
41 Flatbush Avenue,
1st Floor, New York,
NY 11217, USA

Visit us on the World Wide Web at:
www.americanmedicalpublishers.com

ISBN: 978-1-63927-423-9

Cataloging-in-Publication Data

Pediatric cardiology : diagnosis and management / edited by Sara Thornton.
p. cm.
Includes bibliographical references and index.
ISBN 978-1-63927-423-9
1. Pediatric cardiology. 2. Pediatric cardiology--Diagnosis. 3. Heart--Diseases--Treatment. I. Thornton, Sara.
RJ421 .P43 2021
618.921 2--dc23

Table of Contents

Preface

This book has been a concerted effort by a group of academicians, researchers and scientists, who have contributed their research works for the realization of the book. This book has materialized in the wake of emerging advancements and innovations in this field. Therefore, the need of the hour was to compile all the required researches and disseminate the knowledge to a broad spectrum of people comprising of students, researchers and specialists of the field.

Pediatric cardiology is a specialty of pediatrics that is concerned with the diagnosis and treatment of cardiac conditions in children. They may be affected by a number of heart conditions, some of which are structural abnormalities, while others involve impairments in the electrical system which controls the heartbeat. Congenital heart diseases include holes occurring between the heart chambers, abnormal blood vessels, valve defects, and abnormal heart rhythms or arrhythmias. Some of the focus areas in pediatric cardiology are the care of children in the cardiac ICU, heart catheterization and other interventional procedures, advanced cardiac imaging, heart failure, heart transplantation, etc. This book brings forth some of the most innovative concepts and elucidates the unexplored aspects of pediatric cardiology. The objective of this book is to give a general view of the different areas of this discipline. For all readers who are interested in pediatric cardiology, the case studies included herein will serve as an excellent guide to develop a comprehensive understanding.

At the end of the preface, I would like to thank the authors for their brilliant chapters and the publisher for guiding us all-through the making of the book till its final stage. Also, I would like to thank my family for providing the support and encouragement throughout my academic career and research projects.

Editor

1

Outcomes when congenital heart disease is diagnosed antenatally versus postnatally in the UK

Lewis K Peake*, Elizabeth S Draper, Judith LS Budd and David Field

Abstract

Background: For major congenital heart disease, the benefits of antenatal diagnosis on some post-natal measures have been suggested. However, findings have been inconclusive and focus on short term outcome measures alone with little data from a UK population. Our aim is to describe differences in reported outcomes for patients born with isolated Hypoplastic Left Heart Syndrome or Transposition of the Great Arteries in a UK population, following either antenatal or postnatal diagnosis.

Methods: Retrospective population-based study with case note review covering a 15 year period (1st January 1998 to 31st December 2012) in the British county of Leicestershire. Cases were identified from two local registers: the East Midlands and South Yorkshire Congenital Anomaly Register and a list of surgical patient held by the East Midlands Congenital Heart Centre.

Results: In total 52 cases of Hypoplastic Left Heart Syndrome or Transposition of the Great Arteries were identified with 24 (46.2%) diagnosed antenatally. Maximum and minimum follow up was 181 and 16 months respectively. Median follow up was 83 months (IQR: 44–111).

The risk of intubation in the postnatal period (OR: 4.64, 95% CI: 1.40 - 15.32) was greater in cases of Hypoplastic Left Heart Syndrome or Transposition of the Great Arteries diagnosed after birth when compared to those diagnosed antenatally. There was a non-significant increase in the risk of metabolic acidosis in the postnatal period (OR: 12.5, 95% CI: 0.64 - 245.46). No differences in mortality or long-term outcomes were demonstrated between antenatally and postnatally diagnosed cohorts.

Conclusions: These results confirm data from American and European populations that, for a British population, an antenatal diagnosis of a major congenital heart disease can have a favourable impact on some postnatal outcome measures. There appears to be no evidence that time of diagnosis impacts on long-term outcome measures.

Keywords: Heart defects, Congenital, Transposition of great vessels, Hypoplastic left heart syndrome, Prenatal diagnosis

Background

In the UK, one in 180 children is born with Congenital Heart Disease (CHD) [1]. Diagnosis can be made antenatally - something which has become increasingly common since the routine implementation of 20-week fetal anomaly scanning and the development of modern ultrasonography [2] - or following symptom presentation in the post natal period.

It has been suggested that short term outcomes in congenital heart disease would improve with antenatal diagnosis because birth in an appropriate setting can be planned in terms of the timing of delivery and immediate access to specialist staff and facilities [3]. In addition, those neonates without an antenatal diagnosis are at risk of discharge without their condition being identified, despite routine baby checks. Where the child is affected by major congenital heart disease that is essentially unstable, this can lead to haemodynamic compromise and result in emergency admission. Similarly, access to surgical intervention may be delayed, or else undertaken with the patient in a sub-optimal condition [4].

* Correspondence: lkpeake@doctors.org.uk
Department of Health Sciences, University of Leicester, Leicester LE1 6TP, UK

Despite this sound reasoning, and whilst improvements in some postnatal measures with an antenatal diagnosis have been demonstrated [5-8], such benefits have not been identified consistently. Much of the existing literature focuses on reviews that are based within tertiary care centres, thus limiting cases to a highly selective group with the greatest potential to survive. There is little reporting of longer term outcomes and sparse data concerning a relevant British population.

Objectives

The aim of the study was to explore the effect of antenatal diagnosis on congenital heart disease mortality and long term morbidity within a British population.

The specific objectives where to:

- Investigate if an antenatal diagnosis of transposition of the great arteries (TGA) or Hypoplastic left heart syndrome (HLHS) results in improved short term outcomes, i.e. neonatal mortality, risk of metabolic acidosis, Apgar score and need for intubation in the perinatal period.
- Investigate if an antenatal diagnosis of TGA or HLHS correlated with an improvement in long term outcomes, i.e. late mortality, neurodevelopmental deficits, ongoing symptoms and reliance on medication.

Methods

Study design

This study comprised a retrospective analysis of outcome data in patients diagnosed with Hypoplastic Left Heart Syndrome or Transposition of the Great Arteries whose mothers lived within the British county of Leicestershire, which has an annual birth rate of approximately 11,000 per year. From 2010 all pregnant women were offered fetal anomaly scanning at around 20 weeks of gestation. From 1998 to 2010 such scanning was offered to a significant proportion of women but was not universal.

Cases were identified from two separate sources: the East Midlands and South Yorkshire congenital anomalies register (EMSYCAR) and the cardiac surgical database held by the East Midlands Congenital Heart Centre (EMCHC). This cross validation of cases was used to ensure complete ascertainment and facilitate accuracy regarding the epidemiology of major congenital heart disease in Leicestershire. A standardised data collection proforma was used to gather information from the medical records.

Isolated Hypoplastic Left Heart Syndrome (HLHS) and Transposition of the Great Arteries (TGA) were chosen for investigation based on their relatively high case numbers locally, case homogeneity and existing literature suggesting a significant proportion of cases were diagnosed antenatally in pregnancies subject to fetal anomaly scanning.

Setting

All cases of Hypoplastic Left Heart Syndrome and Transposition of the Great Arteries born within the county of Leicestershire between 1st January 1998 and 31st December 2012 were identified. A case note review was then attempted. Identification was primarily through the East Midlands and South Yorkshire Congenital Anomalies Register [9]. This database collects data on all congenital anomalies diagnosed across its constituent counties and is one of a network of 12 regional/disease specific registers that make up the British Isles Network of Congenital Anomaly Registers (BINOCAR) [10]. A database of surgical patients held by the local tertiary care centre (East Midlands Congenital Heart Centre, EMCHC) was used for validation and identification of additional cases.

Participants

A search of the EMSYCAR database was undertaken for diagnoses of ICD-10 Q234 (HLHS) and Q203 (TGA) born in the study period. Cases were limited to those with a Leicestershire postcode at birth.

A separate list of cases was created from the database of surgical patients held by the EMCHC (Glenfield Hospital, Leicester) for the same period. Clinical notes were then reviewed and relevant data extracted. This comprised clinical information only to ensure anonymity and to comply with information governance; no patient identifiers were recorded.

Within the existing literature there is inconsistency in the approach to cases with a chromosomal diagnosis in terms of inclusion/exclusion [11-13]. Ultimately it was decided to exclude all cases with a confirmed chromosomal defect in order to provide a clearer picture of the implications of antenatal diagnosis for isolated defects.

Cases were also excluded if found to have additional cardiac defects outside those typically seen with diagnoses of HLHS or TGA. A ventricular septal defect in a case of TGA (a common association) was not an exclusion criterion. Cases with major extra-cardiac malformations likely to impact on morbidity or mortality were also excluded.

Variables

Data points collected were grouped into three life stages: the birth and postnatal period, the surgical period and the post-surgical period (see Table 1). Items within the surgical period group were incomplete for some cases due to intervention in hospitals outside of the East Midlands Congenital Heart Centre. All data were as documented in the clinical case notes.

Table 1 Collected data items

Birth/Postnatal period	
Birth status	Stillborn, Liveborn, Liveborn later died
Gestational age	Rounded to the nearest week
Delivery method	Vaginal, Assisted Vaginal, Elective C-S, Emergency C-S
Apgar @ 5 mins	
Acidosis in postnatal period	pH < 7.35 on any Arterial Blood Gas within postnatal period
Intubation	Needed mechanical ventilation prior to surgery
Surgical period	
Listed	Yes or No. If no, reason: i.e. Parental or MDT choice
Weight at time of surgery	*Grammes*
Age at time of surgery	*Days*
Cardiopulmonary bypass time	*Minutes*
Cross-clamp time	*Minutes*
Length of post-op ICU stay	*Hours* if <4 days; *days* if >4 days
Surgical mortality	Mortality between induction and post-op ICU discharge.
Post-surgical period	
Ongoing cardiac symptoms	Adjudged at max follow-up. E.g. SOB, decreased exercise tolerance
Ongoing cardiac medications	Adjudged at max follow-up. E.g. β-blockers, Diuretics
Need for re-intervention	
Neurodevelopmental impairment	Referral to specialist service (e.g. SALT) or specific diagnosis (e.g. Cerebral Palsy of Developmental delay)
Mortality	

Summary of the data items collected for each case, split into the postnatal period, surgical period and the post-surgical/long-term period.
SOB: Shortness of Breath. SALT: Speech and Language Therapist.

Study size

As a local population-based study, it was limited by the number of cases of HLHS and TGA born within the available time-frame of 15 years, the period of data collection for the EMSYCAR database.

Statistical methods

Data were collated and analysed with IBM SPSS Statistics 20. Antenatal detection rates for each condition were compared to the 50% target set by the Fetal Anomaly Screening Programme (FASP) [14]. Comparisons between the outcomes detected in the antenatal and postnatal cohorts were made, with odds ratios and 95% confidence intervals calculated. Where data items were missing from the notes, cases were excluded from the specific outcome analysis between cohorts.

Ethics

Ethics permission was provided by the Trent research ethics committee in relation to the East Midlands and South Yorkshire Congenital Anomalies Register.

Results

Participants

Search of both databases identified 32 HLHS and 52 TGA cases. Two of the HLHS cases identified from EMSYCAR were later downgraded to milder cardiac defects (Shone's Complex and Patent Foramen Ovale with Ventricular Septal Defect) and were excluded from analysis. Four HLHS and 11 TGA cases were excluded due to an association with a chromosomal diagnosis or for concurrent cardiac defects (see Figure 1).

At case note review, a further 15 cases (Four HLHS and 11 TGA) had to be excluded as insufficient clinical data could be accessed. Total cases used in the final analysis numbered 22 for HLHS and 30 for TGA. Perinatal outcome analysis was also carried out for both conditions combined. This was based on all 52 cases; 24 in the antenatally detected cohort and 28 in the postnatally detected cohort (see Figure 1).

Descriptive data

Case characteristics are outlined in Table 2. The maximum and minimum follow up periods were 181 and 16 months respectively. Median follow up was 83 months (IQR: 44–111).

In the HLHS group nearly three quarters were antenatally diagnosed. There were no significant differences between the birth weight or gestational age in the antenatally and postnatally detected cohorts and all but one case for each cohort had surgery. For the TGA group, two thirds were postnatally diagnosed and there were no

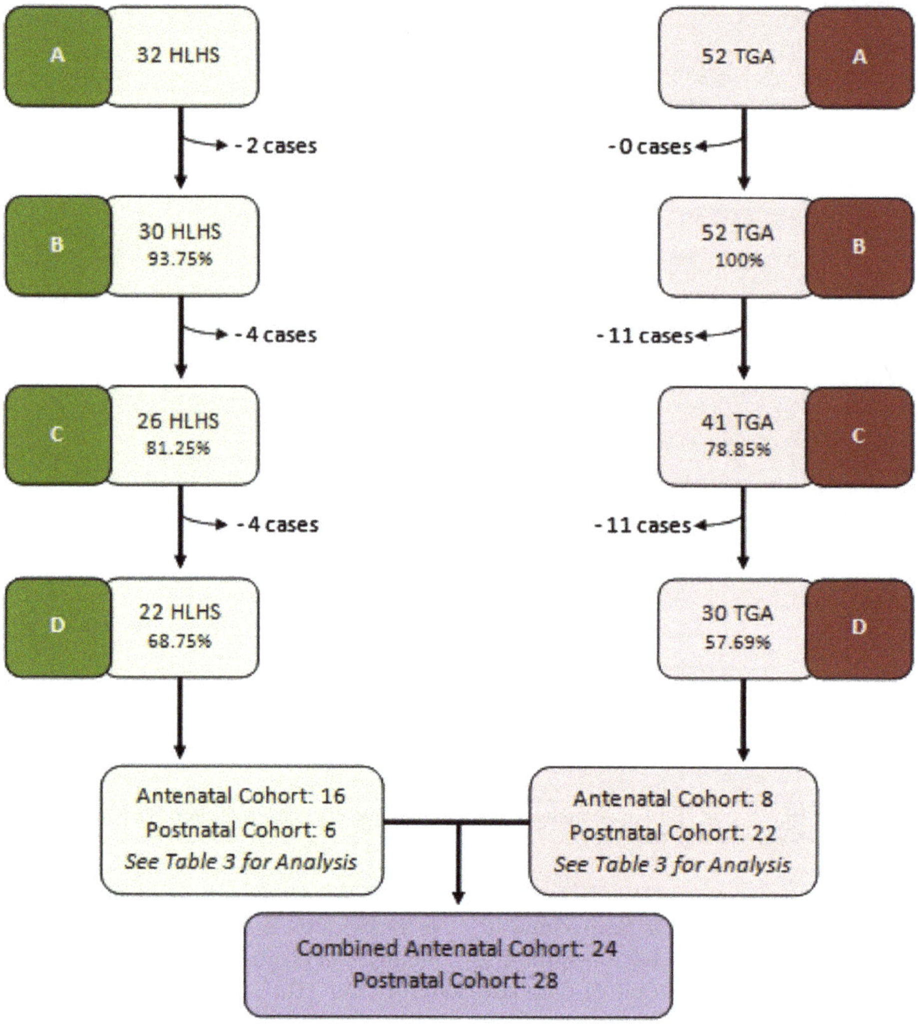

Figure 1 Summary of case inclusion/exclusion. Summary of case numbers of TGA and HLHS and those lost due to exclusion. Antenatal and postnatal cohorts were compared for each diagnosis, then collectively. **A**: Number of cases identified from EMSYCAR and EMCHC database searches. **B**: All cases minus those excluded due to change of diagnosis at birth. **C**: Minus those excluded due to chromosomal diagnosis. **D**: Minus those excluded due to extra-cardiac manifestations or cardiac complexity.

significant differences in birth weight or gestational age between the antenatally and postnatally diagnosed cohorts.

Outcome data

Outcome measures for the antenatal and postnatal cohorts of HLHS and TGA are presented in Table 3 and Table 4.

For HLHS, the major differences between the two cohorts were in the postnatal measures. Of the antenatal cohort, 75% had a recorded metabolic acidosis compared to 100% in the postnatal cohort - OR: 4.68 (95% CI: 0.21 - 100.99). The antenatal cohort was less likely to require intubation and mechanical ventilation in the postnatal period but due to the small numbers the odds ratio did not quite reach significance: 31.3% vs. 83.3% - OR: 11 (95% CI: 1.00 - 120.44). Assessment of the surgical measures was difficult for the HLHS group as many patients received surgery outside of the local tertiary paediatric cardiac care centre. Neither cohort experienced significantly better long-term outcome measures such as ongoing symptoms (Antenatal: 80%, Postnatal: 25% - OR: 0.08 (95% CI: 0.01 - 1.29)), neurodevelopmental issues (Antenatal: 20%, Postnatal: 20%) or long-term mortality (see Table 3).

For the TGA group, there was also a difference in the numbers requiring intubation in the postnatal period. Intubation was documented in just one case (12.5%) of antenatally diagnosed neonates with TGA, compared to 12 (54.5%) of those diagnosed postnatally - OR: 8.40 (95% CI: 0.88 - 80.27). Surgical measures could be assessed for this group, but no difference in age at surgery ($p = 0.39$), weight at surgery ($p = 0.40$) or length of post-op ICU stay

Table 2 Patient characteristics by diagnosis

	HLHS (Ant)	HLHS (Post)	OR (95% CI) or p-value
Number of cases	16	6	
Antenatally diagnosed, %	72.7		
Gender:			
Female, n(%)	11 (68.8)	2 (33.3)	
Male, n(%)	5 (31.2)	4 (66.7)	
Median birth weight, g(IQR)	3042 (2720–3392)	3780 (3490–4100)	p = 0.08
Median gestational age, weeks(IQR)	39 (38–39)	40.5 (38–42)	p = 0.17
C-Section, n(%)	4 (25.0)	2 (33.3)	1.50 (0.20 - 11.54)
Received surgical intervention, n(%)	15 (93.8)	5 (83.3)	3.00 (0.16 - 57.37)
	TGA (Ant)	**TGA (Post)**	**OR (95% CI) or p-value**
Number of cases	8	22	
Antenatally diagnosed, %	36.4		
Gender:			
Female, n(%)	1(12.5)	2 (9.1)	
Male, n(%)	7 (87.5)	20 (90.9)	
Median birth weight, g(IQR)	3525 (3415–3870)	3400 (3200–3600)	p = 0.49
Median gestational age, weeks(IQR)	39 (38–41)	40 (38.5 - 41)	p = 0.37
C-section, n(%)	1 (12.5)	3 (13.6)	1.10 (0.10 - 12.47)
Received surgical intervention, n(%)	8 (100)	21 (95.5)	1.19 (0.04 - 32.08)

This table summarises the case characteristics for HLHS and TGA patients by diagnostic stage. There were no significant differences in birth parameters between the antenatal and postnatal cohort. The strong predominance for Male Transposition of the Great Arteries cases is unexpected and unexplained.

($p = 0.89$) was found. Similarly there were no differences in long-term outcome measures between the two cohorts.

When the two diagnoses were combined (see Table 5), there was a significant difference in the risk of requiring intubation for those diagnosed postnatally - OR: 4.64 (95% CI: 1.40 - 15.32). There was also an increased risk of metabolic acidosis - OR: 12.5 (95% CI: 0.64 - 245.46) but this was not significant. The only patients to die within the first week of life across both diagnoses were diagnosed postnatally.

Discussion

Key results

This study has highlighted two specific outcomes where an antenatal diagnosis is favourable - risk of metabolic acidosis and need for postnatal intubation. The finding is seen most clearly in the combined cohorts and this approach of combining the effect on differing anomalies has been reported previously in the American and European literature for both outcomes [7,8]. Our findings suggest that antenatal diagnosis of HLHS and TGA in the UK results in improved perinatal outcomes. However in relation to the increased risk of intubation in the postnatally diagnosed cohort this could reflect a more cautious approach to treatment in this patient group where, at presentation, there is often a range of diagnostic possibilities. Conversely, where a provisional diagnosis already exists treating clinicians may be prepared to adopt a more conservative approach to management. We noted no difference in later outcomes or in terms of overall survival when comparing antenatally and postnatally diagnosed cases.

Interpretation

The impact of antenatal diagnosis on some perinatal outcomes has been reported previously. Fuchs et al. [5] investigated >250 patients over a 10 year period across four different diagnoses (including TGA), with an 83% antenatal detection rate. The maximum follow up period was 130 months, with a median of 37.8 months. In the prenatally diagnosed cohort, evidence of pre-operative cardiac failure, need for re-surgery and duration of post-operative ICU stay were all found to be significantly favourable ($p\text{-value} \leq 0.05$) compared to those diagnosed postnatally. Long-term, they found no difference in dependency on cardiac medication or long term survival between the two groups. However, being based in a tertiary care centre, they were unable to include patients without a prenatal diagnosis who died before they were transferred to their unit.

Calderon et al. [6] also explored some longer term outcomes, specifically the effect of prenatal detection of

Table 3 Outcome measures for antenatally, postnatally diagnosed HLHS

Hypoplastic left heart syndrome		Antenatal diagnosis	Postnatal diagnosis	OR (95% CI) or p-value
Liveborn cases		16	6	
Case status				
Liveborn - alive:		10	5	
Liveborn - later died:		6	1	
Postnatal	Median Apgar Score	9	9	n/a
	Pre-operative Acidosis, *n(%)*	12 (75.0)	6 (100.0)	4.68 (0.21 - 100.99)
	Intubation, *n(%)*	5 (31.3)	5 (83.3)	11 (1.00 - 120.44)
	Mortality within first week, *n(%)*	0 (–)	1 (16.7)	n/a
Surgical	Attempted Surgery, *n*	15	5	n/a
	Median Age at Surgery (IQR), *days*	3.5 (3–7.5)	7 (5–21.5)	p = 0.16
	Median Weight at Surgery (IQR), *gram*	3060 (2900–3510)	3900 (2360–4200)	n/a
	Median Bypass Time (IQR), *mins*	153 (123.5 - 192.5)	134 (117–151)	n/a
	Length of ICU Stay Post Surgery, *days*	16.5 (7–27.5)	11 (8–14.5)	n/a
Long-term outcome	30 day survival (all Liveborn)	75.0% (12/16)	83.3% (5/6)	0.60 (0.05 - 6.80)
	1 Year survival (all Liveborn)	62.5% (10/16)	83.3% (5/6)	0.33 (0.31 - 3.58)
	3 Year survival (all Liveborn <2010)	76.9% (10/13)	80.0% (4/5)	0.83 (0.66 - 10.60)
	5 Year survival (all Liveborn <2008)	75.0% (6/8)	75.0% (3/4)	n/a
	10 Year Survival (all Liveborn <2003)	- (0/0)	50.0% (1/2)	n/a
	Documented neurodevelopment issues, *n*	4/10	2/5	p = 1.00
	Cases requiring on-going cardiac medication, *n*	9/9	4/4	n/a
	Cases with ongoing cardiac symptoms (All), *n*	8/10	1/4	0.08 (0.01 - 1.29)
	Cases with ongoing cardiac symp. (Fontan), *n*	3/4	1/3	n/a

Comparison between outcomes seen in patients with antenatally and postnatally detected Hypoplastic Left Heart Syndrome over three life periods: postnatal period, surgical period and long-term.
Denominators for long-term outcomes decreased as cases were lost from analysis due to absence of clinical information.

TGA on neurocognitive development. This prospective study showed a correlation between postnatal diagnosis and a less favourable score in "cognitive flexibility" and "social cognition". Both results were statistically significant and highlighted the need for further investigation in terms of how congenital heart disease can impact on neurodevelopment.

Levey et al. [15] looked at a wider range of congenital heart diseases. Their four year retrospective review included 439 cases of varying diagnoses, creating a large heterogeneous group with widely disparate outcomes. They highlighted a reduced risk of preoperative intubation (OR 0.62, $p = 0.033$) and emergency surgery (OR 0.18, $p < 0.001$) in the prenatally diagnosed cohort. No differences were demonstrated in mortality or neonatal measures such as Apgar score or time to surgery.

Limitations

This study aimed to overcome the potential bias of similar papers, identifying cases from a geographically defined population rather than just those referred to a single tertiary centre. In this way, postnatally diagnosed cases that did not undergo surgery were included. Despite this, surgical data could not be gathered for those operated on outside the East Midlands Congenital Heart Centre, which could limit the interpretation of some of the long term outcomes gathered.

The EMSYCAR database relies on case notification from medical professions. Multiple notifications per case are encouraged to ensure high levels of ascertainment, but some degree of incomplete referral is likely. As fetal detection is one key point for referral, the postnatally diagnosed cohorts are the most likely groups to have been subject to such an affect.

External validity

All cases were Leicestershire born. The county has a strong reputation for the treatment of congenital heart disease which may or may not be comparable to other areas of the UK. The impact of this local specialist service on parental decision making regarding maintenance of an antenatally diagnosed CHD pregnancy is unknown. The balance of antenatal and postnatal cohorts may have been affected by this.

Table 4 Outcome measures for antenatally, postnatally diagnosed TGA

Transposition of the great arteries		Antenatal diagnosis	Postnatal diagnosis	OR (95% CI) or p-value
Liveborn cases		8	22	
Case status				
Liveborn - alive:		8	19	
Liveborn - later died:		0	3	
Postnatal	Median Apgar Score *(IQR)*	9 (8–9)	9 (9–9)	n/a
	Pre-operative Acidosis, *n(%)*	8 (100.0)	22 (100.0)	n/a
	Intubation, *n(%)*	1 (12.5)	12 (54.5)	8.40 (0.88 - 80.27)
	Mortality within first week, *n(%)*	0 (0.0)	1(4.5)	1.19 (0.04 - 32.08)
Surgical	Attempted Surgery	8	21	n/a
	Median Age at Surgery (IQR), *days*	12.5 (6–26)	29.5 (10–29)	p = 0.39
	Median Weight at Surgery (IQR), *gram*	3900 (3400–3920)	3450 (3200–4205)	p = 0.40
	Median Bypass Time (IQR), *mins*	170 (144–227)	189 (177–269)	p = 0.50
	Length of ICU Stay Post Surgery, *days*	5 (3.5 - 19)	8 (5–8)	p = 0.89
	Post-Op Complication, *n(%)*	2 / 8 (25.0)	2 / 21 (9.5)	0.32 (0.32 - 2.75)
Long-term outcome	30 day survival (all Liveborn)	100% (8/8)	90.9% (20/22)	2.07 (0.09 - 47.90)
	1 Year survival (all Liveborn)	100% (8/8)	86.3% (19/22)	3.05 (0.14 - 65.78)
	3 Year survival (all Liveborn <2010)	100% (6/6)	83.3% (15/18)	2.94 (0.13 - 65.26)
	5 Year survival (all Liveborn <2008)	100% (5/5)	85.7% (12/14)	2.20 (0.09 - 53.85)
	10 Year Survival (all Liveborn <2003)	100% (2/2)	83.3% (5/6)	n/a
	Documented neurodevelopment issues	1/8	3/19	1.31 (0.12 - 14.93)
	Cases with post-surgical cardiac symptoms	1/8	3/15	1.75 (0.15 - 20.23)
	Cases requiring cardiac medication	2/8	3/15	0.75 (0.10 - 5.77)

Comparison between outcomes seen in patients with antenatally and postnatally detected Transposition of the Great Arteries over three life periods: postnatal period, surgical period and long-term.
Denominators for long-term outcomes decreased as cases were lost from analysis due to absence of clinical information.

Bias

With respect to the neuro-developmental outcomes, a potential source of bias is the increased follow-up afforded to some cases. It is possible that the cases which are more medically unstable (and therefore have more frequent reviews) will be more likely to have a negative outcome diagnosed and recorded if present, than those cases that are reviewed less frequently.

The study utilised two separate patient registers to overcome the potential selection bias of other papers

Table 5 Outcome measures for anteatally, postnatally diagnosed isolated HLHS or TGA

		Antenatal diagnosis	Postnatal diagnosis	OR (95% CI) or p-value
Liveborn cases		24	28	
Case status				
Liveborn - alive:		18	24	
Liveborn - later died:		6	4	
Short term	Median Apgar Score	9	9	*
	Pre-operative Acidosis, *n(%)*	20/24 (83.3)	28/28 (100.0)	12.5 (0.64 - 245.46)
	Intubation, *n(%)*	6/24 (25.0)	17/28 (60.7)	4.64 (1.40 - 15.32)
	Mortality within first week, *n(%)*	0/24 (–)	2/28 (7.1)	4.62 (0.21 - 101.16)
	30 day survival	83.3% (20/24)	89.3% (25/28)	0.60 (0.12 - 3.00)
	1 Year survival	75.0% (18/24)	85.7% (24/28)	0.50 (0.12 0 2.04)

Comparison between cases antenatally and postnatally diagnosed with isolated HLHS or TGA. Short term outcomes only were included due to the appropriateness of analysing long-term outcomes for a disparate group.

with a similar focus, i.e. those based in a specialist centre which focused only on cases which underwent surgery. The majority of cases were already present on both databases, suggesting high levels of reporting.

Conclusion

This small study, based on a geographically defined population, has been able to confirm the findings of previous case series of apparent short term benefits of antenatal over post natal diagnosis. No differences in longer term outcomes were identified and this too is in keeping with previous case series. However both the nature of previous studies and the relatively small number of patients reviewed here means that any effect on long term outcome is uncertain. Rates of adverse neurodevelopmental outcome in babies with major congenital heart disease remain relatively high and merit further investigation to understand fully whether antenatal diagnosis has the potential to improve longer term outcome.

Abbreviations

BINOCAR: British Isles Network of Congenital Anomaly Registers; CHD: Congenital heart disease; EMCHC: East Midlands Congenital Heart Centre, Glenfield Hospital, Leicester, UK; EMSYCAR: East Midlands and South Yorkshire Congenital Anomaly Register; HLHS: Hypoplastic left heart syndrome; TGA: Transposition of the Great Arteries.

Competing interests

The authors declare that they have no competing interests.

Authors' contributions

All authors contributed to the concept and design of the study. LP collected all data and drafted the manuscript. DF, ED and JB helped to revise the paper. All authors read and approved the final manuscript.

Funding

The study was undertaken as part of an Intercalated BSc at the University of Leicester. There was no funding from outside sources.

References

1. Townsend N, Bhatnagar P, Wickramasinghe K, Williams J. Children and young people statistics. 2013. 2013;2013. https://www.bhf.org.uk/~/media/files/research/heart-statistics/g694-bhf-children-and-young-people-statistics-2013.pdf.
2. NICOR. National Institute for Cardiovascular Outcomes Research. [https://nicor4.nicor.org.uk/CHD/an_paeds.nsf/vwContent/Antenatal%20Diagnosis?Opendocument]
3. Brown KL, Sullivan ID. Prenatal detection for major congenital heart disease: a key process measure for congenital heart networks. Heart. 2014;100:359–60.
4. Brown KL, Ridout DA, Hoskote A, Verhulst L, Ricci M, Bull C. Delayed diagnosis of congenital heart disease worsens preoperative condition and outcome of surgery in neonates. Heart. 2006;92:1298–302.
5. Fuchs IB, Muller H, Abdul-Khaliq H, Harder T, Dudenhausen JW, Henrich W. Immediate and long-term outcomes in children with prenatal diagnosis of selected isolated congenital heart defects. Ultrasound Obstet Gynecol. 2007;29:38–43.
6. Calderon J, Angeard N, Moutier S, Plumet MH, Jambaque I, Bonnet D. Impact of prenatal diagnosis on neurocognitive outcomes in children with transposition of the great arteries. J Pediatr. 2012;e1.94–8. e1.
7. Kumar RK, Newburger JW, Gauvreau K, Kamenir SA, Hornberger LK. Comparison of outcome when hypoplastic left heart syndrome and transposition of the great arteries are diagnosed prenatally versus when diagnosis of these two conditions is made only postnatally. Am J Cardiol. 1999;83:1649–53.
8. Landis B, Levey A, Levasseur S, Glickstein J, Kleinman C, Simpson L, et al. Prenatal diagnosis of congenital heart disease and birth outcomes. Pediatr Cardiol. 2013;34:597–605.
9. University of Leicester E. EMSYCAR - East Midlands & South Yorkshire Congenital Anomalies Register. [http://www2.le.ac.uk/departments/health-sciences/research/timms/projects/car]
10. BINOCAR. British Isles Network of Congenital Anomaly Registers. [http://www.binocar.org/]
11. Masuda M, Kado H, Tanoue Y, Fukae K, Onzuka T, Shiokawa Y, et al. Does Down syndrome affect the long-term results of complete atrioventricular septal defect when the defect is repaired during the first year of life? Eur J Cardiothorac Surg. 2005;27:405–9.
12. Formigari R, Michielon G, Digilio MC, Piacentini G, Carotti A, Giardini A, et al. Genetic syndromes and congenital heart defects: how is surgical management affected? Eur J Cardiothorac Surg. 2009;35:606–14.
13. Morris CD, Magilke D, Reller M. Down's syndrome affects results of surgical correction of complete atrioventricular canal. Pediatr Cardiol. 1992;13:80–4.
14. Donna Kirwan, NHS Fetal Anomaly Screening Programme. 18^{+0} to 20^{+6} Weeks Fetal Anomaly Scan National Standards and Guidance for England. 2010.
15. Levey A, Glickstein JS, Kleinman CS, Levasseur SM, Chen J, Gersony WM, et al. The impact of prenatal diagnosis of complex congenital heart disease on neonatal outcomes. Pediatr Cardiol. 2010;31:587–97.

2

Successful treatment of arrhythmia-induced cardiomyopathy in an infant with tuberous sclerosis complex

Noriko Motoki*, Yuji Inaba, Satoshi Matsuzaki, Yohei Akazawa, Takafumi Nishimura, Tetsuhiro Fukuyama and Kenichi Koike

Abstract

Background: Tuberous sclerosis complex (TSC) is an autosomal-dominant tumor suppressor gene syndrome that is characterized by the development of distinctive benign tumors and malformations in multiple organ systems (N Eng J Med 355:1345-1356, 2006). Cardiac rhabdomyomas are intracavitary or intramural tumors observed in 50–70 % of infants with TSC but only cause serious clinical problems in a very small fraction of these patients (N Eng J Med 355:1345-1356, 2006; Pediatrics 118:1146-1151, 2006; Eur J Pediatr 153:155-7, 1994); most individuals have no clinical symptoms and their tumors spontaneously regress. However, despite being clinically silent, these lesions can provoke arrhythmias and heart failure (Pediatrics 118:1146-1151, 2006; Eur J Pediatr 153:155-7, 1994).

Case presentation: We here report the clinical findings of an infant suffering from TSC complicated with dilated cardiomyopathy (DCM) after the regression of cardiac rhabdomyomas. Although his tumors improved spontaneously, tachycardia and irregular heart rate due to frequent premature ventricular and supraventricular contractions persisted from the newborn period and were refractory to several medications. His cardiomyopathy was suspected to have been induced by the tachycardia or arrhythmia. We found carvedilol therapy to be safe and highly effective in treating the cardiomyopathy. To our knowledge, this is the first case report of TSC with DCM after regression of cardiac tumors and its successful treatment.

Conclusion: The patient's clinical course suggests that careful life-long disease management is important, even in TSC patients without apparent symptoms.

Keywords: Tuberous sclerosis complex, Cardiac rhabdomyoma, Dilated cardiomyopathy, Arrhythmia, Carvedilol

Background

Tuberous sclerosis complex (TSC) is an autosomal dominant tumor suppressor gene syndrome that is characterized by the development of benign tumors and malformations in multiple organ systems [1]. Although cardiac rhabdomyomas are observed in approximately 50–70 % of infants with TSC, most patients exhibit no clinical symptoms and their tumors spontaneously regress [1–3]. However, such tumors occasionally cause serious clinical problems, including symptomatic cardiac failure and several kinds of arrhythmia [2, 3]. We here report the successful treatment with carvedilol of an infant with TSC complicated with dilated cardiomyopathy (DCM) which might have been induced by arrhythmia after regression of cardiac rhabdomyomas.

Case presentation

The male patient was born spontaneously at term after an uneventful pregnancy despite the detection of cardiac tumors at 36 weeks by fetal echocardiography. After birth, he was diagnosed as having TSC based on the diagnostic criteria of white leaf-shaped hypomelanotic macules, a subependymal nodule, and a retinal hamartoma [4]. Multiple intramural cardiac tumors of 5–25 mm in diameter were found by transthoracic echocardiography (Fig. 1a, b). Soon after birth, the boy exhibited numerous episodes of premature supraventricular

* Correspondence: nmotoki@shinshu-u.ac.jp
Department of Pediatrics, Shinshu University School of Medicine, Asahi 3-1-1, Matsumoto 390-8621, Japan

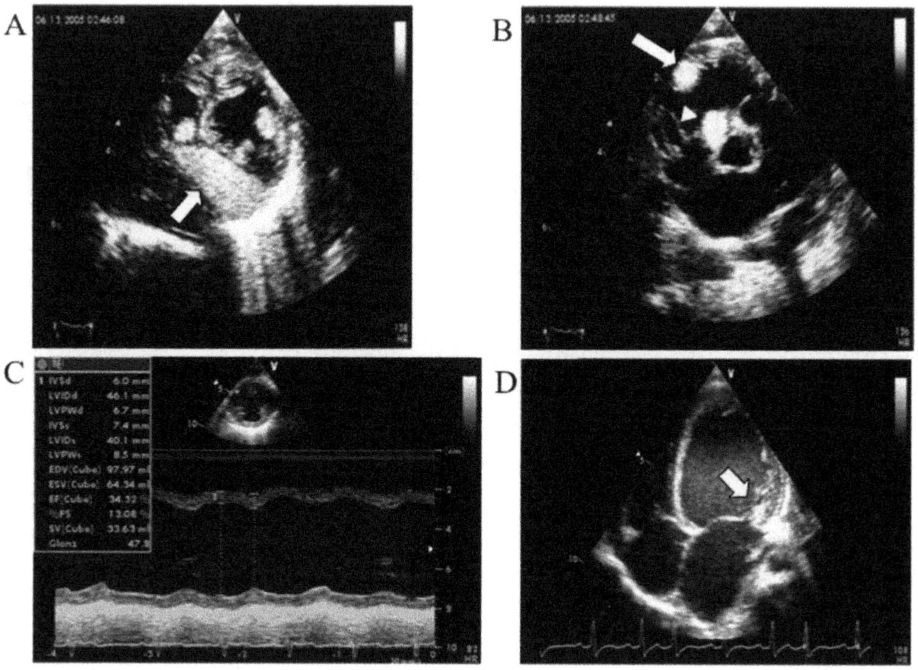

Fig. 1 Echocardiographic findings. At birth, tumors were located on the postero-septal wall of the left ventricle (**a**, *arrow*), right ventricular outflow (**b**, *arrow*), and intraventricular septum (**b**, *arrowhead*) at birth. At the age of 23 months, 2D echocardiography disclosed an enlarged left ventricle (**c**), and M-mode echocardiography revealed poor left ventricular wall contraction (**d**)

contractions (PSVC), multifocal premature ventricular contractions (PVC), and non-sustained ventricular tachycardia (NSVT). Mexiletine treatment was commenced at 1 month of age (Fig. 2a). Since a maximum NSVT of 14 beats at a rate of 269 bpm was detected by Holter electrocardiography (ECG) at the age of 5 months, we added disopyramide to his therapy regime, which resulted in a decline in NSVT frequency. The tumors gradually diminished in size, but his frequent PSVC and tachycardia persisted.

At 20 months of age, the patient's cardiac function was preserved; echocardiography revealed a left ventricular end-diastolic diameter (LVDd) of 30.8 mm (Z-score: 0.5) and a left ventricular fractional shortening (LVFS) of 28 %.

At 23 months of age, he was admitted to our hospital due to cardiac dysfunction. His body height and weight were 85 cm (+0.1 SD) and 11.5 kg (+0.1 SD), respectively. Blood pressure was 88/47 mmHg. Heartbeat was irregular at 134 bpm without extra heart sounds or murmurs. Neither hepatomegaly nor pretibial edema was observed. Laboratory data including blood cell counts, electrolytes, CRP, CK-MB, troponin T, glucose, ammonia, lactic and pyruvic acid, and thyroid function showed no abnormalities. However, brain natriuretic peptide (BNP) and human atrial natriuretic peptide levels were markedly increased at 619 pg/ml (normal range: < 20 pg/ml) and 654 pg/ml (normal range: < 43 pg/ml), respectively. There were no significant increases of viral antibody titers in his serum, including those for the Coxsackie virus, adenovirus, or echovirus. His cardiothoracic ratio was 64 % on a chest radiograph. Twelve-lead ECG revealed irregular tachycardia (139 bpm) and sporadic PSVC without ST abnormality or wide QRS duration (Fig. 3). According to Holter ECG, the patient's total number of heartbeats (THB) was 195,807 per day and mean heart rate was 136 bpm. Frequent multifocal PVC (20,883 beats per day; 10.7 % of THB) and PSVC (29,733 beats per day; 15.2 % of THB) were also noted. Echocardiography revealed cardiac dilatation and diffuse hypokinesis, LVDd of 45.2 mm (Z-score: 3.0), and LVFS of 15 % (Fig. 1c). Severe mitral insufficiency caused by the expansion of the mitral annulus was detected as well. His coronary arteries were normal. Surprisingly, his cardiac tumors had diminished in size and were recognizable as a small bright area in the posterior mitral valve (Fig. 1d).

Diuretics and angiotensin converting enzyme inhibitor were administered as anti-heart failure therapies. To control tachycardia and reduce afterload on the failing heart, we also commenced oral administration of carvedilol at 0.15 mg/day (0.01 mg/kg/day) that was gradually increased to 3.0 mg/day (0.3 mg/kg/day) 3 months later. Although frequent PSVC persisted, the boy's mean HR gradually decreased and the incidence of PVC and its short run became markedly diminished (Fig. 2a). BNP gradually decreased to within normal range. The

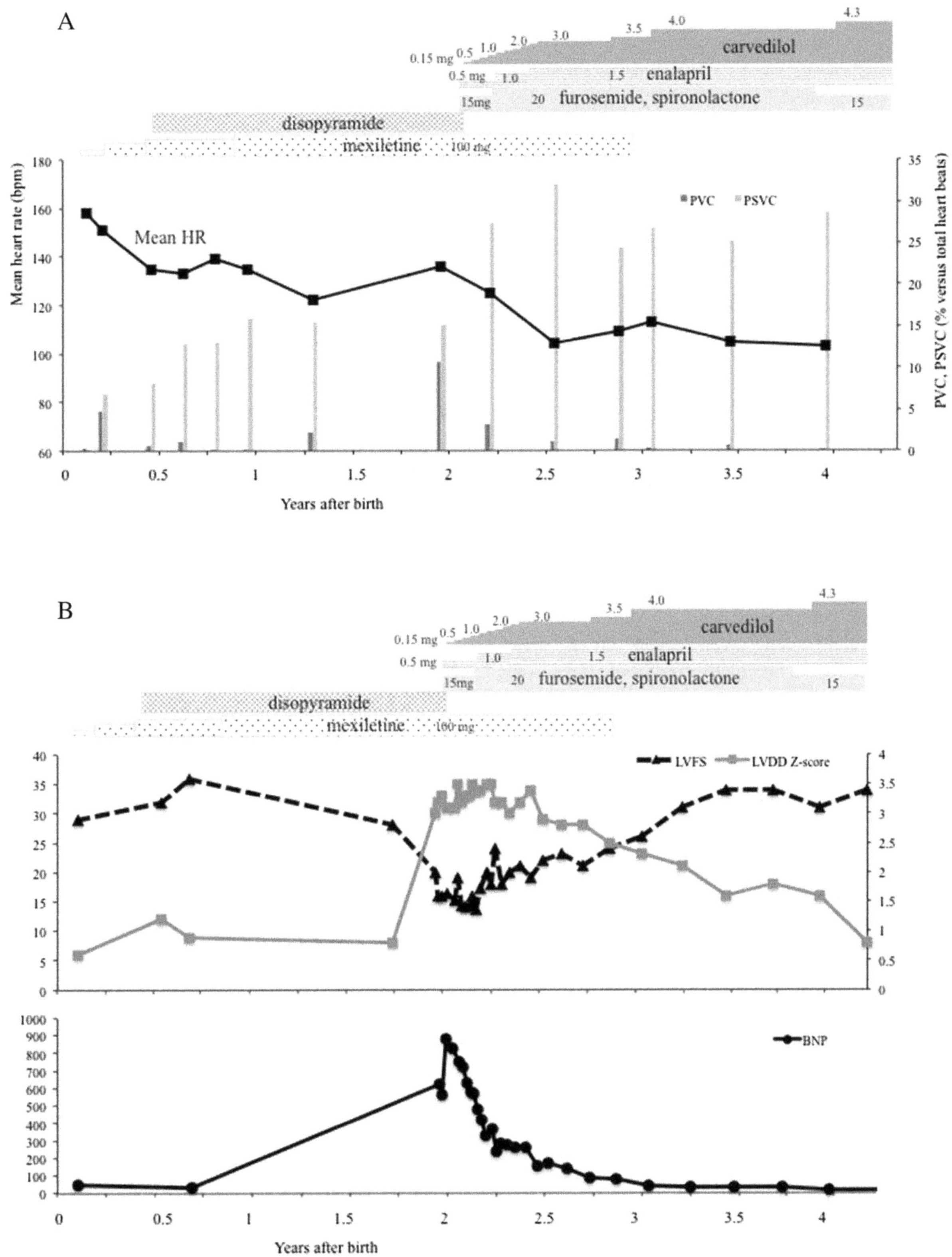

Fig. 2 a, **b** Changes in cardiac function before and during treatment with carvedilol. BNP, Brain natriuretic peptide; LVDd, Left ventricular end-diastolic diameter; LVFS, Left ventricular fractional shortening; HR: Heart rate; PSVC, Premature supraventricular contraction; PVC, Premature ventricular contraction

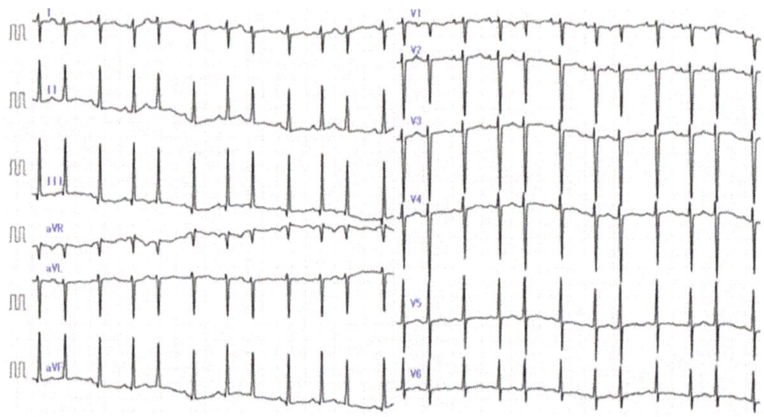

Fig. 3 Electrocardiography findings. Twelve-lead electrocardiography (ECG) revealed irregular tachycardia (139 bpm) and sporadic PSVC without ST abnormality or wide QRS duration

abnormal values of LVFS and LVDd persisted for 1 year after the initiation of carvedilol treatment, but both parameters eventually improved to normal levels (34 % and 35.8 mm [Z-score: 0.8], respectively) by the age of 4 years (Fig. 2b).

Discussion

We here report the clinical findings of an infant boy suffering from TSC complicated with DCM. Although his tumors regressed spontaneously, tachycardia and heart rate irregularity due to frequent PSVC and PVC persisted from the newborn period. After the commencement of carvedilol aimed to control heart rate and reduce afterload in the failing heart, BNP and LV systolic function improved within months and LV volume recovered slowly over several years.

The most frequent cardiac involvement in TSC is multiple cardiac rhabdomyomas, which may spontaneously regress during the first few years. However, TSC is a known cause of heart failure because of myocardial depression and inflow or outflow obstruction by tumors [1–3]. TSC is also classified as one of the secondary causes of cardiomyopathy [5]. Several reports have described DCM as a primary cardiac involvement in patients with TSC [5, 6]. Although 1 case was of TSC and DCM without cardiac tumors, the cause of the cardiomyopathy was unknown [6]. Our patient's cardiac tumors had improved spontaneously by the time of the appearance of cardiac dysfunction. Differential diagnoses for his heart failure included myocarditis, coronary artery abnormality, hormone or metabolic abnormalities, and mitochondrial disease, but it was ultimately difficult to pinpoint its precise nature.

TSC-related cardiac rhabdomyomas can combine with several other kinds of arrhythmias [1–3]. However, the relationship between tachycardia/arrhythmia and cardiomyopathy has not been clearly described in TSC. Here, we consider that tachycardia or arrhythmia was responsible for the patient's cardiomyopathy.

Atrial ectopic tachycardia is the most common arrhythmia in pediatric arrhythmia-induced cardiomyopathy (AIC), for which beta-blockers are frequently used as the first-line therapy [7]. Heart rate irregularity also occurs in pediatric AIC as salvos of tachycardia interspersed with periods of sinus rhythm [8]. Prior reports have described weeks to months for LV systolic functional recovery in AIC, and months to years for reverse remodeling to bring heart rate and rhythm under control [9, 10].

The relationship between arrhythmia and cardiomyopathy can be difficult to characterize because arrhythmias may exist for years before their recognition and the development of cardiomyopathy [8]. Cardiac magnetic resonance imaging may help differentiate AIC from DCM; in many cases, patients with DCM that does not improve exhibit findings in late gadolinium enhancement suggestive of an underlying scar [11].

As a non-selective beta-blocker with additional vasodilating properties, carvedilol has been demonstrated to improve survival in adult patients with severe chronic heart failure [12]. In a multicenter, randomized, double-blind, placebo-controlled trial by Shaddy et al. [13], carvedilol did not significantly affect the primary end point of composite clinical outcomes in children or adolescents with symptomatic heart failure due to systemic ventricular dysfunction. However, a prespecified subgroup analysis noted significant interaction between treatment and ventricular morphology, indicating a possible differential effect between patients with a systemic left ventricle (i.e., beneficial trend) and those whose systemic ventricle was not the left ventricle (i.e., non-beneficial trend). Other studies have shown carvedilol to be effective for chronic heart failure in pediatric patients with systemic left ventricle, such as DCM [14, 15].

Additionally, chronic use of a beta-blocker in conjunction with ACE inhibitor therapy improved clinical status and exercise tolerance in patients with heart failure [16]. The beta-blocking effects of carvedilol may be important because catecholamines induce oxidative stress in the myocardium, and the direct antioxidant effect of this drug may contribute to oxidative stress relief in the failing myocardium [15]. Accordingly, carvedilol-mediated reductions in heart rate and oxidative stress were suspected to have accounted for the improvement in LV dysfunction in our patient. Special attention must be paid to the negative inotropic effect of carvedilol during treatment initiation in patients with severe cardiac dysfunction [14, 17]. We therefore started with a very small dose, and gradually increased it to avoid any adverse effects on cardiac function.

Conclusion

To our knowledge, this is the first reported case of an infant suffering from TSC complicated with DCM after the regression of cardiac rhabdomyomas whose cardiomyopathy was suspectedly induced by arrhythmia. We found that carvedilol therapy was safe and effective for treating the cardiomyopathy despite the patient's very young age. TSC rhabdomyomas generally disappear spontaneously and have a good prognosis. However, the present case exhibited heart failure with severely reduced LV function during the course of illness, suggesting the importance of meticulous life-long follow-up, even in apparently asymptomatic patients with TSC.

Consent

Written informed consent was obtained from the patient's parents for publication of this case report and any accompanying images. A copy of the written consent is available for review by the Editor-in-Chief of this journal.

Abbreviations

AIC: arrhythmia-induced cardiomyopathy; BNP: brain natriuretic peptide; DCM: dilated cardiomyopathy; ECG: electrocardiography; LVDd: left ventricular end-diastolic diameter; LVFS: left ventricular fractional shortening; NSVT: non-sustained ventricular tachycardia; PSVC: premature supraventricular contractions; PVC: premature ventricular contractions; THB: total number of heartbeats; TSC: tuberous sclerosis complex.

Competing interests

The authors declare that they have no competing interests.

Authors' contributions

NM wrote this manuscript under supervision of YI and KK. SM, YA, TN and TF reviewed the clinical data. All authors have read and approved the final manuscript.

Acknowledgements

The authors sincerely thank the patient and his parents for providing all of the clinical and laboratory information and samples.

References

1. Crino PB, Nathanson KL, Henske EP. The tuberous sclerosis complex. N Eng J Med. 2006;355:1345–56.
2. Jóźwiak S, Kotulska K, Kasprzyk-Obara J, Domańska-Pakieła D, Tomyn-Drabik M, Roberts P, et al. Clinical and genotype studies of cardiac tumors in 154 patients with tuberous sclerosis complex. Pediatrics. 2006;118:1146–51.
3. Jóźwiak S, Kawalec W, Dłuzewska J, Daszkowicz-Małek M, Michałowicz R. Cardiac tumors in tuberous sclerosis: their incidence and course. Eur J Pediatr. 1994;153:155–7.
4. Roach ES, Gomez MR, Northrup H. Tuberous sclerosis complex consensus conference; Revised clinical diagnostic criteria. J Child Neurol. 1998;13:624–8.
5. Maron BJ, Towbin JA, Thiene G, Antzelevitch C, Corrado D, Arnett D, et al. Contemporary definitions and classification of the cardiomyopathies: an American Heart Association Scientific Statement from the Council on Clinical Cardiology, Heart Failure and Transplantation Committee; Quality of Care and Outcomes Research and Functional Genomics and Translational Biology Interdisciplinary Working Groups; and Council on Epidemiology and Prevention. Circulation. 2006;113:1807–16.
6. Jain D, Kumar V, Kar DP, Prasad SR. Initial presentation with dilated cardiomyopathy in a patient of tuberous sclerosis: a rare case report. Indian Heart J. 2013;65:84–7.
7. Moore JP, Patel PA, Shannon KM, Albers EL, Salerno JC, Stein MA. Predictors of myocardial recovery in pediatric tachycardia-induced cardiomyopathy. Heart Rhythm. 2014;11:1163–9.
8. Gopinathannair R, Etheridge SP, Marchlinski FE, Spinale FG, Lakkireddy D, Olshansky B. Arrhythmia-induced cardiomyopathies: mechanisms, recognition, and management. J Am Coll Cardiol. 2015;66:1714–28.
9. Gillete PC, Wampler DG, Garson A, Zinner A, Ott D, Cooley D. Treatment of atrial automatic tachycardia by ablation procedures. J Am Coll Cardiol. 1985;6:405–9.
10. Cruz FE, Cheriex EC, Smeets JL, Atie J, Peres AK, Penn OC, et al. Reversibility of tachycardia-induced cardiomyopathy after cure of incessant supraventricular tachycardia. J Am Coll Cardiol. 1990;16:739–44.
11. Hasdemir C, Yuksel A, Camli D, Kartal Y, Simsek E, Musayev O, et al. Late gadolinium enhancement CMR in patients with tachycardia-induced cardiomyopathy caused by idiopathic ventricular arrhythmias. Pacing Clin Electrophysiol. 2012;35:465–70.
12. Packer M, Coats AJ, Fowler MB, Katus HA, Krum H, Mohacsi P, et al. Effect of carvedilol on survival in severe chronic heart failure. N Engl J Med. 2001;344:1651–8.
13. Shaddy RE, Boucek MM, Hsu DT, Boucek RJ, Canter CE, Mahony L, et al. Carvedilol for Children and adrescents with heart failure. JAMA. 2007;298:1171–9.
14. Azeka E, Franchini Ramires JA, Valler C, Bocchi EA. Delisting of infants and children from the heart transplantation waiting list after carvedilol treatment. J Am Coll Cardiol. 2002;40:2034–8.
15. Bajcetic M, Kokic Nikolic A, Djukic M, Kosutic J, Mitrovic J, Mijalkovic D, et al. Effects of carvedilol on left ventricular function and oxidative stress in infants and children with idiopathic dilated cardiomyopathy: A 12-month, two-center, open-label study. Clin Ther. 2008;30:702–14.
16. Abdulla J, Kober L, Christensen E, Torp-Pedersen C. Effect of beta-blocker therapy on functional status in patients with heart failure - A meta-analysis. Eur J Heart Fail. 2006;8:522–31.
17. Blume ED, Canter CE, Spicer R, Gauvreau K, Colan S, Jenkins KJ. Prospective single-arm protocol of carvedilol in children with ventricular dysfunction. Pediatr Cardiol. 2006;27:336–42.

3

A male infant had subdural effusion and paroxysmal supraventricular tachycardia during the febrile episode of Kawasaki disease

Chia-Pei Chou[1], I-Chun Lin[2] and Kuang-Che Kuo[2*]

Abstract

Background: Kawasaki disease is an acute, febrile, self-limiting, inflammatory systemic vasculitis seen in early childhood, most commonly in those below 5 years of age. In Kawasaki disease, the coronary arteries are most commonly affected, which may lead to asymptomatic coronary artery ectasia or formation of an aneurysm. Paroxysmal supraventricular tachycardia(PSVT) is a severe and rare cardiovascular complication of Kawasaki disease. A case of Kawasaki disease presenting with unusual findings, including subdural effusion and PSVT is reported.

Case presentation: This is a 4-month-10-day-old boy presents with anterior fontanelle bulging and moderate bilateral subdural effusion at the acute stage of Kawasaki disease and PSVT at the subacute stage of Kawasaki disease. The subdural effusion was resolution after intravenous immunoglobulin(IVIG) administration. And the PSVT was subsided after administered 3 doses of adenosine, 1 dose of amiodarone loading and Propranolol twice per day use. At 1-year follow-up has made a complete recovery with no arrhythmia episodes, developmental effects or abnormal neurologic findings.

Conclusion: Subdural effusion in the acute stage of Kawasaki disease may be an inflammatory response. It may resolves spontaneously after anti-inflammatory treatment such as IVIG infusion. PSVT is a severe cardiovascular complication of Kawasaki disease. In those who taking aspirin, we need to carefully observe the heart rhythm and PSVT side effects, especially in the first month.

Keywords: Infant, Kawasaki disease, Subdural effusion, Paroxysmal supraventricular tachycardia, Aspirin

Background

Kawasaki disease is an acute, febrile, self-limiting systemic vasculitis seen in early childhood, most commonly in those below 5 years of age. This condition is the leading cause of acquired heart disease in children [1]. There are no specific biomarkers for the diagnosis of Kawasaki disease.

The diagnostic criteria of typical Kawasaki disease include fever lasting for 5 days in addition to 4 of the following 5 clinical features: oropharyngeal changes; non-purulent conjunctivitis; acute cervical lymphadenopathy with lymph node diameter > 1.5 cm; peripheral extremity changes; or a generalized polymorphous rash [2, 3].

In Kawasaki disease, the coronary arteries are most commonly affected, which may lead to asymptomatic coronary artery ectasia or formation of an aneurysm. Rarely, Kawasaki disease may cause myocarditis, pericarditis, or lead to arrhythmias. Ventricular arrhythmia is also an unusual finding in Kawasaki disease in the past case presentation or literature review. Kawasaki disease is a systemic inflammatory disease commonly associated with thrombocytosis, especially after the first week of illness [4]. The incidence of Kawasaki disease with neurological complications is approximately 1.1-3.7 %. Subdural fluid collection is rarely described in association with Kawasaki disease in the previous literature.

* Correspondence: light@cgmh.org.tw
[2]Department of Pediatrics, Kaohsiung Chang Gung Memorial Hospital and Chang Gung University College of Medicine, No.123, Dapi Rd., Niaosong Dist., Kaohsiung City 833, Taiwan, R.O.C
Full list of author information is available at the end of the article

Full doses of intravenous immunoglobulin (IVIG) are the mainstay of treatment. Early administration of IVIG may reduce the risk of cardiac involvement to 5 % [5]. During the clinical course, close monitoring of cardiovascular function and coronary artery diameter is necessary. For coronary artery abnormalities, aspirin is part of the standard treatment [5]. In most children, the heart problems subside after 5 or 6 weeks without lasting damage. However, in some children, the coronary arteries are damaged permanently.

Case presentation

The 4-month-10-day-old boy presented with intermittent fever for 2 days and he was taken to emergency department on February 16, 2014. He had received a 10-valent pneumococcal vaccine (PCV 10), 2 days prior to his visit, in a local clinic and did not have a fever or throat injection at the time. After admission, physical examination revealed injected throat and tonsils, coarse breathing sounds, polymorphous rashes over the trunk, anterior fontanelle bulging, and poor activity while febrile. Laboratory examination revealed leukocytosis (WBC: 28300/uL), segmented predominance (segment: 67 %) and an elevated CRP level (CRP: 69.4 mg/L). Urine analysis showed mild pyuria (WBC: 12/uL) and ketones (ketone: 40 mg/dL). He was admitted to the hospital for suspected bacterial meningitis, and antibiotic therapy with cefotaxime was started. However, his parents declined our suggestion for cerebrospinal fluid (CSF) tapping.

Persistent intermittent fever was noted on February 17, 2014. In addition, he presented with injected and fissured lips, a strawberry tongue, erythema and edema over palms and soles, and bilateral bulbar conjunctival injection. The echocardiography was performed for possible Kawasaki disease on February 17, 2014 and revealed the z-score of the left coronary artery and right coronary artery was 1.25 and 1.83, no coronary artery dilatation complication. Swelling with erythematous change over the Bacillus Calmette-Guérin vaccine (BCG) injection site was noted on February 18, 2014. Brain ultrasound (Fig. 1) was also performed for anterior fontanelle bulging on February 18, 2014 and revealed moderate subdural fluid collection.

Due to persistent intermittent fever for 5 days, on February 18, 2014, IVIG therapy (IVIG 2 g/kg administered over 12 h) was prescribed from that afternoon until the next morning. Aspirin 30 mg once per day was prescribed starting February 19, 2014. Fever subsided gradually from February 21, 2014, following which low-dose aspirin was continued. The symptoms of polymorphous rash, injected and fissured lips, and BCG injection site swelling showed improvement. The patient was discharged without any discomfort or fever on February 25, 2014.

The patient experienced a fever of 38.9 °C again on March 5, 2014 in the early morning hours, and then subsided spontaneously. In addition, a mildly injected lip and distal limbs swelling without desquamation were noted. Tachyarrhythmia (heart rate > 200 beats/min) was present at the afternoon. Electrocardiogram (ECG) (Fig. 2) showed PSVT. The echocardiography revealed tachycardia with the z-score of the left coronary artery and right coronary artery was 2.5 and 1.94, no evidence of coronary artery dilatation, no ischemic change, and no other abnormal findings. Laboratory

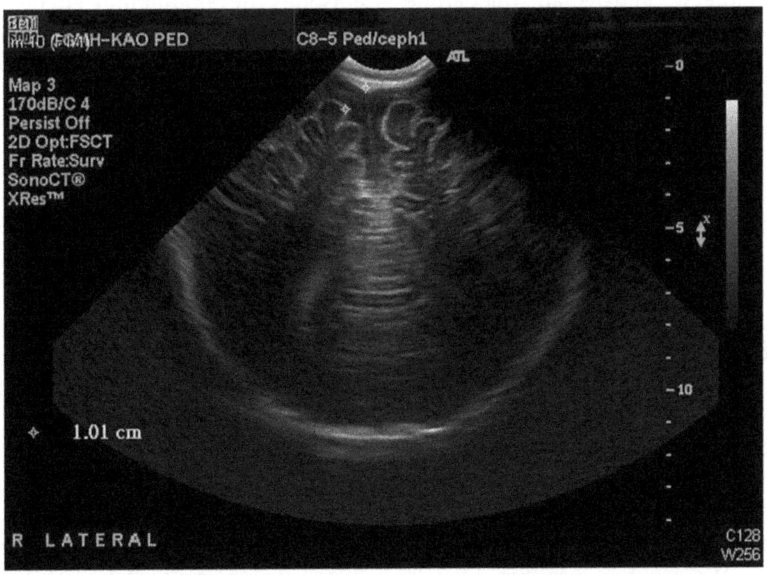

Fig. 1 Brain ultrasound. Initial brain ultrasound on admission with moderate subdural fluid collection(1.01 cm)

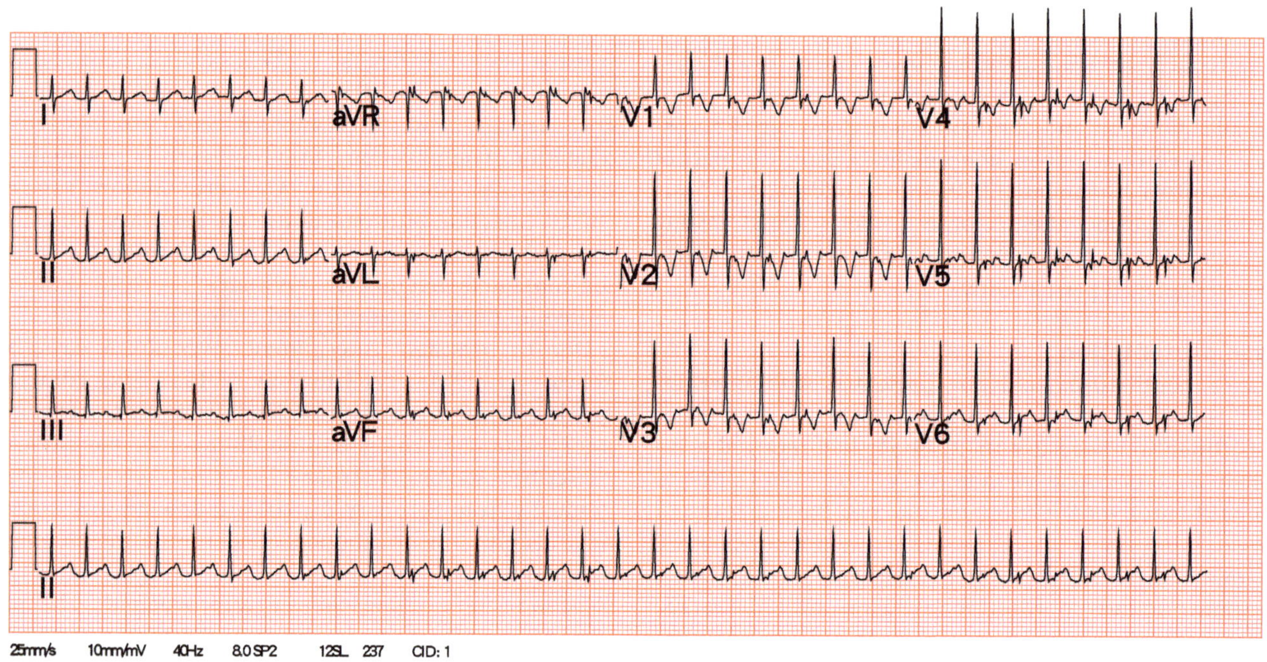

Fig. 2 Electrocardiogram. Initial ECG with paroxysmal supraventricular tachycardia

examination showed leukocytosis (WBC: 17300/uL), thrombocytosis (platelet: 820000/uL), an elevated CRP level (CRP: 117.4 mg/L), an elevated ESR level (ESR: 108 mm/h), and normal cardiac enzymes. The ECG monitor persistently showed PSVT, even when the patient did not have a fever and was not crying. We administered 3 doses of adenosine (1 mg, 1 mg, and 2 mg intravenous push). His heart rate was lowered to 60 beats/min with adenosine administration, but was refractory soon after crying and being in an irritable mood. Therefore, we initiated an amiodarone loading dose of 5 mg/kg (40 mg in 20 ml of D5W) for 1 h. Following this patient's condition improved and was relatively stable; the ECG monitor showed tachyarrhythmia (heart rate 150–160 beats/min) with the P wave. Propranolol 2.5 mg twice per day was also prescribed for control of the arrhythmic heart rate, after which, tachyarrhythmia was improved with a baseline heart rate of 125–135 beats/min. The repeat ECG (Fig. 3) showed a normal sinus rhythm with normal PR and QT intervals and no delta waves.

Brain ultrasound (Fig. 4) performed on March 6, 2014 revealed mild subdural fluid collection. Blood, urine, and CSF cultures were sterile. Because CSF microscopic analysis showed no pleocytosis, with normal sugar, protein, and chloride levels, bacterial meningitis was less likely. Desquamation on tips of fingers and toes appeared on March 8, 2014. The echocardiography performed on March 10, 2014 revealed a normal echocardiogram with normal coronary arteries. We stopped propranolol use on March 14, 2014. The patient was discharged on March 15, 2014, as his general condition had improved, and his vital signs were relatively stable.

The patient had regular follow-up examinations at the pediatric outpatient department. The echocardiography revealed a normal echocardiogram and normal coronary arteries. ECG also showed a normal sinus rhythm. He had taken aspirin for 2 months, which was discontinued on April 21, 2014. Brain ultrasound revealed complete resolution of the subdural effusion. No more arrhythmia episodes, developmental effects or abnormal neurologic findings were detected at the 1-year follow-up.

Discussion

Subdural effusion in Kawasaki disease

The incidence of Kawasaki disease with neurological complications is approximately 1.1-3.7 %. Nervous system complications previously reported include seizure, facial nerve palsy, meningoencephalitis, hemiplegia, ataxia, chorea, ischemia, abnormal vision, disturbed consciousness, behavioral changes, sensorineural hearing loss, and monocyte-predominant pleocytosis in CSF [6, 7]. Subdural fluid collection is rarely described in association with Kawasaki disease. Only 7 equivocal cases of extracerebral fluid collection or subdural effusion in the acute stage of atypical Kawasaki disease have been reported in the literature [8, 9].

Aoki et al. [8] reported the case of a 6-month-old girl in the acute stage of Kawasaki disease, who presented with retinal hemorrhage complications and bilateral

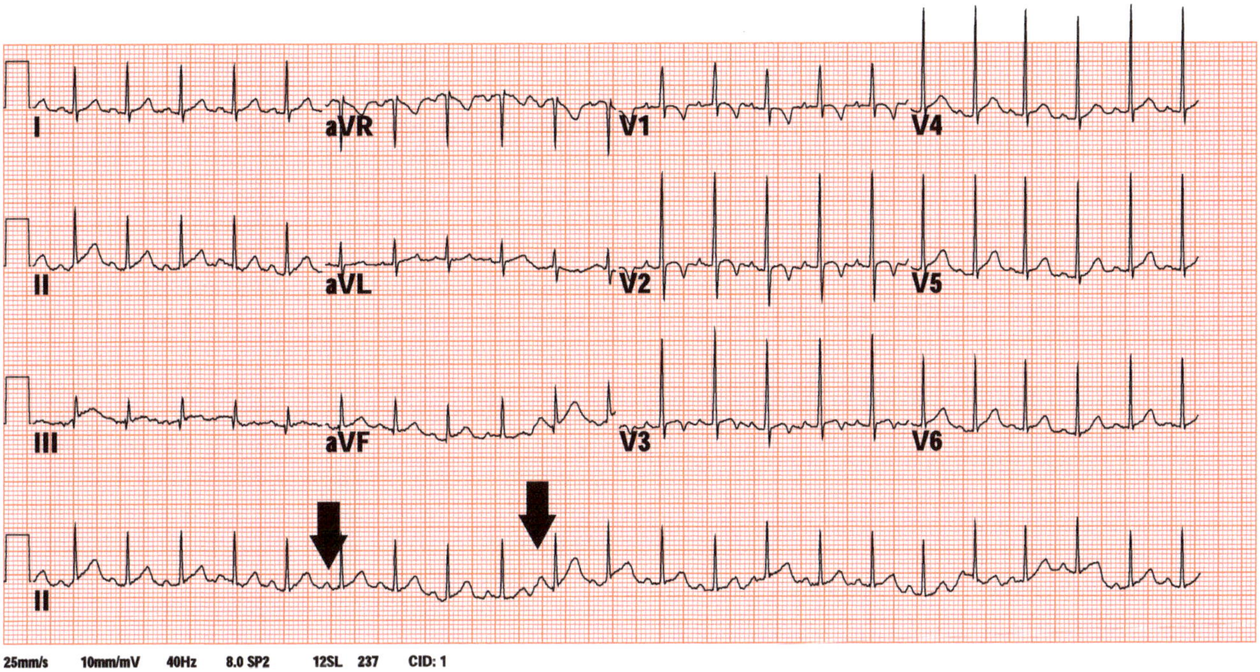

Fig. 3 Electrocardiogram. ECG with normal sinus rhythm after 3 doses of adenosine, amiodarone loading dose of 5 mg/kg, and Propranolol. Arrow mark: P waves

subdural fluid collection with intracranial hypertension. The subdural effusion with intracranial hypertension was controlled using a subdural tap and glycerol administration. Additionally, a computerized tomography (CT) scan confirmed reduction of subdural fluid collection.

Bailie et al. [9] described the case of a 6-month-old boy with possible Kawasaki disease, who had complications related to bilateral subdural collection and prolonged right-sided seizure. He also presented with tachycardia (approximately 120–150 beats/min). The patient had an amazing response to administration of IVIG (2 g/kg) and high-dose aspirin (100 mg/kg/day in 4 divided doses). CT scan showed complete resolution of the subdural collection at the 6-months follow-up.

Our patient is a typical case of Kawasaki disease with moderate bilateral subdural effusion and is the youngest one of all previously reported cases in previous literature. However, our patient only presented with anterior

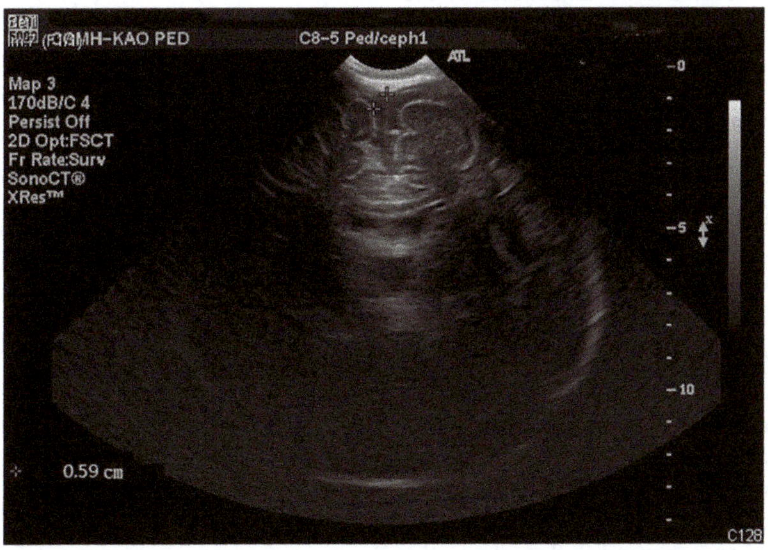

Fig. 4 Brain ultrasound. Follow-up brain ultrasound 2 weeks after IVIG administration showing mild subdural fluid collection(0.59 cm)

fontanelle bulging and poor activity when febrile, without any specific neurological signs or encephalopathy symptoms. This patient underwent only IVIG administration as an anti-inflammatory measure in the acute stage of Kawasaki disease. Brain ultrasound revealed a definite reduction in the volume of subdural effusion 2 weeks post-presentation and IVIG infusion. There was no any lasting damage, and this child demonstrated normal development at the 1-year symptom-free follow-up.

PSVT in Kawasaki disease

The cardiovascular complications of Kawasaki syndrome commonly include symptoms related to coronary artery dilation, coronary aneurysm, myocarditis, or myocardial ischemia. Ventricular arrhythmia is an unusual finding and rare complication in the acute phase of Kawasaki disease; this sign is independent of coronary artery involvement in Kawasaki disease [10].

Haney et al. [11] reported a 2.5-year-old child with ventricular arrhythmia in the acute stage of Kawasaki disease. The arrhythmia was resolved after empirical treatment with oral steroids.

Seymour et al. [12] described the case of a 12-year-old girl with medical history of Kawasaki disease diagnosed at the age 2 years and who received appropriate treatment for this condition. The patient presented with supraventricular tachycardia (SVT) at 180 beats/min. Intravenous access and vagal maneuvers were performed to abate the SVT without success. After 2 doses of adenosine was administered by rapid intravenous bolus, the heartbeat decreased to a sinus rhythm of 88 beats/min. No further damage was noted during an outpatient follow-up.

Our patient is a typical and rare case of Kawasaki disease with PSVT. Tachyarrhythmia (heart rate > 200 beats/min) and PSVT were presented after admission in the subacute stage of Kawasaki disease, and our patient had taken aspirin for only 2 weeks. It was difficult to control his heart rate. We had attempted 3 doses of adenosine (1 mg, 1 mg, and 2 mg intravenous push), and amiodarone loading dose of 5 mg/kg (40 mg in 20 ml of D5W) for 1 h to control the PSVT. Propranolol 2.5 mg twice per day was added to control the arrhythmia. There were no signs of any defects or damage on the ECG and echocardiography at the 1-year follow-up.

IVIG in the subacute stage of Kawasaki disease

The clinical presentation of Kawasaki disease is conventionally divided into 4 stages: acute, subacute, convalescent and chronic. The subacute stage of Kawasaki disease begins when the fever has abated, and it may last for 4–6 weeks. The rate of sudden death is the highest in the subacute stage. Persistence of fever beyond 2–3 weeks in the subacute stage of Kawasaki disease may be an indication of recrudescent Kawasaki disease or persistent Kawasaki disease. This condition requires secondary IVIG therapy [13].

On the other hand, we have defined recurrent Kawasaki disease as a separate episode fulfilling Kawasaki disease criteria after an earlier occurrence has fully resolved, typically at least 2 months later [13]. The recurrence rate was 6.89 per 1000 person-years, with a high incidence within 12 months following the first episode [14]. Recurrent Kawasaki disease requires reevaluation and retreatment with IVIG and aspirin. Patients with recurrent Kawasaki disease are at an increased risk for developing cardiac sequelae.

In our patient, the secondary fever episode subsided after treatment with antipyretics, and the fever episode duration was less than 24 h. It is obvious that the secondary fever episode in our patient was not a case of recrudescent or recurrent Kawasaki disease. Therefore, our patient did not need secondary IVIG infusion or retreatment. The only intervention needed was symptom-control and monitoring of further complications of Kawasaki disease.

Conclusions

We hereby present a young infant with IVIG-responsive subdural effusion and difficult-to-control PSVT complications due to Kawasaki disease.

Subdural effusion in the acute stage of Kawasaki disease may be an inflammatory response. Administration of IVIG relieves acute inflammation. As in our case, there is no need for a subdural tap or any surgical intervention; the subdural effusion resolves spontaneously after anti-inflammatory treatment such as IVIG infusion. Additionally, there is no any lasting defect or damage in patients with Kawasaki disease. PSVT is a severe cardiovascular complication of Kawasaki disease and may be related to sudden death or lasting damage in the case of incomplete symptom control or inadequate treatment. In those who taking aspirin, we need to carefully observe the heart rhythm and PSVT side effects, especially in the first month. A second fever episode in a patient with Kawasaki disease should be differentially diagnosed. If the fever occurs during the subacute stage of Kawasaki disease and persists less than 2–3 weeks, it is not a case of recrudescent Kawasaki disease or recurrent illness. Treatment with secondary IVIG therapy or corticosteroids is therefore not requires.

Abbreviations

BCG: Bacillus Calmette-Guérin vaccine; CSF: cerebrospinal fluid; CT: computerized tomography; ECG: electrocardiogram; IVIG: intravenous immunoglobulin; PSVT: paroxysmal supraventricular tachycardia; SVT: supraventricular tachycardia.

Acknowledgements

The authors sincerely thank the patient and his parents for providing all of the clinical and laboratory information and samples. Thank you to the partly supported by grants from Chang Gung Memorial Hospital, Taiwan (CMRPG8E0481).

Funding
No funding was obtained for this study.

Authors' contributions
C-PC: Dr. Chou drafted the initial manuscript, designed the study, analysis and interpretation of data, literatures collection instruments and approved the final manuscript as submitted. I-CL: Dr. Lin gave the opinions and recommendations for this manuscript. K-CK: Dr. Kuo conceptualized the study, reviewed and revised the manuscript, and approved the final manuscript as submitted. All authors approved the final manuscript as submitted and agree to be accountable for all aspects of the work.

Authors' information
Chia-Pei Chou: Dr. Chou is a resident doctor of department of Family Medicine in Kaohsiung Chang Gung Memorial Hospital.
I-Chun Lin: Dr. Lin is an attending physician of department of Pediatrics in Kaohsiung Chang Gung Memorial Hospital. She is also a Pediatric Cardiologist.
Kuang-Che Kuo: Dr. Kuo is an attending physician of department of Pediatrics in Kaohsiung Chang Gung Memorial Hospital. He is also a Pediatric Infectious Diseases specialist.

Competing interests
The authors declare that they have no competing interests.

Author details
[1]Department of Family Medicine, Kaohsiung Chang Gung Memorial Hospital and Chang Gung University College of Medicine, No.123, Dapi Rd., Niaosong Dist., Kaohsiung City 833, Taiwan, R.O.C. [2]Department of Pediatrics, Kaohsiung Chang Gung Memorial Hospital and Chang Gung University College of Medicine, No.123, Dapi Rd., Niaosong Dist., Kaohsiung City 833, Taiwan, R.O.C.

References

1. Newburger JW, Takahashi M, Gerber MA, Gewitz MH, Tani LY, Burns JC, et al. Diagnosis, treatment, and long-term management of Kawasaki disease: a statement for health professionals from the Committee on Rheumatic Fever, Endocarditis and Kawasaki Disease, Council on Cardiovascular Disease in the Young. American Heart Association Circulation. 2004;110(17):2747–71. doi:10.1161/01.CIR.0000145143.19711.78.
2. Kawasaki T. [Acute febrile mucocutaneous syndrome with lymphoid involvement with specific desquamation of the fingers and toes in children]. Arerugi. 1967;16(3):178–222.
3. Council on Cardiovascular Disease in the Young; Committee on Rheumatic Fever, Endocarditis, and Kawasaki Disease; American Heart Association . Diagnostic guidelines for Kawasaki disease. Circulation. 2001;103(2):335–6.
4. Dajani AS, Taubert KA, Gerber MA, Shulman ST, Ferrieri P, Freed M, et al. Diagnosis and therapy of Kawasaki disease in children. Circulation. 1993; 87(5):1776–80.
5. Yellen ES, Gauvreau K, Takahashi M, Burns JC, Shulman S, Baker AL, et al. Performance of 2004 American Heart Association recommendations for treatment of Kawasaki disease. Pediatrics. 2010;125(2):e234–41. doi:10.1542/peds.2009-0606.
6. Okanishi T, Enoki H. Transient subcortical high-signal lesions in Kawasaki syndrome. Pediatric Neurology. 2012;47(4):295–8. doi:10.1016/j.pediatrneurol.2012.05.022.
7. Tabarki B, Mahdhaoui A, Selmi H, Yacoub M, Essoussi AS. Kawasaki disease with predominant central nervous system involvement. Pediatric Neurology. 2001;25(3):239–41.
8. Aoki N. Subdural effusion in the acute stage of Kawasaki disease (Mucocutaneous lymph node syndrome). Surgical Neurology. 1988;29(3):216–7.
9. Bailie NM, Hensey OJ, Ryan S, Allcut D, King MD. Bilateral subdural collections–an unusual feature of possible Kawasaki disease. European Journal of Paediatric Neurology. 2001;5(2):79–81. doi:10.1053/ejpn.2001.0469.
10. Burns JC, Shike H, Gordon JB, Malhotra A, Schoenwetter M, Kawasaki T. Sequelae of Kawasaki disease in adolescents and young adults. Journal of the American College of Cardiology. 1996;28(1):253–7.
11. Haney I, Beghetti M, McCrindle BW, Gow RM. Ventricular arrhythmia complicating Kawasaki disease. The Canadian Journal of Cardiology. 1995;11(10):931–3.
12. Seymour JJ, Dickinson ET. Delayed cardiovascular sequelae from Kawasaki syndrome. The American Journal of Emergency Medicine. 1998;16(6):579–81.
13. Nakamura Y, Oki I, Tanihara S, Ojima T, Yanagawa H. Cardiac sequelae in recurrent cases of Kawasaki disease: a comparison between the initial episode of the disease and a recurrence in the same patients. Pediatrics. 1998;102(6):E66.
14. Hirata S, Nakamura Y, Yanagawa H. Incidence rate of recurrent Kawasaki disease and related risk factors: from the results of nationwide surveys of Kawasaki disease in Japan. Acta Paediatrica. 2001;90(1):40–4.

4

Differences in GlycA and lipoprotein particle parameters may help distinguish acute kawasaki disease from other febrile illnesses in children

Margery A. Connelly[1*], Chisato Shimizu[2], Deborah A. Winegar[1], Irina Shalaurova[1], Ray Pourfarzib[1], James D. Otvos[1], John T. Kanegaye[2,3], Adriana H. Tremoulet[2,3] and Jane C. Burns[2,3]

Abstract

Background: Glycosylation patterns of serum proteins, such as α1-acid glycoprotein, are modified during an acute phase reaction. The response of acute Kawasaki disease (KD) patients to IVIG treatment has been linked to sialic acid levels on native IgG, suggesting that protein glycosylation patterns vary during the immune response in acute KD. Additionally, the distribution and function of lipoprotein particles are altered during inflammation. Therefore, the aim of this study was to explore the potential for GlycA, a marker of protein glycosylation, and the lipoprotein particle profile to distinguish pediatric patients with acute KD from those with other febrile illnesses.

Methods: Nuclear magnetic resonance was used to quantify GlycA and lipoprotein particle classes and subclasses in pediatric subjects with acute KD ($n = 75$), post-treatment subacute ($n = 36$) and convalescent ($n = 63$) KD, as well as febrile controls ($n = 48$), and age-similar healthy controls ($n = 48$).

Results: GlycA was elevated in acute KD subjects compared to febrile controls with bacterial or viral infections, IVIG-treated subacute and convalescent KD subjects, and healthy children ($P < 0.0001$). Acute KD subjects had increased total and small low density lipoprotein particle numbers (LDL-P) ($P < 0.0001$) and decreased total high density lipoprotein particle number (HDL-P) ($P < 0.0001$) compared to febrile controls. Consequently, the ratio of LDL-P to HDL-P was higher in acute KD subjects than all groups tested ($P < 0.0001$). While GlycA, CRP, erythrocyte sedimentation rate, LDL-P and LDL-P/HDL-P ratio were able to distinguish patients with KD from those with other febrile illnesses (AUC = 0.789–0.884), the combinations of GlycA and LDL-P (AUC = 0.909) or GlycA and the LDL-P/HDL-P ratio (AUC = 0.910) were best at discerning KD in patients 6–10 days after illness onset.

Conclusions: High levels of GlycA confirm enhanced protein glycosylation as part of the acute phase response in KD patients. When combined with common laboratory tests and clinical characteristics, GlycA and NMR-measured lipoprotein particle parameters may be useful for distinguishing acute KD from bacterial or viral illnesses in pediatric patients.

Keywords: Kawasaki disease, Biomarkers, GlycA, Lipoprotein particle number

Abbreviations: ANC, Absolute neutrophil count; AUC, Area under the curve; CAA, Coronary artery aneurysm; CATHGEN, CATHeterization GENetics registry; CRP, C-reactive protein; ESR, Erythrocyte sedimentation rate; HDL-C, High density lipoprotein cholesterol; HDL-P, High density lipoprotein particle number; IQR, Interquartile range;
(Continued on next page)

* Correspondence: connem5@labcorp.com
[1]LipoScience, Laboratory Corporation of America® Holdings, 2500 Sumner Blvd, Raleigh, NC 27616, USA
Full list of author information is available at the end of the article

(Continued from previous page)
IVIG, Intravenous immunoglobulin; JUPITER, Justification for the use of statins in primary prevention: an intervention trial; KD, Kawasaki disease; LDL-P, Low density lipoprotein particle number; NMR, Nuclear magnetic resonance; PMN, Polymorphonuclear cells; PREVEND, Prevention of renal and vascular end-stage disease study; ROC, Receiver operating characteristic; TG, Triglycerides; VLDL, Very low density lipoprotein; WBC, White blood cell count; WHS, Womens Health Study

Background

Kawasaki disease (KD) is a self-limited vasculitis that typically presents in young children as an acute illness with fever and mucocutaneous changes [1, 2]. If KD is incorrectly diagnosed or left untreated, coronary artery aneurysms (CAA) may develop, predisposing KD patients to long-term cardiovascular complications including myocardial ischemia and infarction [3, 4]. Therefore, early diagnosis and treatment in the acute phase of the disease with intravenous immunoglobulin (IVIG) are important to reduce the risk of CAA [5, 6]. Diagnosis of KD, however, is challenging because the clinical signs are shared by other childhood acute rash/fever illnesses and there are no laboratory tests with sufficient specificity or sensitivity for detection of KD [7]. Therefore, additional biomarkers are needed to aid in diagnosis.

GlycA is a novel, nuclear magnetic resonance (NMR)-measured marker of inflammation whose signal arises from the carbohydrate side-chains of circulating proteins [8]. Hence, GlycA is a composite biomarker that integrates both the protein levels and glycosylation states of the most abundant acute phase proteins in serum. GlycA predicted adverse cardiovascular events in subjects in the Women's Health, JUPITER, PREVEND, CATHGEN and Intermountain Heart Collaborative studies, independent of traditional risk factors [9–13]. GlycA also predicted incident diabetes in a population of apparently healthy US women as well as in a large population of men and women in the Netherlands [14, 15]. Elevated GlycA was shown to be associated with disease activity and coronary atherosclerosis in rheumatoid arthritis patients [16]. Little is known, however, about the levels of this novel biomarker in acute pediatric illnesses such as KD. Glycosylation patterns of serum and cell surface proteins are critical determinants of the immune response [17, 18], and response of acute KD patients to IVIG treatment has been linked to sialic acid levels on native IgG [19]. We, therefore, hypothesized that GlycA levels are elevated in pediatric subjects with acute KD and serve as an indicator of acute inflammation.

Recently we reported that pediatric and adult KD subjects evaluated during the late convalescent phase of their illness had a similar lipoprotein profile compared to age-matched, healthy controls [20]. However, there are specific changes in the distribution of lipoprotein particle classes and subclasses in patients with active chronic inflammatory disease [21, 22]. Therefore we posited that the severe systemic inflammation that occurs in acute KD modifies the lipoprotein particle distribution and that these alterations may serve as additional markers of KD.

The aim of this study was to determine the ability of GlycA concentrations and NMR lipoprotein particle measures to distinguish pediatric patients with acute KD from those with other febrile illnesses.

Methods

Study population

Subjects included 75 children diagnosed with KD according to American Heart Association (AHA) criteria and treated at Rady Children's Hospital in San Diego, CA between November 2005 and June 2011. Specimens were obtained during 4 stages of KD: 1) pre-IVIG treatment acute (2–10 days after start of illness; illness day 1 defined as first day of fever), and post-IVIG treatment 2) subacute (13–24 days after start of illness), 3) early convalescent (25–75 days after start of illness) and 4) late convalescent (9–49 months after start of illness). The post-treatment subacute, early and late convalescent KD samples were obtained from subjects enrolled during the acute phase of illness. However, not all subjects provided samples during each of the subsequent stages.

Coronary artery status for acute KD subjects was classified as dilated if the internal diameter normalized for body surface area (Z score) was equal to or greater than 2.5 standard deviation units from the mean for the left anterior descending or right coronary arteries assessed by echocardiography during the first 6 weeks after disease onset. Aneurysms were defined as segments ≥1.5 times the diameter of the adjacent segments. Resistance to IVIG treatment was defined as fever at ≥36 h after the end of the IVIG infusion [7].

Forty-eight age-similar, healthy children undergoing minor orthopedic surgical procedures and 48 febrile children with acute illnesses of viral (adenoviral infection, influenza A or B, and viral syndrome) or bacterial (scarlet fever, cutaneous abscess) origin were also included in the study as healthy or febrile controls (Table 1). Written informed consent and assent when appropriate were obtained from the parents and subjects, respectively. The protocol was approved by the

Table 1 Clinical characteristics of pediatric untreated acute and IVIG-treated subacute and convalescent KD subjects and healthy and febrile controls

Characteristic	Acute KD 2–10 days (*n* = 75)	Subacute KD 13–24 days (*n* = 36)	Early Convalescent KD 25–75 days (*n* = 43)	Late Convalescent KD 9–49 months (*n* = 20)	Acute Febrile Controls Bacterial origin (*n* = 12)	Acute Febrile Controls Viral origin (*n* = 36)	Healthy Controls (*n* = 48)
Male, *n* (%)	39 (52)	20 (56)	26 (60)	11 (55)	10 (83)	21 (58)	–
Age, years	3.6 (1.8–5.0)	2.9 (1.7–4.6)	3.1 (1.7–4.5)	8.0 (6.7–9.2)	6.2 (4.7–8.2)	2.8 (1.6–5.3)	4.7 (3.0–6.6)
Illness day/month	6.0 d (4.5–7.0)	19 d (16–21)	48 d (34–55)	16 m (14–29)	3.5 d (3.0–4.3)	6.0 d (4.0–6.3)	–
Median lab values							
WBC, $\times 10^3/\mu L$	13.7 (10.6–17.3)	7.3 (6.8–9.0)	7.4 (6.0–8.5)	–	12.4 (10.1–14.5)#	8.7 (6.3–11.5)#	–
PMN, %	56 (45–66)	37 (26–50)	37 (27–42)	–	62 (46–70)	40 (23–54)	–
ANC, cells/μL	9646 (6693–12,131)	3025 (1953–3950)	2516 (1823–3525)	–	7014 (5565–9444)	3408 (2071–6764)	–
ESR, mm/h	61 (47–75)	37 (31–57)	17 (9–31)	–	31 (22–40)#	30 (17–39)#	–
CRP, mg/dL	7.4 (4.7–16.7)	0.3 (0.3–0.8)	0.3 (0.3–0.3)	–	2.2 (1.0–8.6)#	4.1 (2.2–5.0)#	–
GlycA, μmol/L	808 (693–919)	440 (382–512)	309 (272–377)	341 (319–395)	595 (571–745)	611 (551–702)	319 (290–354)

Median (IQR = Interquartile Range; 25th-75th percentile); *KD* Kawasaki Disease, *d* days, *m* months, *WBC* white blood cell count, *PMN* polymorphonuclear cells, *ANC* absolute neutrophil count, *ESR* erythrocyte sedimentation rate, *CRP* C-reactive protein; GlycA, NMR-measured marker of systemic inflammation. #Lab data available for WBC 46 subjects, ESR 42 subjects, CRP 31 subjects
Acute KD samples were taken pre-IVIG treatment. All other KD samples were taken post-IVIG treatment

Institutional Review Board at the University of California San Diego.

Inflammatory markers

White blood cell count (WBC), absolute neutrophil count (ANC), percent polymorphonuclear cells (PMN), high sensitivity C-reactive protein (CRP), and erythrocyte sedimentation rate (ESR) were measured as part of clinical care.

NMR analysis

NMR spectra were acquired from EDTA plasma samples as previously described for the *NMR LipoProfile®* (lipoprotein particle) test at LipoScience (now Labcorp, Raleigh, NC) [23]. The NMR Profiler platform is comprised of a 9.4T (400 MHz ^{1}H frequency) spectrometer (Bruker Biospin) with an integrated fluidics sample delivery system. The GlycA signal was quantified as previously described [8]. Lipoprotein particle profiles, triglycerides (TG) and high density lipoprotein cholesterol (HDL-C) were quantified using the LipoProfile-3 algorithm. Briefly, lipoprotein particle classes [very low density lipoprotein (VLDL), low density lipoprotein (LDL) and high density (HDL)] and subclasses [small, medium and large] were quantified using the amplitudes of their spectroscopically distinct lipid methyl group NMR signals [23]. Quantification of TG and HDL-C was accomplished by converting NMR particle numbers to lipid mass concentration units, assuming that the lipoprotein particles have normal lipid content. Previously published data showed that NMR-derived TG and HDL-C values correlate well with chemically measured values [23]. Samples were collected, stored at −80 °C and run in batch in 2014. Stability of GlycA and the lipoprotein analytes in frozen samples are stable for at least 6.5 years when stored at −80 °C [8, 23].

Statistical analysis

Patient characteristics were summarized by group. Medians and interquartile ranges (IQRs) were reported for continuous variables, and frequency counts and percentages were reported for categorical variables. One-way ANOVA and Dunnet's multiple comparison were used to compare the differences between groups, and two-tailed P values <0.05 were considered statistically significant. Spearman rank correlation coefficients (r) were calculated to evaluate interrelations between the inflammatory markers and lipoprotein parameters, and Mann–Whitney tests were used to gauge the significance of the association. Statistical analyses were performed using GraphPad Prism version 6. To assess the performance of these biomarkers as potential diagnostic tools, receiver operating characteristic (ROC) areas under the curve (AUC), likelihood ratios, positive predictive values, negative predictive values and Wald (χ^2) or z-statistics were calculated using Excel Analyse-it® v3.9.01.

Results

Clinical characteristics of treatment naïve pediatric acute KD subjects ($n = 75$) as well as IVIG-treated subjects with subacute (13–24 days; $n = 36$), early convalescent (25–75 days; $n = 43$) and late convalescent KD (9–49 months; $n = 20$), are described in Table 1 along with age-similar healthy pediatric controls ($n = 48$) and pediatric subjects with various acute febrile illnesses of bacterial ($n = 12$) and viral ($n = 36$) origin. Although GlycA levels were similar between healthy controls and convalescent KD patients, levels were higher in children with acute febrile illness and subacute KD than in healthy controls (P <0.0001), or convalescent KD subjects (P <0.0001) (Table 1, Fig. 1) and further elevated in acute KD patients (P <0.0001). Approximately one third of the subjects with acute KD had higher GlycA concentrations than any of the febrile subjects with acute illness (Fig. 1). GlycA concentrations were higher in subjects with acute KD than in those with influenza A or B, scarlet fever or viral syndrome (P <0.0001, 0.01 and 0.0001, respectively) but not in subjects with abscesses or adenoviral infections (Additional file 1: Figure S1). GlycA levels did not differ between acute KD patients who were resistant and those who responded to IVIG treatment (Additional file 2: Figure S2) or between acute KD subjects with CAA or dilated coronary arteries and those with normal echocardiograms (Fig. 1 and Additional file 2: Figure S2).

GlycA was strongly correlated with inflammatory markers such as WBC ($r = 0.43$), ANC ($r = 0.42$) and ESR ($r = 0.42$) (all P <0.001) and weakly correlated with CRP ($r = 0.26$, P <0.05) in acute KD patients (Additional file 3: Table S1). In addition, GlycA correlated strongly with illness day ($r = 0.48$, P <0.0001), while CRP was inversely correlated with this measure ($r = -0.35$, P <0.01) (Additional file 3: Table S1).

Analysis of NMR-measured lipoprotein and lipid parameters revealed that TG and TG-rich lipoprotein particles (VLDL measures) did not differ between healthy controls, pediatric KD patients and children with acute febrile illness (Table 2). There were, however, notable differences in HDL-P, LDL-P (Fig. 2a and b) and their subclasses among the various groups. Acute KD subjects and febrile controls had decreased HDL-C and total HDL-P (P <0.0001). Acute KD subjects and children with viral illnesses had decreased large HDL-P (P <0.0001), while acute KD subjects and children with bacterial illnesses had reduced small HDL-P (P <0.0001) compared to healthy controls and convalescent KD subjects (Table 2). Subjects with acute KD had higher total and small LDL-P (P <0.0001) than subjects in other groups. In addition, they had lower large LDL-P, leading

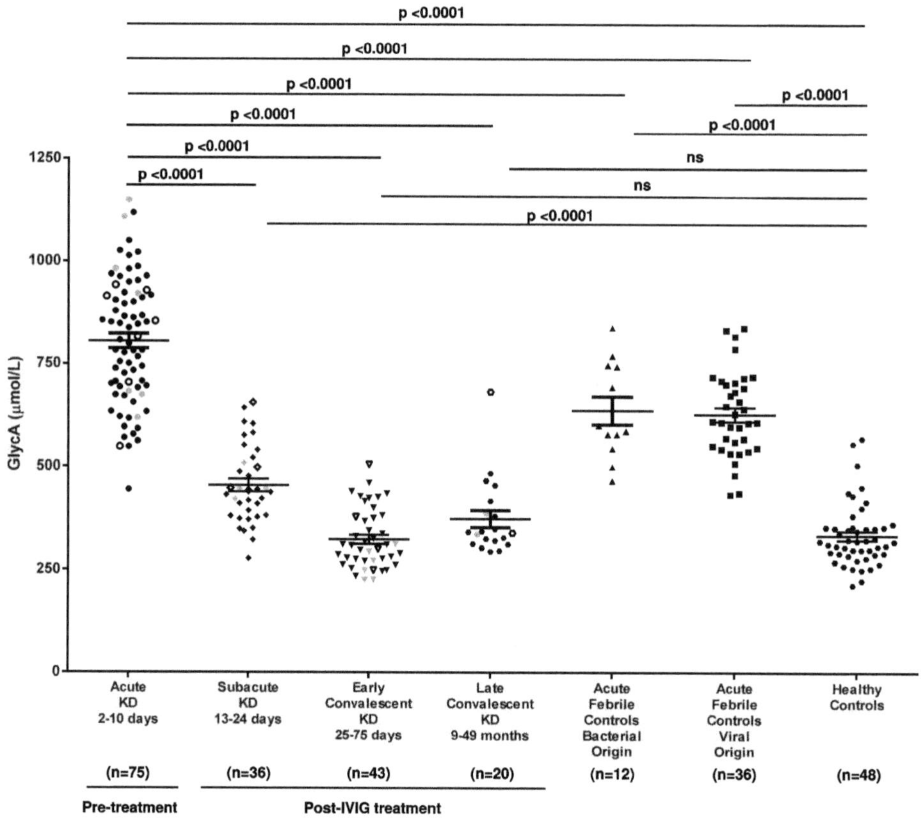

Fig. 1 Plasma concentrations of GlycA (μmol/L) among patients with: acute, subacute, early and late convalescent KD patients, febrile controls of bacterial and viral origin, and healthy controls. KD subjects are identified by coronary artery status: normal acute echocardiogram (*solid black symbol*); CAA (*open symbol*); or dilated coronary artery (*solid gray symbol*). *Horizontal bars* represent median and interquartile range

to a reduction in weighted-average LDL size, compared to all groups except those with acute febrile illness of viral origin (data not shown). Subjects with subacute KD had lipoprotein profiles between those of acute and convalescent illness, with HDL and LDL parameters nearing those of healthy controls (Table 2). Subjects with subacute, early and late convalescent KD had LDL-P/HDL-P ratios that mirrored those of normal healthy controls (Table 2). The LDL-P/HDL-P ratio was higher in acute KD subjects than in the other six groups (P <0.0001), while no significant differences were observed among healthy controls, subacute and convalescent KD subjects, and febrile controls (Fig. 2c).

To further explore the relationships between GlycA, CRP, ESR and the ratio of LDL-P/HDL-P with time, we plotted each biomarker as a function of illness day (Fig. 3). CRP peaked on day 3 and trended downward to approximately 50 % of peak levels by days 5–6, whereas GlycA continued to rise until days 5–6 and remained high through days 9–10 (Fig. 3a). Similar to GlycA, the LDL-P/HDL-P ratio continued to rise until days 7–8 and remained high until after IVIG-treatment (Days 13–15, Fig. 3b). ESR rose early and remained high, but exhibited a high degree of variability (Fig. 3c and d). Notably, GlycA and the LDL-P/HDL-P ratio appeared to distinguish themselves from the other biomarkers between days 6 and 10.

A ROC analysis was performed to evaluate the relative strengths of the NMR-measured biomarkers, CRP and ESR, at differentiating acute KD from combined febrile illness (bacterial and viral origin). The highest ROC AUCs (95 % confidence intervals) were 0.789 (0.707–0.872), 0.820 (0.721–0.918), 0.823 (0.752–0.894) and 0.884 (0.814–0.954) for the LDL-P/HDL-P ratio, CRP, GlycA and ESR, respectively, for illness days 2–10. A ROC analysis restricted to illness days 6–10 revealed AUC values of 0.691 (0.556–0.826), 0.730 (0.587–0.873), 0.842 (0.732–0.952), O.864 (0.765–0.963), 0.879 (0.778–0.979) and 0.891 (0.814–0.967), for total HDL-P, CRP, the LDL-P/HDL-P ratio, total LDL-P, ESR and GlycA, respectively (Additional file 4: Table S2). GlycA added to total LDL-P or the LDL-P/HDL-P ratio, resulted in AUCs (95 % confidence interval) of 0.909 (0.823–0.994) and 0.910 (0.838–0.982), respectively (Additional file 4: Table S2). The Wald test or z-statistics were 3.15, 6.09, 7.22, 7.37, 9.40, 9.99 and 11.65, and the positive likelihood ratios were 8.89, 6.49, 14.15, 6.29, 16.51, 15.33 and 15.92 for CRP, the LDL-P/HDL-P ratio, total LDL-P,

Table 2 Lipid profiles for pediatric untreated acute and IVIG-treated subacute and convalescent KD subjects and healthy and febrile pediatric controls

Characteristic	Acute KD 2–10 days (*n* = 75)	Subacute KD 13–24 days (*n* = 36)	Early Convalescent KD 25–75 days (*n* = 43)	Late Convalescent KD 9–49 months (*n* = 20)	Acute Febrile Controls Bacterial origin (*n* = 12)	Acute Febrile Controls Viral origin (*n* = 36)	Healthy Controls (*n* = 48)
HDL-C, mg/dL	26 (19–33)	44 (39–47)	53 (48–58)	56 (52–65)	37 (32–41)	34 (28–39)	49 (42–54)
TG, mg/dL	78 (66–97)	104 (83–142)	79 (67–105)	68 (65–99)	86 (55–120)	63 (56–75)	93 (73–115)
LDL particles, nmol/L							
Total LDL-P	1513 (1228–1826)	1259 (766–1416)	984 (680–1115)	861 (705–1167)	1186 (934–1273)	1052 (916–1231)	1110 (948–1248)
IDL-P	110 (65–159)	128 (56–176)	100 (44–143)	88 (63–118)	88 (65–117)	78 (55–107)	106 (71–145)
Large LDL-P	116 (29–244)	472 (261–629)	415 (281–497)	339 (290–527)	299 (216–340)	99 (47–215)	558 (426–718)
Small LDL-P	1230 (880–1574)	483 (392–677)	435 (331–532)	456 (291–536)	754 (549–973)	809 (688–996)	394 (190–531)
HDL particles, μmol/L							
Total HDL-P	18 (14–22)	28 (27–32)	32 (30–34)	33 (32–35)	23 (22–24)	23 (20–27)	30 (27–34)
Large HDL-P	2.1 (1.4–3.1)	4.4 (3.3–5.4)	5.9 (4.6–7.6)	6.2 (4.8–8.5)	4.0 (2.8–6.2)	2.2 (1.3–3.2)	4.7 (3.8–5.8)
Medium HDL-P	8.6 (4.7–12.8)	11.4 (9.8–13.9)	11.7 (10.6–14.5)	12.4 (9.6–14.2)	12.9 (9.0–15.9)	10.2 (7.9–12.9)	9.1 (5.8–12.7)
Small HDL-P	6.8 (3.9–9.2)	11.8 (9.5–13.5)	13.6 (12.0–15.0)	13.9 (11.5–15.8)	4.5 (2.6–7.4)	10.5 (7.1–13.1)	16.2 (14.4–18.0)
VLDL particles, nmol/L							
Total VLDL-P	39 (23–62)	56 (30–82)	36 (24–63)	31 (23–56)	57 (21–75)	27 (19–35)	49 (31–69)
Large VLDL-P	0.9 (0.6–1.7)	1.9 (1.2–5.0)	1.2 (0.8–2.1)	1.1 (0.6–1.4)	0.9 (0.4–1.5)	1.3 (0.9–1.5)	1.4 (0.9–2.8)
Medium VLDL-P	4.5 (1.8–10.4)	15.3 (7.3–28.7)	8.8 (3.2–16.5)	5.2 (0.6–1.4)	3.7 (2.5–18.2)	4.1 (2.0–8.1)	9.1 (4.6–19.4)
Small VLDL-P	31 (18–52)	29 (15–45)	31 (18–42)	26 (17–41)	46 (17–57)	19 (12–29)	35 (21–48)
LDL-P/HDL-P	92 (65–119)	41 (28–51)	29 (22–37)	27 (21–34)	50 (37–59)	45 (37–61)	38 (29–42)

Median (IQR = Interquartile Range; 25th-75th percentile). *LDL-C* low density lipoprotein cholesterol, *HDL-C* high density lipoprotein cholesterol, *TG* triglycerides, *LDL-P* low density lipoprotein particle number, *IDL-P* intermediate density lipoprotein particle number, *HDL-P* high density lipoprotein particle number, *VLDL-P* very low density particle number. Acute KD samples were taken pre-IVIG treatment. All other KD samples were taken post-IVIG treatment

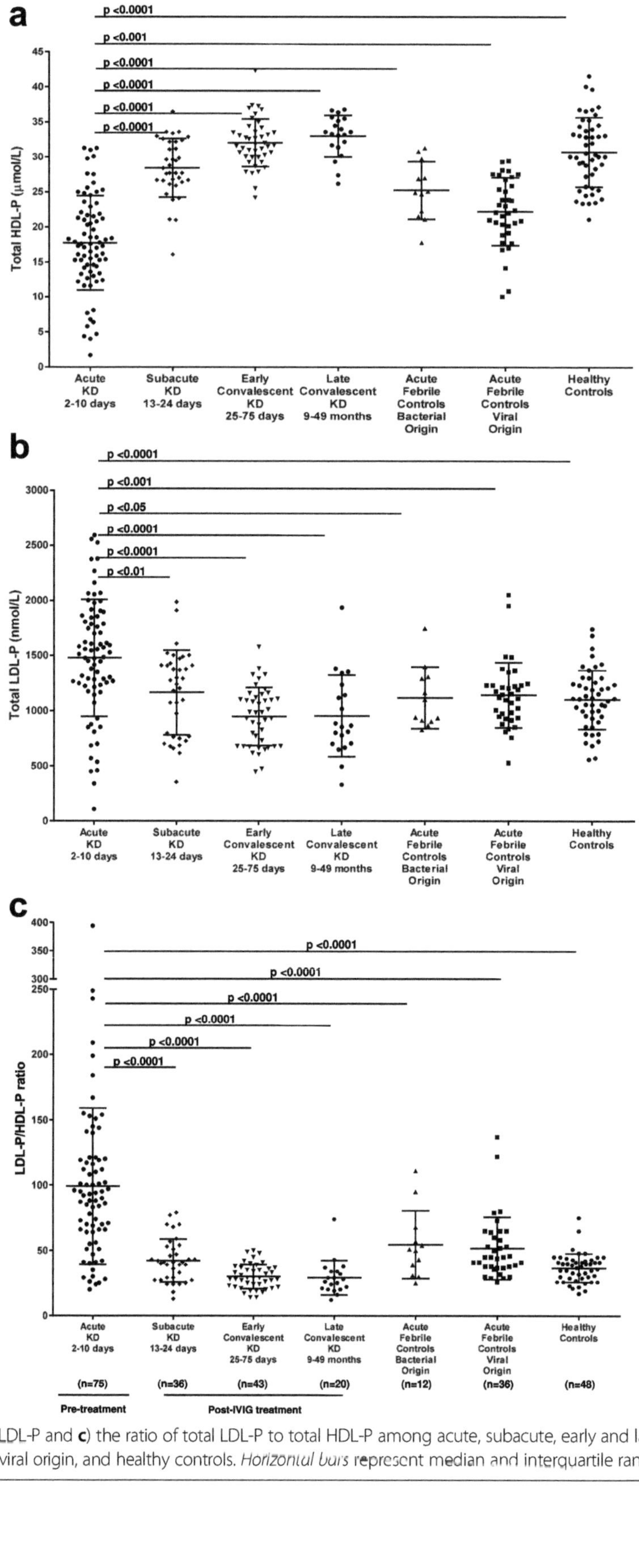

Fig. 2 a) Total HDL-P, **b)** total LDL-P and **c)** the ratio of total LDL-P to total HDL-P among acute, subacute, early and late convalescent KD patients, febrile controls of bacterial and viral origin, and healthy controls. *Horizontal bars* represent median and interquartile range

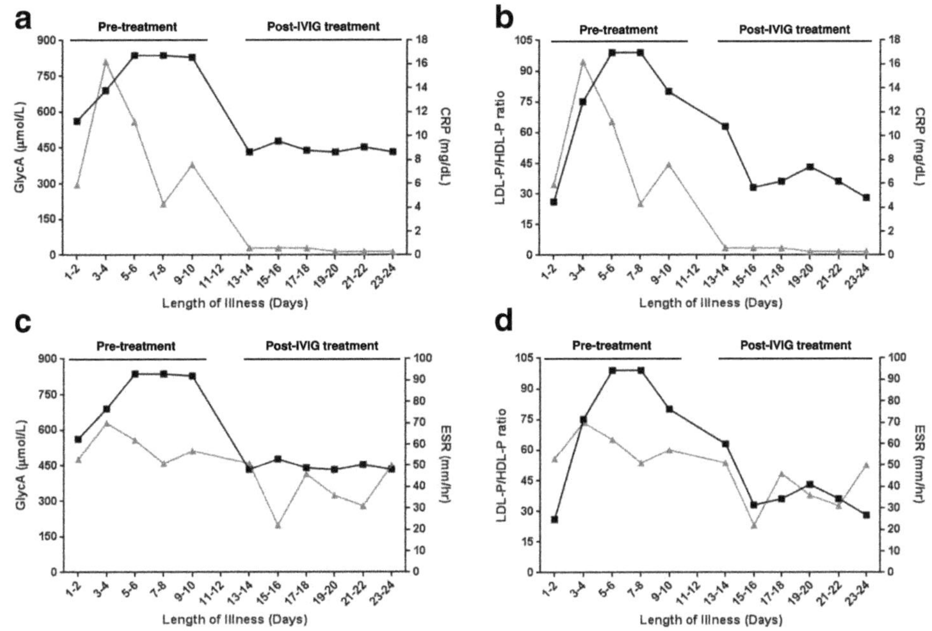

Fig. 3 Time course of biomarkers (median) in KD subjects from acute phase to early convalescence: **a**) GlycA (left y-axis; *black line* and *symbols*) and CRP (right y-axis; *dark gray line* and *symbols*), **b**) LDL-P/HDL-P ratio (left y-axis; *black line* and *symbols*) and CRP (right y-axis; *dark gray line* and *symbols*), **c**), GlycA (left y-axis; *black line* and *symbols*) and ESR (right y-axis; *dark gray line* and *symbols*), **d**) LDL-P/HDL-P ratio (left y-axis; *black line* and *symbols*) and ESR (right y-axis; *dark gray line* and *symbols*) in KD patients plotted as a function of illness day (Illness day 1 = first day of fever). Illness day 1 = first day of fever. Pre-IVIG treatment = days 2–10 and post-IVIG treatment = days 13–24

ESR, GlycA plus total LDL-P, GlycA and GlycA plus LDL-P/HDL-P, respectively (Additional file 4: Table S2). A comparison of the ROC curves for all 6 biomarkers can be found in Fig. 4.

Discussion

In this study, we identified changes in NMR-measured lipoprotein particle parameters and GlycA that may be useful in diagnosing acute KD or in monitoring resolution of inflammation after treatment. GlycA levels were higher in children with acute KD than in those with other febrile illnesses. GlycA levels in acute KD subjects were also higher than levels observed in subjects with chronic inflammatory-mediated illnesses (e.g. cardiovascular disease, rheumatoid arthritis and systemic lupus erythematosus) [9–16, 24]. In addition, lipoprotein particle class and subclass numbers differed between patients with acute KD and those with acute febrile illnesses. Several HDL-P measures were lower in acute KD patients than in healthy, convalescent KD and febrile controls. Total LDL-P and the ratio of LDL-P to HDL-P were higher in acute KD patients than in the other control groups. These changes are consistent with previous observations that acute phase proteins (e.g. α1-acid glycoprotein, serum amyloid A, ceruloplasmin) and lipases (e.g. endothelial lipase, secreted phospholipase A_2-IIa and -V), which are upregulated during inflammation, modify the size distribution and function of lipoprotein particles [25–29].

During acute inflammation, serum levels of CRP and serum amyloid A (SAA) rise and fall within the first few days [30]. In contrast, serum levels of the proteins that give rise to the GlycA NMR signal (e.g. α1-acid glycoprotein, haptoglobin, α1-antitrypsin, α1-antichymotrypsin) rise more slowly, reaching peak concentrations several days after onset of an acute inflammatory reaction, and fall slowly over weeks [30]. Our data support these observations, as CRP levels rose early and fell by day 6 while GlycA levels rose later and remained high through day 10. The finding that GlycA exhibited a strong correlation with illness day, while CRP showed an inverse correlation confirms the results of the kinetic data. Therefore, GlycA and CRP levels may add independent value when evaluating patients with inflammatory illnesses such as KD; especially 6–10 days after illness onset when levels of these two biomarkers varied in relation to one another.

The ROC AUCs of 0.910 and 0.909 for GlycA combined with either the LDL-P/HDL-P ratio or LDL-P, respectively, suggest that these biomarker combinations are better at distinguishing KD from other febrile illnesses than CRP, ESR or any of the 3 biomarkers alone. The results of the Wald and Likelihood Ratio tests, alternative measures of the performance of a diagnostic test, suggest that the combinations of GlycA with LDL-P/HDL-P or LDL-P will correctly distinguish patients with KD from those with febrile illnesses more often than CRP or ESR alone. Thus, NMR-measured biomarkers may be useful in determining

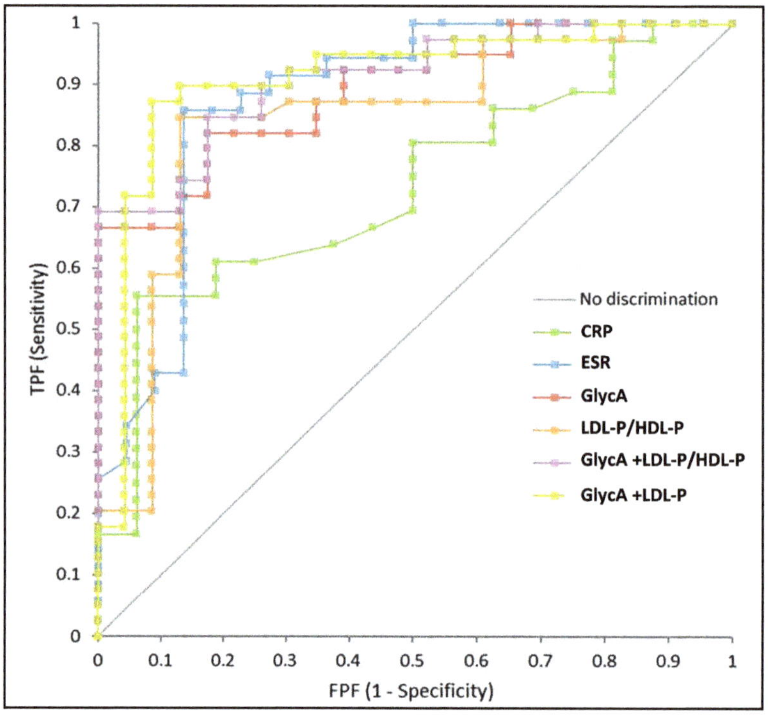

Fig. 4 ROC curves for the discrimination of KD from febrile illnesses during illness days 6–10 by CRP, ESR, GlycA, LDL-P/HDL-P, GlycA and LDL-P/HDL-P and GlycA + LDL-P

antecedent inflammation in patients presenting later (6–10 days) in the course of acute KD. These biomarkers may also be useful in patients whose fever and other mucocutaneous signs have resolved but for whom subsequent periungual peeling prompts evaluation for missed KD. Unfortunately we were unable to test this hypothesis with our data, given that all subjects with acute KD received IVIG-treatment by 10 days after fever onset. Therefore, future studies with samples taken from patients untreated beyond 10 days of fever onset will more accurately determine the kinetics of GlycA and LDL-P/HDL-P ratio as markers of inflammation and will address the question of whether or not these biomarkers will be useful for missed KD.

When used along with the typical clinical characteristics observed in patients with pediatric febrile illnesses and standard diagnostic tools, the combination of GlycA with either LDL-P or the LDL-P/HDL-P ratio may help identify children with KD. GlycA has the advantage of being a more stable biomarker, in terms of within-subject biological variation, than CRP [8]. To illustrate this point we determined the homeostatic set points, the true values of analytes in biological homeostasis, for CRP and GlycA in a cohort of normal, healthy, adult volunteers ($n = 23$) collected for a previously published biological variability study [8]. We calculated that 33 concurrent measurements of CRP would be required to estimate its true value for a single patient, compared to only one for GlycA [8, 31, 32]. In addition, while the ESR is affected by IVIG treatment, GlycA is unaffected by the presence of IgG [8] or IVIG [unpublished results]. Therefore, the combinations of GlycA with either LDL-P/HDL-P or LDL-P are may provide an additional tool for pediatric patient care.

We recognize both strengths and weaknesses in our study. This is the first study to assess glycosylation levels of plasma proteins in a well-characterized cohort of KD and febrile controls who share some clinical features with acute KD patients. However, sample size was limited and would need to be increased in independent cohorts of pediatric subjects in order to test the predictive value of these biomarkers in KD diagnosis. In addition, the kinetic analysis suffered by the limitation that the samples were not taken from the same subjects at each time point. Finally, the study would have benefited by the inclusion of additional samples from patients with scarlet fever, adenoviral infection and juvenile idiopathic arthritis as these illnesses are most likely to cause clinical confusion with KD. Therefore future studies will include samples from these illnesses as well as serious illnesses such as bacterial pneumonia, pyelonephritis and sepsis.

Conclusions

High levels of GlycA confirm enhanced protein glycosylation as part of the acute phase response in KD patients. When combined with common laboratory tests and clinical characteristics, GlycA and NMR-measured lipoprotein particle parameters may be useful for distinguishing acute KD from bacterial or viral illnesses in pediatric patients.

Additional files

Additional file 1: Figure S1. Plasma concentrations of GlycA (μmol/L) in subjects with: acute KD, abscess, adenoviral infection, influenza A or B, scarlet fever or viral syndrome. ns = not statistically significant. Horizontal bars represent median and interquartile range.

Additional file 2: Figure S2. Plasma concentrations of GlycA (μmol/L) in acute KD patients who responded to intravenous immunoglobulin (IVIG) treatment, those who were IVIG-resistant, and healthy controls. Noted are acute KD subjects with a normal echocardiogram (solid black symbol) as well as those who developed a CAA (open symbol) or a dilated coronary artery (solid gray symbol). ns = not statistically significant. Horizontal bars represent median and interquartile range.

Additional file 3: Table S1. Correlations among inflammatory markers in acute KD subjects.

Additional file 4: Table S2. SPerformance characteristics for GlycA, lipoprotein parameters, CRP and ESR restricted to illness days 6-10.

Acknowledgments

This work was supported in part by grants from the National Institutes of Health, Heart, Lung, and Blood Institute (JCB; RO1-HL69413), the iDASH grant U54HL108460 and the Gordon and Marilyn Macklin Foundation (JCB). The authors thank DeeAnna Scherrer and Joan Pancheri, RN for assistance with sample collection.

Authors' contributions

MAC, DAW, IS, RP, and JDO contributed to the testing of the samples at LipoScience (now LabCorp) as well as review of the analyzed data, data interpretation and manuscript review. Although NMR testing was performed free of charge, study samples were tested blinded to any information regarding the study subjects. The study was designed, samples were collected, and data analysis and interpretation was performed by employees at UCSD (CS, JK, AHT, JCB). MAC wrote the initial draft of the manuscript. No honorarium or grant was provided to produce the manuscript. All authors contributed to the manuscript, have seen the final version and have agreed to submit the manuscript for publication. All authors read and approved the final manuscript.

Competing interests

MAC, DAW, IS, RP and JDO are employees of LipoScience (now LabCorp). CS, JTK, AHT, JCB declare that they have no competing interests.

Author details

[1]LipoScience, Laboratory Corporation of America® Holdings, 2500 Sumner Blvd, Raleigh, NC 27616, USA. [2]Department of Pediatrics, University of California, San Diego, CA, USA. [3]Rady Children's Hospital, San Diego, CA, USA.

References

1. Kawasaki T, Kosaki F, Okawa S, Shigematsu I, Yanagawa H. A new infantile acute febrile mucocutaneous lymph node syndrome (MLNS) prevailing in Japan. Pediatrics. 1974;54(3):271–6.
2. Burns JC, Glode MP. Kawasaki syndrome. Lancet. 2004;364(9433):533–44. doi:10.1016/S0140-6736(04)16814-1.
3. Suzuki A, Kamiya T, Kuwahara N, Ono Y, Kohata T, Takahashi O, et al. Coronary arterial lesions of Kawasaki disease: cardiac catheterization findings of 1100 cases. Pediatr Cardiol. 1986;7(1):3–9. doi:10.1007/BF02315475.
4. Gordon JB, Kahn AM, Burns JC. When children with Kawasaki disease grow up: myocardial and vascular complications in adulthood. JACC. 2009;54(21):1911–20. doi:10.1016/j.jacc.2009.04.102.
5. Ogata S, Tremoulet AH, Sato Y, Ueda K, Shimizu C, Sun X, et al. Coronary artery outcomes among children with Kawasaki disease in the United States and Japan. Int J Cardiol. 2013;168(4):3825–8. doi:10.1016/j.ijcard.2013.06.027.
6. Newburger JW, Takahashi M, Beiser AS, Burns JC, Bastian J, Chung KJ, et al. A single intravenous infusion of gamma globulin as compared with four infusions in the treatment of acute Kawasaki syndrome. NEJM. 1991;324(23):1633–9. doi:10.1056/NEJM199106063242305.
7. Newburger JW, Takahashi M, Gerber MA, Gewitz MH, Tani LY, Burns JC, et al. Diagnosis, treatment, and long-term management of Kawasaki disease: a statement for health professionals from the Committee on Rheumatic Fever, Endocarditis and Kawasaki Disease, Council on Cardiovascular Disease in the Young, American Heart Association. Circ. 2004;110(17):2747–71. doi:10.1161/01.CIR.0000145143.19711.78.
8. Otvos JD, Shalaurova I, Wolak-Dinsmore J, Connelly MA, Mackey RH, Stein JH, et al. GlycA: a composite nuclear magnetic resonance biomarker of systemic inflammation. Clin Chem. 2015;61(5):714–23. doi:10.1373/clinchem.2014.232918.
9. Akinkuolie AO, Buring JE, Ridker PM, Mora S. A novel protein glycan biomarker and future cardiovascular disease events. JAHA. 2014;3(5): e001221. doi:10.1161/JAHA.114.001221.
10. Akinkuolie AO, Glynn RJ, Ridker PM, Mora S. Protein glycan side-chains, rosuvastatin therapy, and incident vascular events: an anlysis from the JUPITER trial. Circ. 2014;130(S_2):A17731.
11. Muhlestein JB, Mays H, Winegar D, Rollo J, Connelly M, Otvos J, Anderson J. GlycA and GlycB, novel NMR biomarkers of inflammation, strongly predict future cardiovascular events, but not the presence of coronary artery disease (CAD), among patients undergoing, coronary angiography: the Intermountain Heart Collaborative Study. JACC. 2014;63(12_S):61389.
12. McGarrah R, Craig D, Haynes C, Dowdy ZE, Shah S, Kraus W. GlycA, a novel biomarker of systemic inflammation, improves cardiovascular risk prediction in a high-risk coronary catheterization cohort. JACC. 2015;65(10S):A1606.
13. Gruppen EG, Riphagen IJ, Connelly MA, Otvos JD, Bakker SJ, Dullaart RP. GlycA, a pro-inflammatory glycoprotein biomarker, and incident cardiovascular disease: relationship with C-reactive protein and renal function. PLoS One. 2015;10(9):e0139057. doi:10.1371/journal.pone.0139057.
14. Akinkuolie AO, Pradhan AD, Buring JE, Ridker PM, Mora S. Novel protein glycan side-chain biomarker and risk of incident type 2 diabetes mellitus. ATVB. 2015;35(6):1544–50. doi:10.1161/ATVBAHA.115.305635.
15. Connelly MA, Gruppen EG, Wolak-Dinsmore J, Matyus SP, Riphagen IJ, Shalaurova I, et al. GlycA, a marker of acute phase glycoproteins, and the risk of incident type 2 diabetes mellitus: PREVEND study. Clin Chim Acta. 2015;452:10–7. doi:10.1016/j.cca.2015.11.001.
16. Ormseth MJ, Chung CP, Oeser AM, Connelly MA, Sokka T, Raggi P, et al. Utility of a novel inflammatory marker, GlycA, for assessment of rheumatoid arthritis disease activity and coronary atherosclerosis. Arthritis Res & Ther. 2015;17(1):117. doi:10.1186/s13075-015-0646-x.
17. Amon R, Reuven EM, Leviatan Ben-Arye S, Padler-Karavani V. Glycans in immune recognition and response. Carbohydr Res. 2014;389:115–22. doi:10.1016/j.carres.2014.02.004.
18. Nagae M, Yamaguchi Y. Function and 3D structure of the N-glycans on glycoproteins. Int J Mol Sci. 2012;13(7):8398–429. doi:10.3390/ijms13078398.
19. Ogata S, Shimizu C, Franco A, Touma R, Kanegaye JT, Choudhury BP, et al. Treatment response in kawasaki disease is associated with sialylation levels of endogenous but not therapeutic intravenous immunoglobulin G. PLoS One. 2013;8(12):e81448. doi:10.1371/journal.pone.0081448.
20. Lin J, Jain S, Sun X, Liu V, Sato YZ, Jimenez-Fernandez S, et al. Lipoprotein particle concentrations in children and adults following Kawasaki disease. J Pediatr. 2014;165(4):727–31. doi:10.1016/j.jpeds.2014.06.017.
21. Chung CP, Oeser A, Raggi P, Sokka T, Pincus T, Solus JF, et al. Lipoprotein subclasses determined by nuclear magnetic resonance spectroscopy and coronary atherosclerosis in patients with rheumatoid arthritis. J Rheumatol. 2010;37(8):1633–8. doi:10.3899/jrheum.090639.
22. McInnes IB, Thompson L, Giles JT, Bathon JM, Salmon JE, Beaulieu AD, et al. Effect of interleukin-6 receptor blockade on surrogates of vascular risk in rheumatoid arthritis: MEASURE, a randomised, placebo-controlled study. Ann Rheum Dis. 2013;74(4):694–702. doi:10.1136/annrheumdis-2013-204345.

23. Jeyarajah EJ, Cromwell WC, Otvos JD. Lipoprotein particle analysis by nuclear magnetic resonance spectroscopy. Clinics Lab Med. 2006;26(4):847–70. doi:10.1016/j.cll.2006.07.006.
24. Chung CP, Ormseth MJ, Oeser A, Solus JF, Connelly MA, Otvos JD, Stein CM. GlycA, a novel NMR marker of inflammation, is elevated in systemic lupus erythematosus. Lupus. 2016;25:296–300.
25. G HB, Rao VS, Kakkar VV. Friend Turns Foe: Transformation of anti-inflammatory HDL to proinflammatory HDL during acute-phase response. Cholesterol. 2011:274629. doi:10.1155/2011/274629
26. Jahangiri A. High-density lipoprotein and the acute phase response. Curr Opin Endocrinol Diabetes Obes. 2010;17(2):156–60. doi:10.1097/MED.0b013e328337278b.
27. Lahdesmaki K, Plihtari R, Soininen P, Hurt-Camejo E, Ala-Korpela M, Oorni K, et al. Phospholipase A(2)-modified LDL particles retain the generated hydrolytic products and are more atherogenic at acidic pH. Atherosclerosis. 2009;207(2):352–9. doi:10.1016/j.atherosclerosis.2009.04.031.
28. de la Llera Moya M, McGillicuddy FC, Hinkle CC, Byrne M, Joshi MR, Nguyen V, et al. Inflammation modulates human HDL composition and function in vivo. Atherosclerosis. 2012;222(2):390–4. doi:10.1016/j.atherosclerosis.2012.02.032.
29. Zannis VI, Fotakis P, Koukos G, Kardassis D, Ehnholm C, Jauhiainen M, et al. HDL biogenesis, remodeling, and catabolism. Handb Exp Pharmacol. 2015;224:53–111. doi:10.1007/978-3-319-09665-0_2.
30. Gabay C, Kushner I. Acute-phase proteins and other systemic responses to inflammation. NEJM. 1999;340(6):448–54. doi:10.1056/NEJM199902113400607.
31. Fraser CG. Test result variation and the quality of evidence-based clinical guidelines. Clin Chim Acta. 2004;346(1):19–24. doi:10.1016/j.cccn.2003.12.032.
32. Westgard JO, Darcy T. The truth about quality: medical usefulness and analytical reliability of laboratory tests. Clin Chim Acta. 2004;346(1):3–11. doi:10.1016/j.cccn.2003.12.034.

5

Wasting, underweight and stunting among children with congenital heart disease presenting at Mulago hospital, Uganda

Anthony Batte[1*], Peter Lwabi[2], Sulaiman Lubega[2], Sarah Kiguli[3], Kennedy Otwombe[4], Lucy Chimoyi[5], Violette Nabatte[6] and Charles Karamagi[3,7]

Abstract

Background: Children with congenital heart disease are at increased risk of malnutrition. The aim of this study was to describe the prevalence of wasting, underweight and stunting among children with congenital heart disease attending Mulago National Referral Hospital, Uganda.

Methods: A cross-sectional study among 194 children aged 0–15 years was conducted between August 2013 and March 2014. Anthropometric measurements and clinical assessments were carried out on all children. Anthropometric z-scores based on WHO 2007 reference ranges were generated for each child. Weight-for-height z-scores were generated for children 0–5 years, weight-for-age z-scores for children 0–10 years, and height-for-age and BMI-for-age z-scores for all children. Risk factors associated with malnutrition were determined by Poisson regression.

Results: One hundred and forty five (74.7%) children were aged 0–5 years; and 111 of 194 (57.2%) were female. Forty five of 145 (31.5%) children aged 0–5 years were wasted; 77 of 181 (42.5%) children aged 0–10 years were underweight; 88 of 194 (45.4%) children were stunted; and 53 of 194 (27.3%) children were thin (BMI for age z score < −2). Moderate to severe anaemia (RR 1.11, 95% CI: 1.01–1.22) and moderate to severe heart failure (RR 1.24, 95% CI: 1.13–1.36) were associated with wasting and underweight respectively. Stunting was associated with moderate to severe heart failure (RR 1.11, 95% CI: 1.01–1.21) while thinness was associated with moderate to severe heart failure (RR 1.12, 95% CI: 1.04–1.21) and moderate to severe anaemia (RR 1.15, 95% CI: 1.06–1.25).

Conclusion: Malnutrition is common in children with congenital heart disease, and is associated with anaemia and heart failure. There is need to integrate strategies to identify and manage malnutrition during the care of children with congenital heart disease.

Keywords: Congenital heart disease, Malnutrition, Uganda, Africa

Background

Children with congenital heart disease (CHD) are at an increased risk for wasting, underweight and stunting [1–3]. Malnutrition among these children increases their risk to infections and the risk of death even after corrective surgery [4]. In addition, malnutrition leads to poor growth in children which is associated with delayed mental development, poor school performance and reduced intellectual capacity [4, 5]. These outcomes significantly impair economic productivity in adult life.

Risk factors for malnutrition among children with CHD include heart failure, cyanosis, multiple heart defects, delayed corrective surgery, anaemia and pulmonary hypertension [1, 3, 6]. Furthermore, in children with CHD, poor nutrition is also attributed to inadequate nutritional intake due to feeding difficulties and the increased energy expenditure among these children [7]. In developing countries, corrective surgery for congenital

* Correspondence: abatte2002@yahoo.com
[1]Child Health and Development Centre, Makerere University College of Health Sciences, P.O.Box 6717, Kampala, Uganda
Full list of author information is available at the end of the article

heart defects is delayed and this increases the likelihood of the children developing malnutrition [8].

In Uganda, childhood malnutrition is a public health problem with 33% of children aged under 5 years being stunted, 14% underweight and 5% wasted [9]. Thus malnutrition in children with CHD in Uganda is likely to be common and of multi-factorial origin. A clear understanding of the complex nature of malnutrition in children with CHD is essential to design strategies that will improve outcomes in these children. This study was therefore conducted to determine the prevalence of malnutrition in children with congenital heart disease and the factors associated with wasting, underweight and stunting.

Methods

Study setting and population

The study was carried out at Mulago National Referral Hospital and Uganda Heart Institute, Kampala, from August 2013 to March 2014. Participants were 194 children aged 0–15years with congenital heart disease diagnosed by echocardiography. They were part of a previous study which assessed arrhythmias among children; and the details of the methods and the different heart diseases for each child are described elsewhere [10].

Variables

Data were collected on socio-demographic characteristics and clinical assessments of the children. Weight was measured using a SECA® weighing scale and readings were recorded to the nearest 0.1 kg. Height was measured using a stadiometer (measuring board) and readings recorded to the nearest 0.5 cm. Heights for children below 2 years was taken when the children were lying down while older children had their heights taken when standing. We used the World Health Organisation (WHO) z-scores to classify the nutritional status of the children [11]. A child was classified as underweight if the weight-for-age WHO z-score was < −2 SD, wasted if weight-for-height WHO z-score was < −2 SD (for children aged 0–5 years), thin if BMI-for-age WHO z-score was < −2 SD and stunted if height-for-age z-score was < −2 SD.

All children were assessed for heart failure and the severity of heart failure was graded using the modified Ross score; children were grouped into two categories based on a Ross score 0–6 (mild or no heart failure) and a Ross score >6 (moderate to severe heart failure) [12, 13].

Hemoglobin levels of the children were recorded from complete blood counts that were performed using Celltac E MEK-7222 automatic hematology analyzer. Grading of the severity of anaemia (mild, moderate and severe) was done according to WHO age specific reference ranges [14]. An HIV test was performed on each child using Alere™ HIV-1/2 Determine® as a screen, followed by STAT-PAK® HIV-1/2; the Uni-Gold™ Recombigen® for confirmation. HIV infection in children aged under 18 months who were HIV positive by serology test was confirmed using the HIV DNA PCR test.

Data analysis

Age was categorized into three groups: 0–5, 6–10 and 11–15 years. The demographic and clinical characteristics were stratified by age. Continuous anthropometric measures were stratified using a z-score of < −2 as a cutoff for malnutrition. Overall frequencies were determined for all categorical measures followed by stratification by age. Medians and interquartile ranges of the anthropometric measures were determined overall and by age.

Poisson regression with robust error variances was used to determine factors associated with malnutrition both at the univariate and multivariate level. All the variables with at least one factor having a *p*-value < 0.2 at the univariate level were considered for entry into the multivariate model controlling for age. Statistical analysis was performed using SAS/STAT software version 9.4 (SAS Institute Inc., Cary, NC, USA).

Results

Demographic characteristics of participants

One hundred and forty five of 194 children (74.7%) were aged 0–5 years and 111 of 194 (57.2%) were female. One hundred and thirty eight of 194 children (71.1%) had acyanotic heart disease but only 4 (2.1%) had surgically corrected heart defects (Table 1). Two children (1%) were HIV positive.

Proportion of children wasted, underweight and stunted

Overall, 45 of 145 (31.5%) children aged 0–5 years had weight-for-height z-score < −2 (wasted). The median weight-for-height z-score among these children was −0.89 (IQR: −2.46,-0.10). Of the children aged 0–10 years, 77 of 181 (42.5%) had weight-for-age z-scores < −2 (underweight) and the median weight-for-age z-score among these children was −1.69 (IQR-3.07,-0.69). Fifty three of 194 children (27.3%) had a BMI-for-age z-score < −2 (thin) with a median BMI-for-age z-score of −0.72 (IQR −2.21, 0.17). The number of stunted children was 88 out of 194 (45.4%) with a median height-for-age z-score of −1.67 (IQR −3.21,-0.51). These findings are summarised in Table 2.

Factors associated with malnutrition

Among children under 5 years, children with moderate/severe anaemia (RR: 1.11, 95% CI: 1.01–1.22) had

Table 1 Demographic and clinical characteristics

Variable	Overall	0-5 years ($n = 145$)	6-10 years ($n = 36$)	11-15 years ($n = 13$)
Gender				
Male (%)	83 (42.8)	65 (44.8)	14 (38.9)	4 (30.8)
Female (%)	111 (57.2)	80 (55.2)	22 (61.1)	9 (69.2)
Classification of heart disease				
Cyanotic (%)	56 (28.9)	39 (26.9)	13 (36.1)	4 (30.8)
Acyanotic (%)	138 (71.1)	106 (73.1)	23 (63.9)	9 (69.2)
Heart disease surgically corrected				
Yes (%)	4 (2.1)	2 (1.4)	1 (2.8)	1 (7.7)
No (%)	190 (97.9)	143 (98.6)	35 (97.2)	12 (92.3)
Heart failure				
Moderate/ Severe Heart failure (%)	78 (40.2)	58 (40.0)	16 (44.4)	4 (30.8)
Mild/ no Heart failure (%)	116 (59.8)	87 (60.0)	20 (55.6)	9 (69.2)
Anaemia				
Moderate/ Severe anaemia (%)	68 (35.6)	58 (40.8)	8 (22.2)	2 (15.4)
Mild/ No Anaemia (%)	123 (64.4)	84 (59.2)	28 (77.8)	11 (84.6)

a higher risk of being wasted after controlling for age and heart failure (Table 3). Among children aged 0–10 years, moderate/severe heart failure was associated with being underweight after adjusting for age and anaemia (RR: 1.24, 95% CI: 1.13–1.36) (Table 4). After controlling for age and anaemia, children with moderate/severe heart failure had a higher risk of stunting (RR 1.11, 95% CI 1.01–1.21) (Table 5). After controlling for age, children with moderate/severe heart failure (RR: 1.12, 95% CI: 1.04–1.21) and moderate/severe anaemia (RR: 1.15, 95% CI: 1.06–1.25) had a higher risk of thinness (Table 6).

Discussion

Our study showed that malnutrition in children with congenital heart disease is high. The prevalence of wasting, underweight, thinness and stunting was 31.5%, 42.5%, 27.3% and 45.4% respectively. Malnutrition was more frequent among children with moderate to severe heart failure and moderate to severe anaemia.

Table 2 Proportion of children wasted, underweight and stunted

Variable	Overall	0–5 years ($n = 145$)	6–10 years ($n = 36$)	11–15 years ($n = 13$)
Weight-for-Height z-score				
< −2 (%)	45 (31.5)	45 (31.5)	N/A	N/A
≥ 2 (%)	98 (68.5)	98 (68.5)	N/A	N/A
Median WHZ (IQR)	$n = 143$; −0.89 (−2.46,0.10)	$n = 143$; −0.89 (−2.46,0.10)	N/A	N/A
Weight-for-age z-score				
< −2 (%)	77 (42.5)	65 (44.8)	12 (33.3)	N/A
≥ 2 (%)	104 (57.5)	80 (55.2)	24 (66.7)	N/A
Median WAZ (IQR)	$n = 181$; −1.69 (−3.07,-0.69)	$n = 145$; −1.83 (−3.36,-0.62)	$n = 36$; −1.54 (−2.17,-0.77)	N/A
Height-for-age z-score				
< −2 (%)	88 (45.4)	70 (48.3)	14 (38.9)	4 (30.8)
≥ 2 (%)	106 (54.6)	75 (51.7)	22 (61.1)	9 (69.2)
Median HAZ (IQR)	$n = 194$; −1.67 (−3.21,-0.51)	$n = 145$; −1.91 (−3.34,-0.58)	$n = 36$; −1.62 (−2.47,-0.52)	$n = 13$; −0.93 (−2.57,-0.47)
BMI for age z-score				
< −2 (%)	53 (27.3)	46 (31.7)	4 (11.1)	3 (23.1)
≥ 2 (%)	141 (72.7)	99 (68.3)	32 (88.9)	10 (76.9)
Median BMIZ (IQR)	$n = 194$; −0.72 (−2.21,0.17)	$n = 145$; −0.74 (−2.41,0.33)	$n = 36$; −0.61 (−1.53,-0.15)	$n = 13$; −0.81 (−1.89,0.29)

N/A z-scores for children in this age group cannot be generated using the WHO 2007 z scores

Table 3 Factors associated with wasting among children under 5 years (Weight-for-Height z-score < −2)

Variables	Univariate		Multivariate	
	RR (95% CI)	*P*-Value	RR (95% CI)	*P*-Value
Gender				
Male	Ref			
Female	0.99 (0.90–1.09)	0.844		
Age (years)	0.96 (0.93–0.99)	0.009	0.97 (0.94–1.002)	0.068
Cyanotic heart disease				
No	Ref			
Yes	0.97 (0.88–1.07)	0.598		
Heart failure				
No/mild heart failure	Ref		Ref	
Moderate/ severe heart failure	1.13 (1.03–1.25)	0.012	1.1 (0.997–1.22)	0.058
Anaemia				
No/ mild anaemia	Ref		Ref	
Moderate/severe anaemia	1.13 (1.02–1.24)	0.017	1.11 (1.01–1.22)	0.03

The prevalence of wasting among children aged under 5 years with congenital heart disease in our study was higher than the 7.5% global prevalence of wasting in children under 5 years [15]. In addition, our findings show that children with congenital heart disease are six times more likely to be wasted compared to their counterparts in Uganda [9]. Our study found a high proportion of underweight, stunted and thin children relative to those previously described globally [15, 16] and in Uganda [9, 17]. Other studies have also demonstrated that children with congenital heart disease are at higher risk of malnutrition compared to those without heart disease [1, 18, 19].

Okoromah and colleagues reported prevalence of wasting, stunting and underweight of 41.1%, 28.8% and 20.5% respectively in children with congenital heart disease attending an outpatient tertiary hospital in Nigeria [1]. Although they noted a higher prevalence of wasting, and the proportions of stunted and underweight children were lower than those seen in our study. Furthermore, in comparison to our study, a higher prevalence of malnutrition among children

Table 4 Factors associated with underweight

Variables	Univariate		Multivariate	
	RR (95% CI)	*P*-Value	RR (95% CI)	*P*-Value
Gender				
Male	Ref			
Female	0.99 (0.91–1.09)	0.905		
Age (years)				
0–5	Ref		Ref	
6–10	0.93 (0.84–1.04)	0.187	0.93 (0.84–1.03)	0.206
11–15	N/A			
Cyanotic heart disease				
No	Ref			
Yes	1.03 (0.93–1.15)	0.537		
Heart failure				
No/mild heart failure	Ref		Ref	
Moderate/ severe heart failure	1.24 (1.13–1.36)	<0.001	1.24 (1.13–1.36)	<0.001
Anaemia				
No/ mild anaemia	Ref		Ref	
Moderate/severe anaemia	1.09 (0.99–1.20)	0.092	1.09 (0.99–1.20)	0.086

Table 5 Factors associated with stunting

Variables	Univariate		Multivariate	
	RR (95% CI)	*P*-Value	RR (95% CI)	*P*-Value
Gender				
Male	Ref			
Female	0.995 (0.91–1.09)	0.919		
Age (years)				
0–5	Ref		Ref	
6–10	0.94 (0.84–1.05)	0.295	0.94 (0.84–1.05)	0.292
11–15	0.90 (0.77–1.05)	0.175	0.91 (0.78–1.07)	0.264
Cyanotic heart disease				
No	Ref			
Yes	1.01 (0.91–1.12)	0.85		
Heart failure				
No/mild heart failure	Ref		Ref	
Moderate/ severe heart failure	1.11 (1.01–1.22)	0.026	1.11 (1.01–1.21)	0.037
Anaemia				
No/ mild anaemia	Ref		Ref	
Moderate/severe anaemia	1.07 (0.97–1.18)	0.161	1.06 (0.96–1.17)	0.231

with congenital heart disease was described in India; wasting (55.9%) and underweight (59%) [20]. Lower prevalence of wasting (23.8%) and underweight (14.3%) was reported in Egypt among children under 6 years of age [21]. These studies indicate that the prevalence of malnutrition is high in children with congenital heart disease in various countries. However, heterogeneity exists from country to country implying differences in risk factors for malnutrition among children, in the different settings.

Similar to our findings, various studies have reported an association between malnutrition and heart failure in children with congenital heart disease [1, 20, 21] which is attributed to increased metabolic needs of these children yet they have low energy intake due to their inability to tolerate a high volume of feeds [7, 22].

Table 6 Factors associated with low BMI z-score

Variables	Univariate		Multivariate	
	OR (95% CI)	*P*-Value	OR (95% CI)	*P*-Value
Gender				
Male	Ref			
Female	1.01 (0.94–1.08)	0.825		
Age (years)				
0–5	Ref		Ref	
6–10	0.89 (0.83–0.96)	0.0013	0.91 (0.84–0.97)	0.006
11–15	0.95 (0.83–1.09)	0.47	0.993 (0.86–1.14)	0.91
Cyanotic heart disease				
No	Ref			
Yes	0.97 (0.90–1.04)	0.40		
Heart failure				
No/mild heart failure	Ref		Ref	
Moderate/ severe heart failure	1.12 (1.03–1.21)	0.006	1.12 (1.04–1.21)	0.004
Anaemia				
No/ mild anaemia	Ref		Ref	
Moderate/severe anaemia	1.16 (1.07–1.27)	0.0005	1.15 (1.06–1.25)	0.001

Anaemia has also been reported to be associated with malnutrition in children with congenital heart disease [1, 21]. This is similar to our findings where children with moderate or severe anaemia were more likely to be wasted and thin. Children with malnutrition commonly have anaemia which is attributed to bone marrow hypoplasia, iron, vitamin B12, vitamin A and folate deficiency [23, 24]. Even though we did not assess for these causes of anaemia in our study, we think that these could explain the association between anaemia and malnutrition among children with congenital heart disease noted from our study.

Delayed time to surgical correction of the heart defects has been associated with malnutrition among the children with congenital heart disease [1, 3, 20]. In our study, only 4 children had received surgical correction of their heart defects, and therefore we could not assess this relationship due to small numbers. There was no significant association between cyanotic heart disease and malnutrition, a finding that is contrary to other studies. It may be that a different outcome would have been achieved by a larger sample size.

Although, Uganda has a number of policies and guidelines on promotion of nutrition among children, there is limited emphasis on congenital heart diseases as an underlying risk factor for malnutrition [25, 26]. Hence there is a need to develop interventions such as early surgical repair for heart defects and institutionalisation of other measures to prevent and manage malnutrition in these children.

Limitations

We did not assess other factors that are known to contribute to malnutrition in these children with congenital heart disease such as genetic disorders [27], pulmonary hypertension [3] and social economic status of the households. However, socio-economic status is better assessed in community studies than hospital based studies.

Children with cyanotic congenital heart disease tend to have polycythemia resulting in higher haemoglobin levels [28]. In our study, we used the WHO age specific reference haemoglobin levels to define anaemia [14]. In children with cyanotic heart disease, these reference ranges may not be the best markers for anaemia. However, there are no standardised haemoglobin reference levels for these children and the variations in their haemoglobin levels are not uniform. The sample size of the children in our study is also relatively small but this may not have significantly affected our results.

Conclusion

Children with congenital heart disease had high prevalence rates of wasting, underweight, stunting and thinness. Wasting was associated with moderate to severe anaemia. Stunting and underweight were associated with moderate to severe heart failure, while thinness was associated with moderate to severe heart failure and moderate to severe anaemia. With these high rates of malnutrition in children with congenital heart disease, there is need to integrate strategies to identify and manage malnutrition during their care.

Abbreviations

BMIZ: Body mass index-for-age z score; CHD: Congenital heart disease; HAZ: Height-for-age z score; WAZ: Weight-for-age z score; WHO: World Health Organisation; WHZ: Weight-for-height z score

Acknowledgements

We acknowledge the support and input from the staff and administration of Mulago Hospital, Uganda Heart Institute and Child Health and Development Center, Makerere University. We are also grateful to the patients and caretakers who participated in this study.

Funding

Research reported in this publication was supported by the Fogarty International Center, the National Heart Lung and Blood Institute, and the Common Fund of the National Institutes of Health under Award Number 5R24 TW008861. The content is solely the responsibility of the authors and does not necessarily represent the official views of the National Institutes of Health.

Authors' contribution

AB, PL, SL, SK, VN and CK participated in the design of the study. AB supervised patients' enrolment and coordinated the study. AB, PL, SL, SK, KO, LC, VN and CK participated in data analysis, interpretation of results and writing of the manuscript. All authors read and approved the final manuscript.

Authors' information

Anthony Batte, MBChB, Mmed (Pediatrics), is a Lecturer and Paediatric Nephrologist at Child Health and Development Centre, Makerere University, Uganda. Peter Lwabi, MBChB, Mmed (Pediatrics), Dip Cardiology, is a Pediatric Cardiologist at Uganda Heart Institute. Sulaiman Lubega - MBChB, MMed (Pediatrics), Dip Cardiology, is a Pediatric Cardiologist at Uganda Heart Institute. Sarah Kiguli - MBChB, Mmed (Pediatrics), MHPE is a Professor of Pediatrics and Child Health Makerere University. Kennedy Otwombe B.Ed (Science), M.Sc. (Stats), is a Biostatistician at the Perinatal HIV Research Unit, Faculty of Health Sciences, University of the Witwatersrand, Johannesburg, South Africa. Lucy Chimoyi B.Sc (Biochem), M.Sc (Env Sci), M.Sc. (Epid& Biostat), is a Researcher in the Epidemiology Unit at The Aurum Institute, Johannesburg, South Africa. Violette Nabatte - MBChB, M.med (Pediatrics) is a Pediatrician at Nakaseke Hospital, Uganda. Charles Karamagi, MBChB, Mmed (Pediatrics), PhD is an Associate Professor of Pediatrics and Child health also working with the Clinical Epidemiology Makerere University.

Competing interests

The authors declare that they have no competing interests.

Author details
[1]Child Health and Development Centre, Makerere University College of Health Sciences, P.O.Box 6717, Kampala, Uganda. [2]Uganda Heart Institute, P.O. Box 7051, Kampala, Uganda. [3]Department of Pediatrics and Child Health, Makerere University College of Health Sciences, P.O.Box 7072, Kampala, Uganda. [4]Perinatal HIV Research Unit, Faculty of Health Sciences, University of the Witwatersrand, Johannesburg, South Africa. [5]The Aurum Institute, Johannesburg, South Africa. [6]Nakaseke Hospital, Nakeseke, Uganda. [7]Clinical Epidemiology Unit, Makerere University College of Health Sciences, P.O.Box 7072, Kampala, Uganda.

References

1. Okoromah CA, Ekure EN, Lesi FE, Okunowo WO, Tijani BO, Okeiyi JC. Prevalence, profile and predictors of malnutrition in children with congenital heart defects: a case-control observational study. Arch Dis Child. 2011;96(4):354–60.
2. Mitchell I, Logan R, Pollock J, Jamieson M. Nutritional status of children with congenital heart disease. Br Heart J. 1995;73(3):277–83.
3. Varan B, Tokel K, Yilmaz G. Malnutrition and growth failure in cyanotic and acyanotic congenital heart disease with and without pulmonary hypertension. Arch Dis Child. 1999;81(1):49–52.
4. Medoff-Cooper B, Ravishankar C. Nutrition and growth in congenital heart disease: a challenge in children. Curr Opin Cardiol. 2013;28(2):122–9.
5. Grantham-McGregor S, Baker-Henningham H. Review of the evidence linking protein and energy to mental development. Public Health Nutr. 2005;8(7a):1191–201.
6. De Staebel O. Malnutrition in Belgian children with congenital heart disease on admission to hospital. J Clin Nurs. 2000;9(5):784–91.
7. Menon G, Poskitt E. Why does congenital heart disease cause failure to thrive? Arch Dis Child. 1985;60(12):1134–9.
8. Vaidyanathan B, Roth SJ, Rao SG, Gauvreau K, Shivaprakasha K, Kumar RK. Outcome of ventricular septal defect repair in a developing country. J Pediatr. 2002;140(6):736–41.
9. Uganda Bureau of Statistics (UBOS) and ICF International Inc. Uganda Demographic and Health Survey 2011. Kampala: UBOS and Calverton, Maryland: ICF International Inc; 2012.
10. Batte A, Lwabi P, Lubega S, Kiguli S, Nabatte V, Karamagi C. Prevalence of arrhythmias among children below 15 years of age with congenital heart diseases attending Mulago National Referral Hospital, Uganda. BMC Cardiovasc Disord. 2016;16(1):1.
11. World Health Organisation. Anthropometric reference data for international use. http://www.who.int/childgrowth/publications/deonis_habicht_1996/en/. Accessed 18 Jul 2016.
12. Ross RD, Bollinger RO, Pinsky WW. Grading the severity of congestive heart failure in infants. Pediatr Cardiol. 1992;13(2):72–5.
13. Reithmann C, Reber D, Kozlik-Feldmann R, Netz H, Pilz G, Welz A, Werdan K. A post-receptor defect of adenylyl cyclase in severely failing myocardium from children with congenital heart disease. Eur J Pharmacol. 1997;330(1):79–86.
14. World Health Organization. Haemoglobin concentrations for the diagnosis of anaemia and assessment of severity. Geneva: Vitamin and Mineral Nutrition Information System; 2011.
15. International Food Policy Research Institute. Global Nutrition Report 2016. Washington, DC: From Promise to Impact: Ending Malnutrition by 2030; 2016.
16. Manyanga T, El-Sayed H, Doku DT, Randall JR. The prevalence of underweight, overweight, obesity and associated risk factors among school-going adolescents in seven African countries. BMC Public Health. 2014;14(1):1.
17. Lwanga F, Kirunda BE, Orach CG. Intestinal helminth infections and nutritional status of children attending primary schools in Wakiso District, Central Uganda. Int J Environ Res Public Health. 2012;9(8):2910–21.
18. Chen CW, Li CY, Wang JK. Growth and development of children with congenital heart disease. J Adv Nurs. 2004;47(3):260–9.
19. Daymont C, Neal A, Prosnitz A, Cohen MS. Growth in children with congenital heart disease. Pediatrics. 2013;131(1):e236–42.
20. Vaidyanathan B, Nair SB, Sundaram KR, Babu UK, Shivaprakasha K, Rao SG, Kumar RK. Malnutrition in children with congenital heart disease (CHD) determinants and short term impact of corrective intervention. Indian Pediatr. 2008;45(7):541–6.
21. Hassan BA, Albanna EA, Morsy SM, Siam AG, Al Shafie MM, Elsaadany HF, Sherbiny HS, Shehab M, Grollmuss O. Nutritional status in children with un-operated congenital heart disease: an Egyptian center experience. Front Pediatr. 2015;2015:3.
22. Rogers EJ, Gilbertson HR, Heine RG, Henning R. Barriers to adequate nutrition in critically ill children. Nutrition. 2003;19(10):865–8.
23. Özkale M, Sipahi T. Hematologic and bone marrow changes in children with protein-energy malnutrition. Pediatr Hematol Oncol. 2014;31(4):349–58.
24. Müller O, Krawinkel M. Malnutrition and health in developing countries. Can Med Assoc J. 2005;173(3):279–86.
25. National Planning Authority. Uganda Nutrition Action Plan 2011–2016. Kampala: National Planning Authority; 2011.
26. National Planning Authority. National nutrition planning guidelines for Uganda. Kampala: National Planning Authority; 2015.
27. Knirsch W, Zingg W, Bernet V, Balmer C, Dimitropoulos A, Prêtre R, Bauersfeld U, Latal B. Determinants of body weight gain and association with neurodevelopmental outcome in infants operated for congenital heart disease. Interact Cardiovasc Thorac Surg. 2010;10(3):377–82.
28. Territo MC, Rosove MH. Cyanotic congenital heart disease: hematologic management. J Am Coll Cardiol. 1991;18(2):320–2.

6

Prevalence and risk factors of congenital heart defects among live births: a population-based cross-sectional survey in Shaanxi province, Northwestern China

Leilei Pei, Yijun Kang, Yaling Zhao and Hong Yan*

Abstract

Background: Nearly half of the population of Northwest China live in Shaanxi province, but population-based data on the epidemiologic characteristics of congenital heart defects (CHD) in this population is limited. The study aimed to investigate the prevalence and epidemiologic characteristics of the CHD among infants born between 2010 and 2013 in Shaanxi province.

Methods: Infants born between 2010 and 2013 in Shaanxi province were surveyed using a stratified multi-stage sampling method. Participant characteristics were recorded by questionnaire, medical records were reviewed and CHD was diagnosed using a specialized neonatal echocardiography. A Poisson regression model was applied to assess the association between any CHD and possible risk factors.

Results: A total of 29098 live infants were surveyed with an overall prevalence of 76.0 (95% CI: 66.3, 86.7) per 10000 live infants. The prevalence of major and minor CHD were 26.1 and 49.8 per 10000 live infants, respectively, in surveyed areas. Poisson regression analysis indicated that, compared with singleton infants, the prevalence rate ratio of CHD was higher in twin and multi-fetal infants (PRR:3.1, 95% CI:1.6, 6.1). Using southern Shaanxi as a reference, the PRR of CHD were lower in northern (PRR:0.4, 95% CI:0.3, 0.6) and central Shaanxi province (PRR:0.5, 95% CI:0.4, 0.7). PRR was higher in mothers over 30 years of age than in those under 25 years (PRR:1.6, 95% CI:1.0, 2.5), and in mothers with ≥3 parity than that in mothers with only one parity (PRR:2.2, 95% CI:1.2, 4.2). The risk for CHD among live infants was positively associated with family history of CHD (PRR: 9.8, 95% CI: 5.3, 18.1). Additionally, CHD was less common in the floating population than the permanent population (PRR: 0.6, 95% CI: 0.4, 0.9).

Conclusion: The CHD among live infants seemed to be a serious health problem in Shaanxi province as well as in Northwestern China. Our research have important policy implications for recommendations on CHD intervention in Northwest China.

Keywords: Congenital heart defects, Epidemiologic characteristics, Northwestern China

* Correspondence: yhpaper605@sina.com
Department of Epidemiology and Health Statistics, School of Public Health, Xi'an Jiaotong University Health Science Center, Xi'an, Shaanxi 710061, People's Republic of China

Background

Congenital heart defects (CHD) are one of the most prevalent and serious birth defects, and are the leading causes of birth defects-associated morbidity, mortality, and medical expenditures [1–3]. Many studies in developed Western countries have estimated that approximately 40 to 100 per 10000 live births suffer from CHD, and 26 to 44 per 10000 births from major defects, defined as defects requiring catheter or surgical intervention during the first year of life [1, 4–7]. As complex congenital heart defects can cause spontaneous abortion or stillbirth, the reported incidence of CHD among fetuses (146.0 per 10000 fetuses) may be underestimated [8]. In China, CHD is the most prevalent birth defect, accounting for over 10% of cases of infant mortality in 2008 [9, 10], and surgical treatment of infants with CHD is reported to cost 12 billion Yuan each year in China [11].

In Sparsely populated Northwestern China, economic condition are worse and health services are less developed than in Eastern and Coastal areas of China. Nearly half the population of this region, 37 million people, reside in Shaanxi province. In a population-based cross-sectional survey of the whole province conducted in 2013, we have found that the prevalence of birth defects among alive infants is high in Shaanxi province of Northwest China and cardiovascular system malformations are the most common [12]. Until recently, however, limited population-based data on the main epidemiologic characteristics of CHD in Shaanxi province or Northwest China were available. The objective of the study was to investigate the prevalence and epidemiologic characteristics of CHD among live infants born between 2010 and 2013 in Shaanxi province. We expect the results to provide the most updated information on the rate of CHD among infants in Shaanxi province, Northwest China.

Methods

Study design and participants

A large population-based cross-sectional survey was conducted between August and November 2013 in Shaanxi province, northwest China. Infants born between 2010 and 2013, who were alive at the time of sampling, were evaluated in the study. Considering the imbalanced population distribution between rural and urban areas in the province, a stratified multi-stage sampling method was employed. In rural areas, counties, townships and villages are administered individually, while in urban areas the three administrative districts are districts, streets and communities. Twenty counties in rural areas were selected randomly throughout the province. In each county, 6 townships were chosen and 6 villages from each chosen township were sampled randomly. To account for differences in population density and fertility level between rural and urban areas, 10 districts in urban areas were randomly selected, 3 streets in the chosen districts and 6 communities in the chosen streets, were selected randomly.

Finally, approximately 30 mothers and their babies in each chosen village and 60 mothers and their babies in each chosen community were selected using a completely random sampling method. According to the 2010 sixth census, the population of Shaanxi was approximately 37 million, and the fertility rate was 9.7‰ [13]. A total of 29098 live infants were eventually enrolled in the study, representing a relative sampling size of nearly 9.00% of the total infant population.

Data collection

In the survey, all questionnaires including birth defects questionnaire, family questionnaire, reproductive history questionnaire and family history questionnaire were designed by Xi'an Jiaotong University Health Science Center (Additional file 1: Questionnaire). A pilot study was carried out to pretest all questionnaires and procedures, and detailed interviewer guides were developed. Field surveys and data collection were carried out by the trained field staff from Xi'an Jiaotong University Health Science Center. Ten investigation teams from Xi'an Jiaotong University Health Science Center were established for these counties or districts. Each team consisted of 10 to 12 investigators, a supervisor and a doctor from a local maternal and child health hospital. During the survey, all fieldworkers were closely monitored by their supervisors and randomly examined. When errors and/or missing values were detected, participants were re-interviewed immediately. All the information was collected in the local village clinics and community health service centers. Meanwhile, our work was supported by the local hospitals and health administrative departments and the Ministry of Health in Shaanxi province.

After this study was fully explained to participants, the informed consent was obtained. A face-to-face interview was conducted to collect socioeconomic and demographic characteristics of mothers and their children using the family questionnaires. A multistage process determined the presence of a congenital heart defect in each child. First, the infants were screened for CHD by a doctor from the local maternal and child health hospital. Isolated patent foramen ovale and patent ductus arteriosus among neonates <28 days of life were excluded because they are normal neonatal findings.

For those affected by CHD, an in person interview was conducted with their mothers and medical records reviews were reviewed by a trained physician. Parents were also required to recall the CHD diagnosis process and the time of diagnosis, diagnosing hospital, type of CHD were recorded from medical records. For the new cases of suspected CHD, a specialized neonatal echocardiography and electrocardiography was conducted at the first affiliated hospital of Xi'an Jiaotong University Health Science Center, and participants were diagnosed accordingly.

Main study variables

To present an accurate picture of the burden of CHD, we classified CHD as major or minor. Defects were classified as major when the gross structural complexity was of functional significance, e.g. hypoplastic left heart syndrome (HLHS), atrioventricular septal defect (AVSD), coarctation of the aorta (CoA), and large ventricular septal defects (VSD), large atrial septal defect (ASD), and surgical repair or catheter intervention was likely to be required. The most common major heart defects (e.g. AVSD, VSD, HLHS, ASD) were further grouped as simple or complex. A simple heart defect was defined as one without additional cardiac defects, e.g. AVSD or HLHS, while a complex heart defect was one with additional heart defects, e.g. HLHS with additional coarctation of the aorta. Defects were classified as minor when no intervention was likely to be required, e.g. mild ventricular septal defects (VSD), mild atrial septal defect (ASD), mild pulmonary valve stenosis (PS). Due to less impacts of the defects on infants' life and the privacy of infants, some parents of infants with minor CHD refused to have their infants further checked. Therefore, the type of some minor CHD did not be determined and they were classified as unspecified CHD.

The socioeconomic status of the households was assessed using the Demographic and Health Survey wealth index [14]. Principal component analysis was used to combine the variables representing families' economic level. On the basis of the first principal component, then, the socioeconomic status of the families was classified into the tertiles representing poor, medium and rich families. According to the residence during the pregnancy, women were categorized into two groups (permanent or floating). The floating population included women who lived in surveyed areas for less than three months during pregnancy. Permanent residents were those who lived in surveyed areas for more than three months during pregnancy. Other characteristics of the participants were also entered into the multivariate analysis, including number of ultrasound examination, infant gender (male or female), fetal number (singleton or twin and multi-fetal), family history of CHD among first-degree relatives (yes or no), registered permanent residence (urban or rural), mother's education (no education, primary, junior high, senior high, or college and above), mother's age (<25, 25–29 or ≥30 years groups), parity (1, 2 or ≥3), and areas (north, central or south).

Statistical analysis

Data was entered into Epidata 3.1 by double entry (CDC, Atlanta, GA, USA) and all statistical analysis was performed using STATA version 12.0 software (STATA Corporation, College Station, TX, USA). Baseline characteristics were compared across different areas using analysis of variance (ANOVA) and χ^2 test. Prevalence rate (per 10000 live births) and its 95% confidence intervals (95% CI) of CHD based on Poisson distribution across different areas in the province were also presented. Any congenital heart defects were considered unique outcome variables in the multivariate analysis. The Poisson regression model was applied to assess the association between the outcome variable and covariates, including number of ultrasound examination, infant gender (male as a reference or female), fetal number (singleton as a reference or twin and multi-fetal), family history of CHD among first-degree relatives (no as a reference or yes), registered permanent residence (urban as a reference or rural), residence during the pregnancy (permanent as a reference or floating), mother's education (no education, primary, junior high, senior high, and college and above as a reference), mother's age (<25 as a reference, 25–29 and ≥ 30 years groups), parity (1 as a reference, 2 and ≥ 3), and areas (north, central and south as a reference). A prevalence rate ratio (PRR) was quoted as the output from Poisson regression and could indicate the magnitude of change, which would not be negative and <1 for a decrease and >1 for an increase.

Results

Baseline characteristics of the participants

A total of 1605 villages were sampled within 272 townships in Shaanxi province and 29098 live infants were studied. The average age of children was 16.9 ± 11.3 months (range 0–46 months). The baseline characteristics of the participants across different areas in Shaanxi province were summarized in Table 1. The proportions of the participants from north, central and south of Shaanxi, were 25.7, 53.9 and 20.3% respectively. More than half of participants resided in rural areas, and 11.3% were characterized as floating.

Of the participants, 98.8% were singletons and boys accounted for 54.4%. It should be noted that approximately 0.6% of participants had a family history of CHD among first-degree relatives. Participants were evenly divided between poor, medium and rich households. The mean age of mothers was 28.0 ± 4.9 years and the proportion of women who had attended senior high school and above was close to 38.2%. Amongst the mothers, the average of the parity was 1.7 ± 0.8. Enrolled mothers underwent approximately 2.6 prenatal ultrasound examinations during pregnancy. Almost all the baseline characteristics of the study population differed between the three areas in Shaanxi province.

Table 1 Baseline characteristics of study population by different areas in Shaanxi province [a]

Baseline characteristics	Northern Shaanxi n (%)	Central Shaanxi n (%)	Southern Shaanxi n (%)
Number of ultrasound examination[b]	2.54 (0.8)	2.63 (0.7)	2.58 (0.9)
Infant Gender[b]			
Male	4222 (56.4)	8303 (53.5)	3189 (54.0)
Female	3263 (43.6)	7295 (46.5)	2722 (46.0)
Fetal number			
Singleton	7396 (98.7)	15522 (98.8)	5662 (98.9)
Twin and multi-fetal	100 (1.3)	184 (1.2)	65 (1.1)
Mother's education[b]			
College and above	1044 (13.9)	3860 (24.6)	398 (6.7)
Senior high school	1156 (15.4)	3616 (23.0)	1045 (17.7)
Junior high school	3649 (48.7)	7242 (46.2)	3541 (60.0)
Primary school	1307 (17.4)	839 (5.3)	821 (13.9)
No education	336 (4.5)	133 (0.8)	92 (1.6)
Mother's age, year[b]			
< 25	2209 (29.8)	3227 (20.9)	1792 (30.8)
25–29	3313 (44.6)	6866 (44.5)	2148 (36.9)
≥ 30	1899 (25.6)	5348 (34.6)	1874 (32.2)
Parity[b]			
1	3770 (50.6)	9514 (60.8)	3423 (58.4)
2	3291 (44.2)	5673 (36.2)	2292 (39.1)
≥ 3	393 (5.3)	463 (3.0)	150 (2.6)
Wealth index[b]			
Poor	2740 (36.5)	5199 (33.1)	1706 (28.8)
Medium	2322 (31.0)	5461 (34.8)	1890 (31.9)
Rich	2435 (32.5)	5048 (32.1)	2331 (39.3)
Family history of CHD[b]			
No	7403 (99.2)	15559 (99.4)	5883 (99.7)
Yes	59 (0.8)	92 (0.6)	19 (0.3)
Residence during the pregnancy[b]			
Permanent	6913 (93.2)	13640 (87.2)	5120 (86.7)
Floating	502 (6.8)	1996 (12.8)	785 (13.3)
Household registration[b]			
Urban	1632 (21.8)	3957 (25.2)	423 (7.1)
Rural	5865 (78.2)	11751 (74.8)	5504 (92.9)
Total	7497 (25.7)	15708 (53.9)	5927 (20.3)

[a]Values are given as mean (SD) or the number (percentage) of the study population by socio-demographic characteristics across different areas
[b]denotes significantly differences in characteristics of study population across different areas by $\chi 2$ test or analysis of variance

The prevalence of congenital heart defects

Among the live infants surveyed, we identified 221 cases of CHD, and an overall prevalence of 76.0 (95% CI: 66.3, 86.7) per 10000 infants. To clarify the category of CHD among live infants in Shaanxi province, CHD were subcategorized as major (76 cases) and minor (145 cases). The most common categories of major CHD were large atrial septal defect (ASD; 8.9 per 10000 [95% CI: 5.8, 13.1]), large ventricular septal defect (VSD; 6.9 per 10000 [95% CI: 4.2, 10.6]) and atrioventricular septal defect (AVSD; 4.1 per 10000 [95% CI: 2.1, 7.2]). Moreover, there were 5 cases with tetralogy of Fallot (ToF) and 5 cases with pulmonary valve stenosis (PS). Of the minor CHD, there were 47 unspecified congenital heart diseases. The prevalence of any CHD in the south of Shaanxi province was significantly higher than in north or central Shaanxi province (Tab. 2).

Table 2 Prevalence and categories of CHD among infants by different areas in the Shaanxi province[a]

Defects[b]	Northern Shaanxi		Central Shaanxi		Southern Shaanxi		Total	
	n	per 10000 (95% CI)	*n*	per 10000 (95% CI)	*n*	per 10000 (95% CI)	*n*	per 10000 (95% CI)
Major CHD	18	24.1 (14.3, 38.0)	36	22.9 (16.1, 31.7)	22	37.2 (23.3, 56.3)	76	26.1 (20.6, 32.7)
ASD,total	6	8.0 (2.9, 17.5)	15	9.6 (5.3, 15.8)	5	8.4 (2.7, 19.7)	26	8.9 (5.8, 13.1)
ASD,simple	3	4.0 (0.8, 11.7)	5	3.2 (1.0, 7.4)	3	5.1 (1.0, 14.8)	11	3.8 (1.9, 6.8)
ASD,complex	3	4.0 (0.8, 11.7)	10	6.4 (3.1, 11.7)	2	3.4 (0.4, 12.2)	15	5.2 (2.9, 8.5)
VSD,total	5	6.7 (2.2, 15.6)	11	7.0 (3.5, 12.5)	4	6.8 (1.8, 17.3)	20	6.9 (4.2, 10.6)
VSD,simple	3	4.0 (0.8, 11.7)	6	3.8 (1.4, 8.3)	2	3.4 (0.4, 12.2)	11	3.8 (1.9, 6.8)
VSD,complex	2	2.7 (0.3, 9.7)	5	3.2 (1.0, 7.4)	2	3.4 (0.4, 12.2)	9	3.1 (1.4, 5.9)
AVSD,total	2	2.7 (0.3, 9.7)	5	3.2 (1.0, 7.4)	5	8.4 (2.7, 19.7)	12	4.1 (2.1, 7.2)
AVSD,simple	2	2.7 (0.3, 9.7)	5	3.2 (1.0, 7.4)	4	6.8 (1.8, 17.3)	11	3.8 (1.9, 6.8)
AVSD,complex	0	0.0 (0.0, 4.9)	0	0.0 (0.0, 2.3)	1	1.7 (0.1, 9.4)	1	0.3 (0.1, 1.9)
ToF	1	1.3 (0.1, 7.4)	2	1.3 (0.2, 4.6)	2	3.4 (0.4, 12.2)	5	1.7 (0.6, 4.0)
PS	3	4.0 (0.8, 11.7)	0	0.0 (0.0, 2.3)	2	3.4 (0.4, 12.2)	5	1.7 (0.6, 4.0)
HLHS	1	2.7 (0.1, 7.4)	2	0.6 (0.2, 4.6)	1	1.7 (0.1, 9.4)	4	1.4 (0.4, 3.5)
CoA	0	0.0 (0.0, 4.9)	1	0.3 (0.1, 3.5)	1	1.7 (0.1, 9.4)	2	0.7 (0.2, 2.5)
EA	0	0.0 (0.0, 4.9)	0	0.0 (0.0, 2.3)	2	3.4 (0.4, 12.2)	2	0.7 (0.2, 2.5)
Minor CHD	19	25.4 (15.3, 39.7)	83	52.9 (42.1, 65.5)	43	72.6 (52.6, 97.9)	145	49.8 (42.1, 58.6)
Mild ASD	8	10.7 (4.6, 21.1)	31	19.7 (13.4, 28.0)	17	28.7 (16.7, 46.0)	56	19.2 (14.5, 25.0)
Mild VSD	5	6.7 (1.6, 11.7)	19	12.1 (7.3, 18.9)	8	13.5 (5.8, 26.6)	32	11.0 (7.5, 15.5)
Mild PS	1	1.3 (0.0, 4.9)	7	4.5 (1.8, 9.2)	2	3.4 (0.4, 12.2)	10	3.4 (1.6, 6.3)
Unspecified CHD	5	6.7 (2.2, 15.6)	26	16.6 (10.8, 24.3)	16	27.0 (15.5, 43.9)	47	15.8 (11.9, 21.5)
Any CHD	37	49.5 (34.8, 68.2)	119	75.8 (62.8, 90.7)	65	109.8 (84.8, 140.0)	221	76.0 (66.3, 86.7)

[a]Values are the number and proportion (95% CI) of CHD in the study population across different areas
[b]*Abbreviation*: *AVSD*, atrioventricular septal defect, *ASD* atrial septal defect, *VSD* Ventricular septal defect, *HLHS* hypoplastic left heart syndrome, *CoA* Coarctation of the aorta, *ToF* Tetralogy of Fallot, *PS* Pulmonary valve stenosis, *EA* Ebstein's anomaly

Predictors of congenital heart defects

Poisson regression analysis, adjusted for all the possible risk factors, indicated that twin and multi-fetal infants were more likely to suffer from CHD than singleton infants (PRR:3.1, 95% CI:1.6, 6.1; Tab. 3). CHD was more prevalent in the children of mothers aged over 30 years than those under 25 years of age (PRR:1.6, 95% CI:1.1, 2.5). The prevalence rate ratio of CHD among mothers with more than 3 parity were much higher than that in mothers with only one parity (PRR:2.2, 95% CI:1.2, 4.2). Furthermore, family history of CHD could increase the risk of CHD among participants (PRR:9.8, 95% CI:5.3, 18.1), while the number of ultrasound examinations mothers underwent was not associated with rate of CHD.

The rate of CHD was lower in the floating population (PRR: 0.6, 95% CI: 0.4, 0.9) than permanent population, and in north (PRR: 0.4, 95% CI:0.3, 0.6) and central Shaanxi province (PRR: 0.5, 95% CI: 0.4, 0.7) than in south Shaanxi province. However, urban-rural difference and gender gap in CHD rate among the participants had not been found in surveyed areas.

Discussion

The large population-based cross-sectional study conducted in Shaanxi province, northwest China, investigated the prevalence and epidemiological characteristics of CHD among infants born live between 2010 and 2013. We found that the prevalence of CHD was approximately 76.0 per 10000 live infants, and major defects may be a serious problem in the study. Furthermore, rate of CHD differed significantly with baseline characteristics among the participants in the surveyed areas.

In our study, 221 of 29098 participant infants were diagnosed with CHD. In 2007 a large population-based study in Beijing of fetuses and neonates screened for CHD by echocardiography, reported an incidence rate of 81.6 per 10000 births [15]. In four areas surrounding Shanghai, a previous surveillance program identified 75 cases of CHD among the 4006 fetuses and neonates who were scanned prenatally or neonatally, corresponding to an overall observed prevalence of 187.2 (95% CI: 14.8, 23.5) per 10000 births [7]. A population-based survey in Inner Mongolia reported a CHD prevalence of around 17.1 per 10000 births in 2008 [16]. A total of 1005052

Table 3 Predictors of any CHD among infants alive in Shaanxi province using a poisson regression

Predictors[c]	Univariate analysis[a] PRR (95% CI)	Multivariate analysis[b] PRR (95% CI)
Infant Gender		
Male	Reference	Reference
Female	0.9 (0.7, 1.1)	0.9 (0.7, 1.2)
Fetal number		
Singleton	Reference	Reference
Twin and Multi-fetal	4.3 (2.4, 7.9)*	3.1 (1.6, 6.1)*
Mother's education		
College and above	Reference	Reference
Senior high school	0.9 (0.6, 1.3)	0.8 (0.5, 1.3)
Junior high school	0.9 (0.7, 1.3)	0.7 (0.5, 1.2)
Primary school	0.8 (0.5, 1.3)	0.6 (0.3, 1.1)
No education	1.3 (0.6, 3.0)	1.1 (0.4, 2.8)
Mother's age, year		
<25	Reference	Reference
25-29	1.2 (0.9, 1.8)	1.2 (0.8, 1.8)
≥30	1.6 (1.1, 2.4)*	1.6 (1.1, 2.5)*
Parity*		
1	Reference	Reference
2	1.1 (0.9, 1.5)	1.1 (0.8, 1.6)
≥3	2.6 (1.6, 4.3)*	2.2 (1.2, 4.2)*
Wealth index		
Poor	Reference	Reference
Medium	0.9 (0.6, 1.2)	0.9 (0.6, 1.3)
Rich	0.8 (0.6, 1.1)	0.9 (0.6, 1.3)
Family history of CHD*		
No	Reference	Reference
Yes	10.9 (6.2, 19.1)*	9.8 (5.3, 18.1)*
Residence during the pregnancy		
Permanent	Reference	Reference
Floating	0.6 (0.4, 0.8)*	0.6 (0.4, 0.9)*
Household registration		
Urban	Reference	Reference
Rural	0.9 (0.7, 1.3)	0.9 (0.6, 1.4)
Areas*		
Southern area	Reference	Reference
Central area	0.7 (0.5, 0.9)*	0.5 (0.4, 0.7)*
Northern area	0.5 (0.3, 0.7)*	0.4 (0.3, 0.6)*
Number of ultrasound examination	1.1 (0.9, 1.3)	1.1 (0.6, 1.4)

[a]Only one variable is entered into the poisson regression model
[b]All possible risk factors are entered into the poisson regression model
[c]Prevalence Rate Ratio (PRR) and 95% confidence interval are given to indicate the magnitude of change
*$P < 0.05$

births reported to the Birth Defects Monitoring Network of Guangdong province indicated an overall CHD prevalence of 52.4 per 10000 births (95% CI: 51.0, 53.8) [17]. Cross sectional studies indicated that the prevalence of CHD varied substantially between populations, from 82.8 per 10000 in Belgium to 12.2 per 10000 in Colombia [18, 19]. The prevalence of CHD in our study (76.0 per 10000 live births) is higher than that recently reported in Inner Mongolia (17.1 per 10000), Guangdong (52.4 per 10000), Colombia (12.2 per 10000), and similar to the rates reported in Beijing (81.6 per 10000) and Belgium (82.8 per 10000), but lower than that in Shanghai (187.2 per 1000 births). In our study population, we may have underestimated the rate of CHD as early death was not recorded, and minor CHD may have gone undetected. Therefore, we speculated that the prevalence of CHD in Shaanxi province may be much higher than 76.0 per 10000 live births.

In this study the prevalence of major and minor CHD were 26.1 and 49.8 per 10000 live infants, respectively. The most prevalent major categories of CHD were large atrial septal defect (ASD), large ventricular septal defect (VSD) and atrioventricular septal defect (AVSD). One study of CHD in areas near Shanghai, Eastern China reported a prevalence of 30.0 and 157.3 per 10000 births, respectively, for major and minor defects. The proportion of VSD (62.7%) was the highest among major defects in areas surrounding Shanghai, followed by ASD (18.7%) and ToF (5.3%) [7]. In Norway, research revealed a prevalence of 33.3 and 113.0 per 10000 fetuses for major and minor defects, respectively, and AVSD was the dominant category of major heart defects [5]. In our survey, only infants medically indicated for CHD underwent further diagnostic tests, so minor asymptomatic defects may have gone undetected. Furthermore, we used hospital records or congenital defects registers to identify cases of CHD. Due to asymptomatic or undetected conditions, however, many minor defects were likely overlooked, and nor reported in hospital records or congenital defects registers. Consequently, the percentage of major defects in our study was similar to that in other studies, while the proportion of minor defects was lower than in other studies.

In this study CHD prevalence varied between maternal age groups, and the risk for CHD in surveyed areas increased with maternal age after controlling for other risk factors using Poisson regression. Our results were consistent with previous reports [20–22]. Miller et al. reported that infants born to mothers older than 35 years were more likely to suffer from CHD than those born to younger mothers [21], and Reefhuis and Honein [22] also observed a positive association between maternal age and heart defects. In this study, higher maternal parity was also associated with CHD. A previous study conducted in Texas also revealed a slightly larger rate of birth defects among infants born to mothers with three or more prior births than those born to first-time mothers between 1999 and 2003 [23]. Simultaneously, twin and multi-fetal infants were positively associated with the increased risk of congenital heart disease. It was commonly considered that an excessive number of parturitions may lead to reproductive organ damage and dysfunction and increase the risk of CHD [24]. Further studies will be required to corroborate these findings and, if confirmed, to elucidate possible reasons for these associations.

Previous studies indicate that the relative risk of birth defects was increased in women with a history of similar defects in first-degree relatives [25]. For women with CHD, the prevalence of CHD among their offspring is approximately 10 times higher than that reported in the general population [26, 27]. Similarly, family history of CHD was also identified to an important predictor in our study. Many studies have suggested that sufficient maternal healthcare utilization, such as prenatal care and postnatal care, can efficiently reduce pregnancy-related diseases and newborn morbidity and mortality [28, 29]. Higher numbers of ultrasound examinations during pregnancy could indicate more accurate and early CHD diagnosis, which may have contributed to termination for significant CHD, however in this study we did not find rate of CHD to be associated with number of ultrasound examination. Thus, the role of periceonceptional ultrasound examination in CHD diagnosis should continue to be investigated in the surveyed areas.

In this study we also did not observe a significant difference between the rate of CHD in rural and urban areas. However, we found a significantly lower rate of CHD in floating populations than permanent populations, potentially due to differences in lifestyles and behaviors between these populations in Shaanxi province. The floating population were less likely to experience sustained environmental pollution and occupational exposure than the permanent population in the surveyed areas. However, the root causes of these differences remain unknown.

We also found that CHD incidence varied geographically in the surveyed population. The prevalence of CHD in north and central Shaanxi was lower than in south Shaanxi. Regional differences in CHD prevalence may be due to variations both in incidence and in mortality. In our study, parents in south Shaanxi were more likely to have access to antenatal scans, and hence the number of ultrasound examination was higher in south Shaanxi than in other areas. These interventions likely improved the rate of CHD detection in south Shaanxi, increasing the prevalence. Meanwhile, the discrepancy in rates of early termination of pregnancy between these areas may also have contributed to regional differences in rates of CHD. Another possible explanation is variations in the composition of the population in these study regions. In our study, south Shaanxi province has a larger proportion of floating and rural population than the other two areas, and, as previously noted, the prevalence of CHD was higher in the floating population. In a neighboring province, Inner Mongolia, the risk of birth defects was found to be higher in families living in rural areas than in urban areas [16]. Hence, region discrepancies in CHD could exist in Shaanxi province with a higher prevalence in south Shaanxi. These factors could explain in part the regional discrepancies in CHD prevalence across Shaanxi province. However, further studies will be required to clarify the contributions of these factors.

Here we report a large population-based cross-sectional survey conducted in Shaanxi province, in 30 counties or districts using a multi-stage sampling method, which reliably represents the recent prevalence of CHD in Shaanxi province. However, conclusions are limited by the scope of the study. Firstly, as a cross-sectional survey, only prevalence can be determined, and no conclusions can be drawn on the causes of CHD in this population. Secondly, all cases of CHD could not be included due to the limitations of our surveyed methods. For example, defects causing only undetectable symptoms are difficult to identify in early childhood; Hence, we suspect that our data underestimates the prevalence and burden of CHD. Nevertheless, the current study is the largest survey in Northwestern China, providing the most up-to-date data on CHD, and filling a gap in the knowledge of this geographical region.

Conclusions

In conclusion, CHD among live infants is a serious health problem in Shaanxi province, Northwestern China, particularly in south Shaanxi. Twin and multi-fetal infants, family history among first-degree relatives and higher maternal age and parity were all positively correlated with CHD prevalence among live infants in the study areas. In addition, risk for CHD was lower in the floating population than in the permanent population. These findings may have an important public health policy implications for CHD intervention in northwest China.

Abbreviations

AVSD: Atrioventricular septal defect; CHD: Congenital heart defects; CoA: Coarctation of the aorta; HLHS: Hypoplastic left heart syndrome; PRR: Prevalence rate ratio; Tetralogy of Fallot (ToF): Pulmonary valve stenosis (PS), Analysis of variance (ANOVA).; VSD: Ventricular septal defects

Acknowledgements

We would like to thank all participants and investigators in this study.

Funding
All the work was supported by the National Science Foundation of China (81541069, 81230016, 81602928) and the Research Support Program for Young Teachers in Xi'an Jiaotong University (DWSQc130000033).

Authors'contributions
LP designed the prescription study, conducted the data analysis and prepared the manuscript; YK, YZ and LP collected the data and reviewed the manuscript. HY contributed to the design and analysis of the study and the preparation of the manuscript. All authors read and approved the final manuscript.

Competing interests
The authors declare that they have no competing interests.

References

1. Reller MD, Strickland MJ, Riehle-Colarusso T, Mahle WT, Correa A. Prevalence of congenital heart defects in metropolitan Atlanta, 1998–2005. J Pediatr. 2008;153:807–13.
2. Yang Q, Chen H, Correa A, Devine O, Mathews TJ, Honein MA. Racial differences in infant mortality attributable to birth defects in the United States, 1989–2002. Birth Defects Res A Clin Mol Teratol. 2006;76:706–13.
3. Gilboa SM, Correa A, Botto LD, Rasmussen SA, Waller DK, Hobbs CA, Cleves MA, Riehle-Colarusso TJ, National Birth Defects Prevention Study. Association between prepregnancy body mass index and congenital heart defects. Am J Obstet Gynecol. 2010;202:51.
4. Hoffman JI, Kaplan S. The incidence of congenital heart disease. J Am Coll Cardiol. 2002;39:1890–900.
5. Acharya G, Sitras V, Maltau JM, Dahl LB, Kaaresen PI, Hanssen TA, Lunde P. Major congenital heart disease in Northern Norway: shortcomings of pre- and postnatal diagnosis. Acta Obstet Gynecol Scand. 2004;83:1124–9.
6. Schultz AH, Localio AR, Clark BJ, Ravishankar C, Videon N, Kimmel SE. Epidemiologic features of the presentation of critical congenital heart disease: implications for screening. Pediatrics. 2008;121:751–7.
7. Zhang Y, Riehle-Colarusso T, Correa A, Li S, Feng X, Gindler J, Lin H, Webb C, Li W, Trines J, Berry RJ, Yeung L, Luo Y, Jiang M, Chen H, Sun X, Li Z. Observed prevalence of congenital heart defects from a surveillance study in China. J Ultrasound Med. 2011;30:989–95.
8. Tegnander E, Williams W, Johansen OJ, Blaas HG, Eik-Nes SH. Prenatal detection of heart defects in a non-selected population of 30,149 fetuses-detection rates and outcome. Ultrasound Obstet Gynecol. 2006;27:252–65.
9. Maternal and child health and community health division of the ministry of health. The national annual report and communication of maternal and child health surveillance, 2011; 6. http://wenku.baidu.com/link?url=3szV193S7MpVfRtsepAON0GkKsuKho96H7t0yGe9SpgCX2-EL0p-SvgXjAq-LgaPUxyUUWDAVb-E7dKJKdhjpDhbgzoRV3MjMiyNahu2ITS. Accessed 29 Apr 2015.
10. National Health and Family Planning Commission of the People's Republic of China. The Report of prevention and treatment of births defects in China, 2012. http://www.gov.cn/gzdt/att/att/site1/20120912/1c6f6506c7f811bacf9301.pdf. Accessed 29 Apr 2015.
11. Song X, Li N, Liu J, Chen G, Zhang L, Li C, Zheng X. Depression and its influencing factors among mothers of children with birth defects in china. Matern Child Health J. 2010;16:1–6.
12. Pei L, Kang Y, Cheng Y, Yan H. The Association of Maternal Lifestyle with Birth Defects in Shaanxi Province, Northwest China. PLoS One. 2015;10:e0139452.
13. National Bureau of Statistics of the People's Republic of China. The bulletin of sixth national census in Shaanxi province in 2010. http://www.stats.gov.cn/tjsj/tjgb/rkpcgb/dfrkpcgb/201202/t20120228_30402.html. Accessed 29 Apr 2015.
14. Filmer D, Pritchett LH. Estimating wealth effects without expenditure data–or tears: an application to educational enrollments in states of India. Demography. 2001;38:115–32.
15. Yang XY, Li XF, Lu XD, Liu YL. Incidence of congenital heart disease in Beijing, China. Chin Med J (Engl). 2009;122:1128–32.
16. Zhang X, Li S, Wu S, Hao X, Guo S, Suzuki K, Yokomichi H, Yamagata Z. Prevalence of birth defects and risk-factor analysis from a population-based survey in Inner Mongolia, China. BMC Pediatr. 2012;12:125.
17. Wu L, Li B, Xia J, Ji C, Liang Z, Ma Y, Li S, Wu Y, Wang Y, Zhao Q. Prevalence of congenital heart defect in Guangdong province, 2008–2012. BMC Public Health. 2014;14:152.
18. Moons P, Sluysmans T, De Wolf D, Massin M, Suys B, Benatar A, Gewillig M. Congenital heart disease in 111225 births in Belgium: birth prevalence, treatment and survival in the 21st century. Acta Paediatr. 2009;98:472–7.
19. Baltaxe E, Zarante I. Prevalence of congenital heart disease in 44,985 newborns in CoLombia. Arch Cardiol Mex. 2006;76:263–8.
20. Forrester MB, Merz RD. Precurrence risk of birth defects in Hawaii. Congenit Anom (Kyoto). 2008;48:40–4.
21. Miller A, Riehle-Colarusso T, Siffel C, Frías JL, Correa A. Maternal age and prevalence of isolated congenital heart defects in an urban area of the United States. Am J Med Genet A. 2011;155A:2137–45.
22. Reefhuis J, Honein MA. Maternal age and non-chromosomal birth defects, Atlanta—1968–2000: Teenager or thirty-something, who is at risk? Birth Defects Res A Clin Mol Teratol. 2004;70:572–9.
23. Messer LC, Luben TJ, Mendola P, Carozza SE, Horel SA, Langlois PH. Urban-rural residence and the occurrence of cleft lip and cleft palate in Texas, 1999–2003. Ann Epidemiol. 2010;20:32–9.
24. Luo YL, Cheng YL, Gao XH, Tan SQ, Li JM, Wang W, Chen Q. Maternal age, parity and isolated birth defects: a population-based case-control study in Shenzhen, China. PLoS One. 2013;8:e81369.
25. Oyen N, Boyd HA, Poulsen G, Wohlfahrt J, Melbye M. Familial recurrence of midline birth defects–a nationwide danish cohort study. Am J Epidemiol. 2009;170:46–52.
26. Nelle M, Raio L, Pavlovic M, Carrel T, Surbek D, Meyer-Wittkopf M. Prenatal diagnosis and treatment planning of congenital heart defects-possibilities and limits. World J Pediatr. 2009;5:18–22.
27. Fernandes SM, Arendt KW, Landzberg MJ, Economy KE, Khairy P. Pregnant women with congenital heart disease: cardiac, anesthetic and obstetrical implications. Expert Rev Cardiovasc Ther. 2010;8:439–48.
28. Campbell OM, Graham WJ, Lancet Maternal Survival Series steering group. Strategies for reducing maternal mortality: getting on with what works. Lancet. 2006;368:1284–99.
29. Liu X, Zhou X, Yan H, Wang D. Use of maternal healthcare services in 10 provinces of rural western China. Int J Gynaecol Obstet. 2011;114:260–4.

7

Near-infrared spectroscopy as a predictor of clinical deterioration: a case report of two infants with duct-dependent congenital heart disease

Mirthe J. Mebius[1*], Gideon J. du Marchie Sarvaas[3], Diana W. Wolthuis[2], Beatrijs Bartelds[3], Martin C. J. Kneyber[2,4], Arend F. Bos[1] and Elisabeth M. W. Kooi[1]

Abstract

Background: Some infants with congenital heart disease are at risk of in-hospital cardiac arrest. To better foresee cardiac arrest in infants with congenital heart disease, it might be useful to continuously assess end-organ perfusion. Near-infrared spectroscopy is a non-invasive method to continuously assess multisite regional tissue oxygen saturation.

Case presentation: We report on two infants with duct-dependent congenital heart disease who demonstrated a gradual change in cerebral and/or renal tissue oxygen saturation before cardiopulmonary resuscitation was required. In both cases, other clinical parameters such as heart rate, arterial oxygen saturation and blood pressure did not indicate that deterioration was imminent.

Conclusions: These two cases demonstrate that near-infrared spectroscopy might contribute to detecting a deteriorating clinical condition and might therefore be helpful in averting cardiopulmonary collapse and need for resuscitation in infants with congenital heart disease.

Keywords: Congenital heart disease, Near-infrared spectroscopy, Newborn infants, Cardiac arrest, Cardiopulmonary resuscitation, Intensive care, Case report

Background

Some infants with congenital heart disease (CHD) are at risk of cardiac arrest during hospitalization [1]. In-hospital cardiac arrest occurs in approximately 2% to 6% of children admitted to paediatric intensive care units [2, 3]. Through earlier recognition, cardiac arrest may be prevented and outcomes and survival may be improved [4].

Monitoring end-organ perfusion might help recognizing clinical deterioration at an early stage. Near-infrared spectroscopy (NIRS) is a non-invasive clinical tool to continuously assess multisite regional tissue oxygen saturation (rSO_2) [5]. It is based on the relative transparency of biological young tissue (bone, skin, soft tissue) and the ability to differentiate oxygenated hemoglobin from deoxygenated hemoglobin as they have distinct absorption spectra. The ratio between oxygenated and total hemoglobin represents the regional tissue oxygen saturation [6]. In infants with CHD, multiple studies have investigated tissue oxygenation at various moments during early life [7–14]. Most studies addressed the intraoperative and postoperative period [7–10], but cerebral rSO_2 was also assessed preoperatively in some studies [11–14]. To our knowledge, however, multisite tissue oxygen saturation as a predictor of clinical deterioration in neonates with CHD has not been described before.

We discuss two cases in which continuous monitoring of multisite tissue oxygen saturation using NIRS indicated a deteriorating clinical condition which eventually led to cardiac arrest.

* Correspondence: m.j.mebius01@umcg.nl
[1]University Medical Center Groningen, Beatrix Children's Hospital, Division of Neonatology, University of Groningen, Hanzeplein 1, 9713 GZ Groningen, The Netherlands
Full list of author information is available at the end of the article

Case presentation

Both cases in this report were part of a prospective observational cohort study (registration number NTR5233), which was conducted between May 2014 and August 2016. Parental informed consent was obtained in both cases. We measured cerebral and renal rSO_2 using INVOS 5100c near-infrared spectrometers (Somanetics Corporation, Troy, Michigan, USA) in combination with neonatal sensors (Somanetics Corporation). Nurses were not instructed to act on certain rSO_2 values, as they were not measured for clinical purposes.

Case 1

A boy diagnosed prenatally with pulmonary atresia with an intact ventricular septum was born at our hospital at a gestational age of 37.3 weeks. After birth, the patient was admitted to the neonatal intensive care unit (NICU) with continuous positive airway pressure (CPAP) at seven cmH_2O with a maximum of 40% O_2 and infusion with prostaglandin E_1 (0.025 ug/kg/min) to maintain pulmonary circulation. Prenatal diagnosis and ductal patency were confirmed by the pediatric cardiologist. The patient appeared to be hemodynamically stable with transcutaneous oxygen saturations (SpO_2) between 70% and 90% and mean arterial blood pressures between 46 and 73 mmHg. As the patient was clinically stable, further hemodynamic parameters were not available for this case.

Four hours after birth the boy developed three apneas. The third apnea was followed by loss of cardiac output. Cardiopulmonary resuscitation was initiated immediately according to protocol. Cardiac output and heart rate, however, remained insufficient and the boy died 6 h after birth.

Autopsy confirmed the diagnosis of a pulmonary atresia with a hypoplastic right ventricle and an intact ventricular septum. Furthermore, autopsy revealed a single coronary ostium, multiple ventricular-coronary fistulas and a right ventricle dependent coronary blood flow with bridging of a branch of the right coronary artery. There were signs of recent myocardial ischemia, such as loss of cardiomyocytes. In addition, there was a left-sided open ductus arteriosus between the brachiocephalic trunk and the pulmonary artery. Based on autopsy findings, the most likely cause of death was considered to be massive myocardial ischemia which is not uncommon for this type of anatomy and physiology. Other causes such as a primary intraventricular hemorrhage or infarction cannot be ruled out completely since there was no permission for cerebral autopsy.

Near-infrared spectroscopy case 1

Baseline cerebral and renal rSO_2 were relatively low (around 40%) and decreased rapidly approximately 40 min before cardiopulmonary resuscitation was necessary (Fig. 1). This rapid decrease in cerebral and renal rSO_2. was probably due to a sudden decrease in arterial oxygen saturation. All clinical parameters spontaneously recovered from this incident. Cerebral rSO_2, however, started decreasing again from approximately 40% to 15% 25 min before cardiopulmonary resuscitation was necessary, while other hemodynamic parameters did not alarm the attending staff. Within 10 min, cerebral rSO_2 had already decreased 50% from its original baseline value (40%) to approximately 20%. We cannot fully explain why cerebral rSO_2 decreased before renal rSO_2 and SpO_2.

Case 2

A girl diagnosed prenatally with double outlet right ventricle, transposed great arteries, a ventricular septal defect and a hypoplastic aortic arch was born prematurely at our hospital at a gestational age of 34.9 weeks.

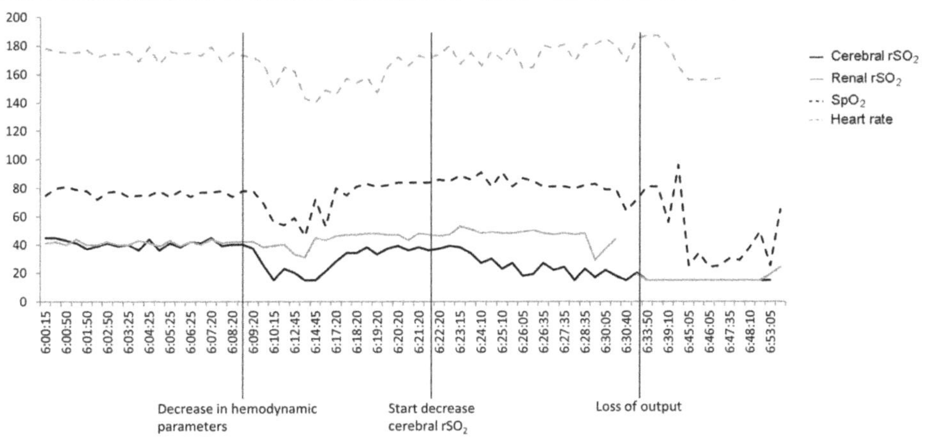

Fig. 1 The course of hemodynamic parameters and cerebral and renal oxygen saturation of the first case. SpO_2, transcutaneous arterial oxygen saturation; rSO_2, regional tissue oxygen saturation

She was admitted to the NICU with CPAP 10cmH_2O with a maximum of 40% O_2 due to respiratory distress/delayed transition. Initially, she had a wide-open ductus arteriosus. Eighteen hours after birth her clinical condition deteriorated with signs of a duct-dependent systemic circulation. Therefore, prostaglandin E_1 infusion was administered (0.025 ug/kg/min) to maintain ductal patency. During the first days after birth there was a fragile balance between pulmonary and systemic blood flow.

At the sixth day after birth, she underwent bilateral pulmonary banding with the intention of controlling an ever increasing pulmonary blood flow. Peri-operatively, hypotension was treated successfully with multiple volume expansions and noradrenalin. Postoperatively, she was on Bi-level Positive Airway Pressure (BiPAP)-assist and prior to loss of output there were no clinical signs of primary respiratory failure (e.g. inadvertent extubation). Arterial pH was 7.34, arterial saturation was 90%, pCO_2 was 4.8 kPa, hemoglobin was 8.0 mmol/l and lactate was 1.5 mmol/l. At that time, arterial blood pressure was 70/30 mmHg and she had normal diuresis. One hour later, she suddenly developed bradycardia followed by loss of cardiac output. Cardiopulmonary resuscitation was initiated immediately according to protocol. Infusion with prostaglandin E_1 was transferred from a peripheral venous site to a central line and was increased in dosage. An echocardiogram suggested an open ductus arteriosus, revealed a poor contractility and an inadequate cardiac output. After 40 min of cardiopulmonary resuscitation, the sternum was re-opened. The heart, however, was almost non-contractile and the girl died 7 days after birth.

Autopsy confirmed the diagnosis and concluded that the lumen of the ductus arteriosus was small with a diameter of less than three millimeter. Whether this was too small to maintain systemic circulation and whether prostaglandin E_1 infusion was inadequate at the time of collapse, remains unknown. Furthermore, autopsy revealed an immature lung parenchyma, atelectasis of part of the basal lobes and small inflammatory areas in both lungs. These pulmonary findings might also have contributed to the cardiopulmonary collapse.

Near-infrared spectroscopy case 2

We observed an increase in cerebral rSO_2 and a decrease in renal rSO_2 1 h before loss of output (Fig. 2). Renal rSO_2 returned to baseline, while cerebral rSO_2 remained approximately 10% above baseline. This incident might have been caused by a closing ductus arteriosus due to insufficient Prostaglandin E_1 administration or an insufficient response to adequate Prostaglandin E_1 administration. Especially the rapidly decreasing renal rSO_2 was indicative of a closing ductus arteriosus. Due to the coarctation of the aorta, renal blood flow was dependent on an open ductus arteriosus. The increase in cerebral rSO_2 was less easy to explain, but could be caused by an increase in cerebral blood flow. Due to the closing ductus arteriosus, the descending aorta might have become narrower, leading to an increased arterial pressure above the coarctation and subsequently increased cerebral blood flow. Thirty minutes before cardiopulmonary resuscitation, cerebral rSO_2 started decreasing from 55% to approximately 20% and renal rSO_2 decreased from 40% to 15%. Renal rSO_2 decreased more rapidly compared with cerebral rSO_2 and approximately 15 min before loss of output, renal rSO_2 was less than 50% from its original baseline value. The more rapid decrease of renal rSO_2 in comparison with cerebral rSO_2 also supports the theory of insufficient systemic circulation due to a closing ductus arteriosus. Apart from a slowly increasing heart rate from 160 bpm to 180 bpm, hemodynamic parameters such as

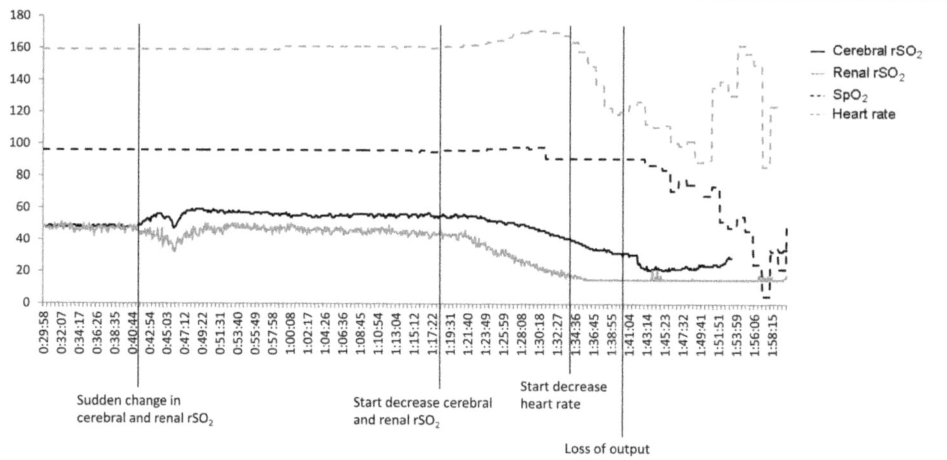

Fig. 2 The course of hemodynamic parameters and cerebral and renal oxygen saturation of the second case. SpO_2, transcutaneous arterial oxygen saturation; rSO_2, regional tissue oxygen saturation

SpO_2 and arterial blood pressure remained stable until several minutes before cardiopulmonary resuscitation was necessary (Fig. 2).

Discussion

These cases demonstrate that continuous monitoring of multisite near-infrared spectroscopy might be helpful in early identification of clinical deterioration in infants with congenital heart disease. In both cases, cerebral and/or renal rSO_2 changed 30 min or more before loss of output while other hemodynamic parameters did not indicate that deterioration was imminent until a few minutes before cardiopulmonary resuscitation was necessary.

Cerebral rSO_2 decreased 30–35% from baseline before loss of output. McNeill et al. found that cerebral rSO_2 values varied 15% or more from baseline rSO_2 values during less than 1% of the day in preterm infants [15]. Furthermore, Bernal et al. demonstrated an average cerebral rSO_2 of 77% with a standard deviation of 6.1% within patients during the first week after birth [16]. As a decrease of 30–35% exceeds this intra-individual variability, it seems more likely that the decrease in cerebral rSO_2 observed in the two cases was a consequence of a deteriorating clinical condition and a subsequent reduction of cerebral perfusion, rather than the normal intra-individual variability of NIRS.

In the current cases we did not respond to changes in cerebral and renal rSO_2, as they were measured in the context of a prospective observational cohort study and not for clinical purposes. In retrospect, these cases indicate that large changes in cerebral and/or renal rSO_2 in infants with duct-dependent CHD should be considered a red flag and warrant a complete check-up of the infant, including physical examination, echocardiography and basic blood tests. The time-interval of 15 to 30 min might give some extra time to prevent clinical deterioration in infants with CHD. Potential therapeutic strategies depend on the reason of the change in cerebral and/or renal rSO_2, but could include mechanical ventilation, pharmaceutical therapy (e.g. inotropes), volume expansion or perhaps emergency surgery. Furthermore, it might be useful to use predefined upper and lower limits of cerebral and renal oxygen saturation, a principle that was recently suggested in a large trial with preterm infants [17]. Due to the heterogeneity of the cardiac population, it is difficult to apply normal ranges of cerebral and renal rSO_2. In this population it might be more useful to use limits below which histological and biochemical changes in tissue have been reported, i.e. below 44% [18].

Conclusions

In conclusion, in infants with duct-dependent congenital heart disease, a significant change in cerebral and/or renal oxygen saturation from baseline as measured by NIRS may be an early indicator of a sudden, unexpected clinical deterioration, which eventually could lead to cardiac arrest and death. Increased awareness and thorough scrutiny of the patient are required when such changes in cerebral and/or renal oxygen saturation are observed.

Abbreviations

BiPAP-assist: Bi-level Positive Airway Pressure - assist; CHD: Congenital heart disease; CPAP: Continuous positive airway pressure; NICU: Neonatal intensive care unit; NIRS: Near-infrared spectroscopy; rSO_2: Regional tissue oxygen saturation; SpO_2: Transcutaneous arterial oxygen saturation

Acknowledgements

We would like to thank the nurses and staff of the neonatal intensive care unit and the pediatric intensive care unit for their help with the NIRS measurements.

Funding

This study was part of the research program of the Graduate School of Medical Sciences, Research Institutes BCN-BRAIN and GUIDE, University of Groningen. M.J. Mebius was financially supported by the Junior Scientific Master Class of the University of Groningen.

Authors' contributions

MJM made substantial contributions to the conception and design of the study, drafted the initial manuscript, revised the manuscript after feedback from co-authors, and approved the final manuscript as submitted. GJdMS was one of the pediatric cardiologists involved in the second case, made substantial contributions to the interpretation of data, critically reviewed the manuscript, and approved the final manuscript as submitted. DWW was the attending staff member in the second case, made substantial contributions to acquisition of data, critically reviewed the manuscript, and approved the final manuscript as submitted. BB was one of the pediatric cardiologists involved in the first case, made substantial contributions to acquisition of data, critically reviewed the manuscript, and approved the final manuscript as submitted. MCJK made substantial contributions to the interpretation of data, critically reviewed the manuscript, and approved the final manuscript as submitted. AFB made substantial contributions to the conception and design of the study, critically reviewed the manuscript, and approved the final manuscript as submitted. EMWK was the attending staff member in the first case, made substantial contributions to the conception and design of the study and the interpretation of data, critically reviewed the manuscript, and approved the final manuscript as submitted.

Authors' information

Not applicable

Competing interests

The authors declare that they have no competing interests.

Financial disclosure

None reported

Author details
[1]University Medical Center Groningen, Beatrix Children's Hospital, Division of Neonatology, University of Groningen, Hanzeplein 1, 9713 GZ Groningen, The Netherlands. [2]University Medical Center Groningen, Beatrix Children's Hospital, Division of Pediatric Intensive Care, University of Groningen, Groningen, The Netherlands. [3]University Medical Center Groningen, Center for Congenital Heart Diseases, Pediatric Cardiology, Beatrix Children's Hospital, University of Groningen, Groningen, The Netherlands. [4]Critical Care, Anesthesiology, Peri-operative & Emergency medicine (CAPE), the University of Groningen, Groningen, The Netherlands.

References

1. Ortmann L, Prodhan P, Gossett J, Schexnayder S, Berg R, Nadkarni V, et al. Outcomes after in-hospital cardiac arrest in children with cardiac disease: a report from Get With the Guidelines-Resuscitation. Circulation. 2011;124: 2329–37.
2. Berg MD, Nadkarni VM, Berg RA. Cardiopulmonary resuscitation in children. Curr Opin Crit Care. 2008;14:254–60.
3. Suominen P, Olkkola KT, Voipio V, Korpela R, Palo R, Rasanen J. Utstein style reporting of in-hospital paediatric cardiopulmonary resuscitation. Resuscitation. 2000;45:17–25.
4. Peddy SB, Hazinski MF, Laussen PC, Thiagarajan RR, Hoffman GM, Nadkarni V, et al. Cardiopulmonary resuscitation: special considerations for infants and children with cardiac disease. Cardiol Young. 2007;17 Suppl 2:116–26.
5. Wahr JA, Tremper KK, Samra S, Delpy DT. Near-infrared spectroscopy: theory and applications. J Cardiothorac Vasc Anesth. 1996;10:406–18.
6. Pellicer A, Bravo Mdel C. Near-infrared spectroscopy: a methodology-focused review. Semin Fetal Neonatal Med. 2011;16:42–9.
7. Simons J, Sood ED, Derby CD, Pizarro C. Predictive value of near-infrared spectroscopy on neurodevelopmental outcome after surgery for congenital heart disease in infancy. J Thoracic Cardiovasc Surg. 2012;143:118–25.
8. Kussmann BD, Wypij D, Laussen PC, Soul JS, Bellinger DC, DiNardo JA, et al. Relationship of intraoperative cerebral oxygen saturation to neurodevelopmental outcome and brain magnetic resonance imaging at 1 year of age in infants undergoing biventricular repair. Circulation. 2010;122:245–54.
9. Chakravarti SB, Mittnacht AJ, Katz JC, Nguyen K, Joashi U, Srivastava S, et al. Multisite near-infrared spectroscopy predicts elevated blood lactate level in children after cardiac surgery. J Cardiothorac Vasc Anesth. 2009;23:663–7.
10. Zulueta JL, Vida VL, Perisinotto E, Pittarello D, Stellin G. Role of intraoperative regional oxygen saturation using near infrared spectroscopy in the prediction of low output syndrome after pediatric heart surgery. J Card Surg. 2013;28:446–52.
11. Toet MC, Flinterman A, Laar I, Vries JW, Bennink GB, Uiterwaal CS, et al. Cerebral oxygen saturation and electrical brain activity before, during, and up to 36 hours after arterial switch procedure in neonates without pre-existing brain damage: its relationship to neurodevelopmental outcome. Exp Brain Res. 2005;165:343–50.
12. Uebing A, Furck AK, Hansen JH, Nufer E, Scheewe J, Dütschke P, et al. Perioperative cerebral and somatic oxygenation in neonates with hypoplastic left heart syndrome or transposition of the great arteries. J Thorac Cardiovasc Surg. 2011;142:523–30.
13. Kurth CD, Steven JL, Montenegro LM, Watzman HM, Gaynor JW, Spray TL, et al. Cerebral oxygen saturation before congenital heart surgery. Ann Thorac Surg. 2001;72:187–92.
14. Mebius MJ, Van der Laan ME, Verhagen EA, Roofthooft MTR, Bos AF, Kooi EMW. Cerebral oxygen saturation during the first 72 h after birth in infants diagnosed prenatally with congenital heart disease. Early Hum Dev. 2016; 103:199–203.
15. McNeill S, Gatenby JC, McElroy S, Engelhardt B. Normal cerebral, renal and abdominal regional oxygen saturations using near-infrared spectroscopy in preterm infants. J Perinatol. 2011;31:51–7.
16. Bernal NP, Hoffman GM, Ghanayem NS, Arca MJ. Cerebral and somatic near-infrared spectroscopy in normal newborns. J Pediatr Surg. 2010;45:1306–10.
17. Pellicer A, Greisen G, Benders M, Claris O, Dempsey E, Fumagalli M, et al. The SafeBoosC phase II randomised clinical trial: a treatment guideline for targeted near-infrared-derived cerebral tissue oxygenation versus standard treatment in extremely preterm infants. Neonatology. 2013;104:171 –8.
18. Kurth CD, Levy WJ, McCann J. Near-infrared spectroscopy cerebral oxygen saturation thresholds for hypoxia-ischemia in piglets. J Cereb Blood Flow Metab. 2002;22:335–41.

8

Assessment of cardiac function in children with congenital adrenal hyperplasia

J . Tony Nengom[1*], S. Sap Ngo Um[1,2], D. Chelo[1,2], R. Mbono Betoko[1], J. Boombhi[1,3], F. Mouafo Tambo[1,4], A. Chiabi[1,4], S. Kingue[1,3] and P. Koki Ndombo[1,3]

Abstract

Background: High level of androgens found in congenital adrenal hyperplasia (CAH) seems to have a deleterious effect on heart function. We therefore evaluate cardiac function of children with CAH in comparison with a healthy group.

Methods: We carried out a case-control study in the single endocrinology unit of the Mother and Child Center of Chantal Biya's Foundation. Cases were matched for age and genotypic sex to 2 healthy controls. We analyzed the ejection fraction (LVEF), fractional shortening and left ventricular mass; output and cardiac index; E and A waves velocities, E/A ratio and the mitral deceleration time and diameter of the left atrium; tricuspid annular plane systolic excursion and pulmonary artery systolic pressure were also measured.

Results: We included 19 patients with a median age of 6.26 ± 3.75 years and 38 controls stackable distribution. The left ventricular mass of cases was greater than that of controls. A case of reversible cardiomyopathy on hormone replacement therapy was found.
For the cases, the average ejection fraction was 71.95 ± 7.88%; the average fractional shortening was 40.67 ± 7.02%. All these values were higher than those of controls, although the difference was not statistically significant. Diastolic left ventricular function was more impaired among the cases.
Right ventricular function was similar in both groups. These abnormalities were highly correlated to the late age at diagnosis and duration of treatment.

Conclusion: This study shows an altered cardiac function in CAH compared to healthy control and highlights importance of an early diagnosis of cases, a tight control of androgens levels and a regular monitoring of cardiac function.

Keywords: Cardiac function, Congenital adrenal hyperplasia, Children

Background

Children with Congenital Adrenal Hyperplasia (CAH), are exposed to high levels of androgens [1] leading to virilization of affected fetus. Besides their control of sexual function, androgens have multiple physiological functions including a major cardiovascular role [2, 3]. There is increasing evidence that patients with classical CAH have multiple vascular risk factors and that they are at increased risk for cardiovascular disease in adulthood [4–6]. Monitored measurements show that these patients also manifest elevated 24-h ambulatory blood pressure which can even lead to heart failure [7–9]. Various studies in children with CAH, show ventricular hypertrophy and impaired left ventricular function precisely the diastolic one by significant prolongation of both iso volumetric relaxation time and mitral deceleration time [9–11]. In Cameroon, there is very little data regarding the cardiovascular status and cardiac function of children followed up for CAH. This justify the present study with the aim of assessing cardiac function in affected children in Cameroon and compare them to a group of healthy children.

* Correspondence: tnengom@gmail.com
[1]Faculty of Medicine and Biomedical Sciences of Yaounde I University, P.O Box: 14855, Yaounde, Cameroon
Full list of author information is available at the end of the article

Methods

This was a matched case-control study, performed over a 9 months' period (October 2015 to July 2016). We included all recorded children affected with CAH in the national registry and followed in the single service of pediatric endocrinology of the country: the Mother and Child Center of the Chantal Biya Foundation (MCC/CBF). Cases aged 10 months to 15 years were matched for age and genotypic sex to 2 healthy controls. We used paired and unbalanced sampling (1 case per 2 controls) to increase the potency of the results and to limit the bias related to the sample size. The controls were recruited in children coming for a routine visit or vaccination. We excluded controls with another chronic condition, a known cardiovascular disease or acute illness modifying cardiac function (anemia, severe infection).

After an informed consent obtained from parents and assent from children aged >12 years, diagnosis circumstances, morphology (pelvic ultrasound, bone age) and lab results (17 hydroxyprogesterone, karyotype and biomolecular diagnosis when available) at diagnosis were noted. Height and weight were measured to the nearest 0.1 cm and 0.1 kg. Three blood pressures were measured and the mean noted for each case and control, with an electronic sphygmomanometer (Omron HEM 712C, Kyoto, Japan). The blood pressure was derived in percentile for height and genotypic sex. A general cardiac examination was done by a senior cardiologist.

Thereafter, a standard echocardiography in time mode motion, two-dimensional and Doppler [12, 13] was performed in both cases and controls with Siemens Acusson Cypress® (Siemens, Munich Germany) ultrasound machine.

The variables analyzed were:

- For the left ventricle: ejection fraction, fractional shortening, stroke volume and left ventricular mass; cardiac output and index; the E and A waves velocities, the E/A wave ratio and the mitral deceleration time;
- For the right ventricle: tricuspid annular plane systolic excursion (TAPSE). The pulmonary artery systolic pressure was also measured.

Height$^{2.7}$ (in meters) has been validated as an indicator of lean body mass and has been recommended for indexing LVM. Use of height$^{2.7}$ to index LVM also minimizes the effect of age, gender and race [14–17]. Stroke volume was indexed by the body surface area [18].

Statistical analyses were done using Microsoft® Excel 2013 and SPSS 20 software from IBM. Average and proportions served to describe quantitative and qualitative data. Comparison was done with the T test of Student (for normally distributed variable and homogeneity of variances) and a suitable non-parametric test Kruskall Wallis. Multivariate analysis was done to evaluate correlation between variables (Spearman). A *p* value <0.05 was statistically significant.

The study received ethical approval from institutional board review of Faculty of medicine and biomedical sciences of Yaounde.

Results

We included 19 cases and 38 controls aged 10 months to 15 years with an average age of 6.26 ± 3.75 years. The most represented age was 4 years, with a proportion of 21% of cases. Among cases, 5 were boys and 14 girls. After the karyotype, only one was actually genotypically male (XY). As diagnosis circumstances, abnormal genitalia was the most represented (84.2%).The average age at diagnosis was 3.7 years (1 month to 12 years) (Tables 1 and 2).

Advance bone age was found in all patients at diagnosis. The most enzyme deficiency found was that of 11-βOH (11 Beta-hydroxylase), 78.9% of cases. Achondroplasia was found in 2 cases and one patient present with dilated cardiomyopathy diagnosed at 1 year of life, reversible on hormone replacement therapy (Table 2).

Blood pressure was significantly higher in cases than controls, either systolic or diastolic ($p = 0.025$) (Figs. 1 and 2).

Concerning systolic function of the left ventricle, cases' average ejection fraction (LVEF) was 71.95 ± 7.88%, VS 69.29 ± 7.95% in controls. The average fractional shortening (LVFS) was 40.67 ± 7.02% and 37.25 ± 5.64% for cases and controls respectively. In addition, mean stroke volume (SV) was 47.56 ± 13.58 ml/m^2 and 43.15 ± 10.83 ml/m^2 in cases and controls, respectively. The average cardiac output of cases was 3.76 ± 1.54 L/min. Mean cardiac index was 4.40 ± 1.07 L/min/m^2 for cases and 4.38 ± 0.94 L/min/m^2 for controls. Although cases values were above controls, the differences were not statistically significant (Table 3).

Diastolic left ventricular function was more impaired among the cases. Thus, we found an average E wave velocity of 0.80 ± 0.32 m/s, lower than that of controls; an A wave velocity of 0.76 ± 0.35 m/s, higher than that of the controls, an average E/A ratio of 1.38 ± 0.96 less than the value of controls and a longer deceleration time, 147.58 ± 42.81(milliseconds) ms (Table 4).

Table 1 General characteristic of study population

Variable	Cases	Controls
N	19	38
Phenotype (girls/boys)	14/5	36/2
Genotype (XX/XY)	18/1	-
Age (years)	6 ± 4	6 ± 4
Weight (kg)	23.8 ± 13.4	23 ± 11.6
Height (cm)	113.3 ± 26.2	118.5 ± 24.2
BMI	17.1 ± 2.9	15.4 ± 2
Heart rate (beats/min)	94.9 ± 20.2	100 ± 15.6

BMI Body Mass Index

Table 2 Clinical, biomolecular presentation of cases

		Number	Percent
Diagnosis circumstances	Abnormal genitalia	16	84.2
	Absence of testis	2	10.5
	Breast development	1	5.3
Age at diagnosis Median(range)	3.7 years (1 month-12 years)	-	-
Advance bone age Y/N	Yes/No	19/0	100/0
Salt wasting syndrome	Yes/No	4/15	21.1/78.9
Type of enzyme deficiency	11 β Hydroxylase deficiency	15	78.9
	21 Hydroxylase deficiency	4	21.1

In terms of the systolic function of the right ventricle, there was no statistically significant difference between the systolic excursion of the plan of the tricuspid annulus (TAPSE) of cases and controls. In contrast, pulmonary pressures were within normal values while significantly higher in controls. However, we noted a case of CAH with a systolic pulmonary arterial hypertension (Table 5).

The left ventricular mass index (LVMI) of cases was statistically greater than that of controls with an average value of 46.02 ± 17.14 g/m$^{2.7}$. The end diastolic and systolic diameters of the left ventricle and the left atrium were almost identical in the two groups (Table 6).

While analyzing correlation, we found that age at diagnosis does not influence the left ventricular mass index. A relationship was found between the diameter of the left atrium and age at diagnosis. For the diameter of the aorta, the correlation was very strong with age at diagnosis ($p = 0.00$) (Table 7). The duration of treatment does not influence the LVEF and LVFS (Table 8).

Discussion

Our study focused on the evaluation of cardiac function among Cameroonian children with congenital adrenal hyperplasia. The aim was to evaluate through standard echocardiography the most common settings for heart function and compared it to a group of healthy children matched for age and sex. With a sample of 57 children (1 case for 2 controls), we found an impaired diastolic function in cases compared to controls and increased values of systolic function in cases. Right cardiac function was similar in the 2 groups.

This pilot study was monocentric but included all patients diagnosed and followed in the country. The lack of references curves of echocardiographic values in the literature for black children [12, 13] makes the interpretation of the values found difficult. The children of this study were not matched according to the fitness level and body composition including the percentage of fat mass, whose importance in cardiovascular health is not negligible [11, 19]. We used the anthropometric parameters and did not take into account the body composition which could influence the interpretation of these results. However, given that none of the children in this study had a body mass index >3 z score, they could all be expected to have normal body fat mass. Moreover, the age of cases and controls (6 years on average) places them at a hyperactive period of life and limits the sedentary lifestyle.

Nonetheless the present study brings relevant data among this particular population.

I. **General characteristics**

Our study population was younger than that of Sowande and al in Nigeria 2009 [20] who included

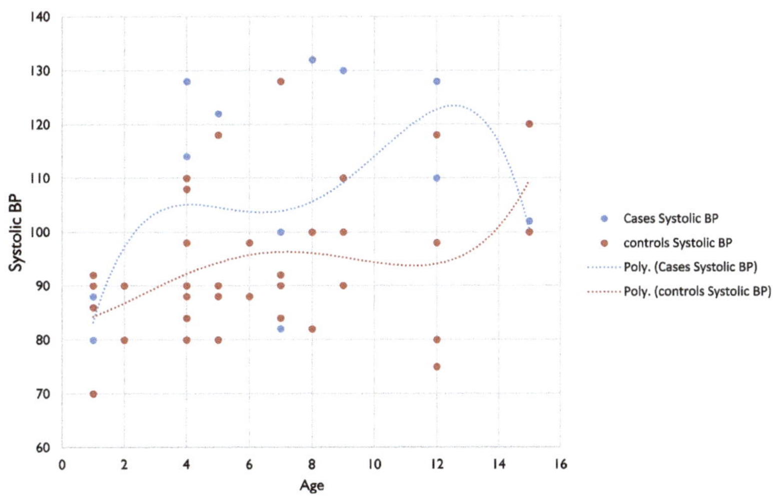

Fig. 1 Systolic blood pressure of the study population

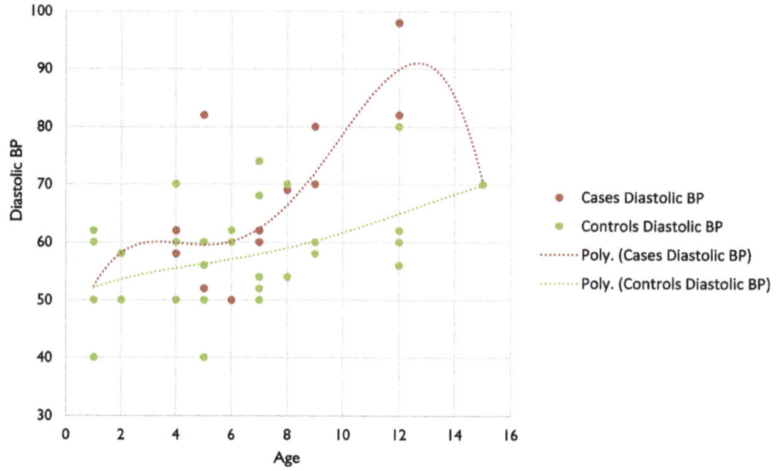

Fig. 2 Diastolic blood pressure of the study population

adolescent and young adults (range 5 weeks to 19 years). Sex rearing proportion was 26.31% (5/19) boys and 73.68% (14/19) girls, and after the karyotype, boys represented 5.26% (1/19). These gender assignment errors were found by Rodrigues and al in 20% of cases in Brazil in 2015 [21], in 30% by Sowande and al in Nigeria in 2009 [20]. In Sudan, Abdullah and al in 2011 [22] in a retrospective study over 5 years involving 122 children, had a higher prevalence of female gender after completion of the karyotype and 19% had to change sex with a preference for males. In Western countries where neonatal diagnosis is made, these sex attribution errors are not found in literature.

Concerning diagnosis circumstances, the most frequent reason for consultation was abnormal genitalia (clitoris hypertrophy). Sowande and al in 2009 in Nigeria, in their retrospective study on disorders of sexual differentiation, had 6 cases attributed to the CAH and all had as a dominant clinical presentation, clitoromegaly [20].

The average age at diagnosis was greater than that of Rodrigues and al (2 months) [21]. Awareness of medical teams concerning abnormal genitalia is greater in Latin America, explaining the present difference. The diagnosis is still delayed in developing countries because of limited access to para clinical test for all patients.

On initial clinical presentation, advanced bone age found in all the patients is related to the late age at diagnosis. Garcia and al in Brazil in 2013 [23], had advanced bone age in 71.43% (10 out of 14) in a population diagnosed and treated before age of 4 months. This highlights the fact that even under treatment, risk of excess androgens circulating is still high. This seems to be controlled in 3 daily doses of hydrocortisone [24].

The most found type of enzyme deficiency was 11β-OH in 78.9%, which is in contradiction to literature where the deficit in 21-OH (21 Hydroxylase) is recognized as the most common, with a prevalence more than 90% [25, 26]. Indeed in absence of neonatal screening, many children with 21-OH deficiency died during the neonatal period. This also explains the low number of boys in our study population.

A child in our study had dilated cardiomyopathy diagnosed at 1 year and a clinical improvement was observed upon initial hormone replacement therapy. A similar case was described in Kuwait. Al Jarallah and al in 2004 [27], published a case of rapidly reversible dilated cardiomyopathy. The congestive

Table 3 Average comparisons of left ventricular ejection fraction, stroke volume, cardiac output, cardiac index, fractional shortening

	Cases	Controls	*P* value
LVEF % mean (range, SD)	71.95 (60–83, 7.8)	69.29 (51–92, 7.9)	0.238
SV ml/m^2, mean (range, SD)	47.56 (20.1–72.6, 13.58)	43.15 (24.5–72.6, 10.83)	0.190
LVFS % mean (range, SD)	40.67 (31.10–51.16, 7.02)	37.25 (25.78–49.61, 5.64)	0.052
Cardiac output L/min, mean (range, SD)	3.376 (0.87–7.06, 1.54)	3.58 (1.55–5.88, 1.11)	0.620
Cardiac index, mean (range, SD) L/min/m^2	4.40 (2.23–6.10, 1.07)	4.38 (2.63–6.55, 0.94)	0.939

LEVF Left Ventricular Ejection Fraction, *SV* Stroke Volume, *LVFS* left ventricular fractional shortening, *SD* Standard Deviation

Table 4 Average comparisons of E and A waves velocities, E/A ratio and mitral deceleration time

	Cases	Controls	*P* value
E wave velocity mean (range, SD) m/s	0.80 (0.33–1.27, 0.32)	0.99 (0.76–1.37, 0.13)	0.081
A wave velocity mean (range, SD) m/s	0.76 (0.36–1.53, 0.35)	0.57 (0.38–0.74, 0.10)	0.082
E/A RATIO mean (range, SD)	1.38 (0.37–3.53, 0.96)	1.80 (1.27–2.61, 0.33)	0.069
Mitral deceleration time ms mean (range, SD)	147.48 (78–228, 42.81)	137.47 (66–222, 40.3)	0.406

heart failure and dilated ventricles declined with the introduction of hydrocortisone.

II. **Blood pressure and Cardiac function**

Blood pressure was higher in cases than controls, either systolic or diastolic. Various studies found similar results: Rodrigues and al [21] and Subbarayan and al [28], found a systolic blood pressure higher among cases.

Reasons for increase in cardiovascular risk of CAH patients are not totally elucidated. Could high levels of androgens have a vasoconstrictor effect? [29–31]. Moreover, the deficit type involved (11-β OH) has a mineralocorticoid effect by the accumulation of 11-deoxycorticosterone [25, 32]. The likely involvement of treatment with glucocorticoids, resulting in a compromise between the advantages and disadvantages [21]. In 2014, AMR and al in Egypt have shown a rise in cardiovascular risk in CAH patients, but no correlation was found between the different variables and the average daily dose of hydrocortisone. The hypothesis of a cumulative effect of steroid treatment over the years was issued [21, 33]. But our study population is young and treated with doses according to recommendations [1, 25].

1. **Systolic function of the left ventricle**

The variables studied to assess left ventricular systolic function were all within normal values for average, but higher in cases than in controls. Although the differences were not statistically significant. The small differences in means between controls and patients could be potentially due to differences in body composition or fitness level. Metwalley and al in Egypt in 2015 [10] studied the left ventricular dysfunction and subclinical atherosclerosis in children and adolescents with classic CAH. He did not found difference between the systolic function of the cases and the controls. However the LVEF of 70.5 ± 3.6 and the LVFS% of 39.2 ± 2.1 were higher than those of controls as in our study.

LVEF expresses the degree of emptying of the left ventricle. It quantifies the capacity of it and arteries to maintain adequate cardiac output under changing

Table 5 Comparison of averages TAPSE and pulmonary artery systolic pressure between the two groups

	Cases	Controls	*P* value
TAPSE mean (range, SD) mm	19.86 (12.9–25.8, 3.44)	20.18 (1.9–32.2, 4.49)	0.785
Systolic pulmonary pressure mean (range, SD) m/s	13.16 (7–25, 4.68)	15.56 (8.5–24.5, 3.96)	0.047

TAPSE Tricuspid Annular Plane Systolic Excursion

Table 6 Comparison of left ventricle's diastolic and systolic diameters, left atrium diameter and left ventricular mass

	Cases	Controls	*P* value
LVDd mean (range, SD) mm/m^2	35.99 (19.4–47.3,7.9)	35.46 (24.1–47.1, 4.94)	0.755
LVSd mean (range, SD) mm/m^2	21.31 (9.7–28, 4.90)	22.22 (13.8–32.2, 3.55)	0.427
LAD mean (range, SD) mm/m^2	23.41 (13.6–32.7, 4.62)	22.71 (16.3–31.7, 3.64)	0.534
LVMI mean (range, SD) g/m$^{2.7}$	46.02 (25–84.67, 17.14)	31.64 (20.2–46.9, 7.64)	**0.000**

LVDd Left Ventricular Diastolic diameter, *LVSd* Left Ventricular Systolic diameter, *LAD* Left Atrial Diameter, *LVMI* Left Ventricular Mass Index
The bold texts represent the result with a statistically significant differences

Table 7 Correlation between cardiac function parameters and age at diagnosis

Parameters	correlation coefficient (Spearman)	*P* value
LVEF	-0.1	0.685
SV	0.382	0.106
LVFS	0.004	0.988
LVMI	0.148	0.544
Cardiac output	0.441	0.059
Cardiac index	0.202	0.408
E/A Ratio	0.247	0.307
E wave velocity	0.191	0.434
A wave velocity	−0.257	0.289
Mitral deceleration time	0.371	0.118
LAD	**0.492**	**0.033**
TAPSE	0.447	0.055
Systolic pulmonary pressure	−0.057	0.817
Aortic diameter	**0.825**	**0.000**

LEVF Left Ventricular Ejection Fraction, *SV* Stroke Volume, *LVFS* Left Ventricular Fractional Shortening, *LVMI* Left Ventricular Mass Index, *LAD* Left Atrial Diameter, *TAPSE* Tricuspid Annular Plane Systolic Excursion
The bold texts represent the result with a statistically significant differences

Table 8 Correlation between the parameters of cardiac function and the duration of treatment

Parameters	Correlation coefficient (Spearman)	*P* value
LVEF	0.31	0.239
SV	0.169	0.531
LVFS	0.34	0.19
LVMI	-0.049	0.857
Cardiac output	0.48	0.061
Cardiac index	−0.09	0.739
E/A ratio	−0.34	0.188
E wave velocity	−0.42	0.098
A wave velocity	0.11	0.68
Mitral deceleration time	**0.51**	**0.04**
LAD	0.44	0.086
TAPSE	**0.72**	**0.002**
Systolic pulmonary pressure	−0.45	0.075
Aortic diameter	0.37	0.159

LEVF Left Ventricular Ejection Fraction, *SV* Stroke Volume, *LVFS* Left Ventricular Fractional Shortening, *LVMI* Left Ventricular Mass Index
The bold texts represent the result with a statistically significant differences

load conditions and / or contractility [34]. Its prognosis value comes from the functional reserves and adaptability to hemodynamic conditions it expresses. This increase in systolic left ventricular activity found among cases may reflect a myocardial stimulation by androgens [3].

2. **Diastolic function of the left ventricle**
The E wave velocity and E / A ratio were higher in controls than in cases. In contrast the A wave velocity was higher in cases than in controls. There was no statistically significant difference. The cases deceleration time varied between 78 and 228 ms, which is higher than the controls. This reflects an impaired relaxation function of the left ventricle of cases compared to controls. Metwalley in Egypt, found similar results [10]: an E / A ratio lowered and an extension of time of mitral deceleration and iso volumetric relaxation, indicating left ventricular dysfunction with very significant values $p < 0.001$. In our study this difference was not statistically significant probably because our children were younger. This situation resulted from longer exposure to androgens whose stimulatory activity on the heart was seen with the rise of systolic settings, an abnormal relaxation of the most sought muscle [3, 35].
3. **Right ventricular function**
In our study it was assessed mainly by systolic excursion of the plan of the tricuspid annulus. No differences were found between cases and controls for TAPSE. Systolic pulmonary pressure was statistically higher in cases than controls with a mean of 19.86 ± 3.44 mm. Alteration of right ventricular function is usually secondary to left heart failure. However, it can be isolated when it is due to certain lung diseases, right heart or pericardial diseases. Assessment of right ventricular function is, in terms of daily practice, extrapolated over the measures taken left [36]. The echocardiography of the right ventricle faces several difficulties, the main ones being represented by its size and its position in the thorax and especially by its special geometry shaped distorted prism [36]. This explains the difficulties of studying right ventricular function in daily practice and a lack of work on this subject allowing us to compare our results with those of other authors [12].
4. **Cardiac cavities**
The left ventricle mass index of the cases was statistically higher than controls. This reflects left ventricular hypertrophy which could be explained by the recognized trophic effect of androgens on cardiomyocytes. All this leading also to an abnormal relaxation of the cardiac muscle [35, 37].

III. **Correlation between cardiac function parameters and disease determinants**
A strong correlation was found between the diameter of the left atrium and age at diagnosis. A delayed age at diagnosis, lead to a prolonged exposure to high levels of androgens with their hypertrophic effect on the myocardium [35, 37]. The correlation is even stronger with the diameter of the aorta, coefficient = 0.825 and p = 0.00. This could be due to a vasodilator effect at high doses of androgens established in some studies [31].
Through inhibition of depolarizing calcium influx, it has been established that in humans, their injection at physiological and supra physiological concentrations induces expansion (up to 4.5%) of the coronary artery and improves coronary flow (up 17.5%) in subjects with arteriosclerotic coronary lesions [3].
A negative significant correlation would have been expected between the duration of the treatment and the cardiac mass, but it is not the case in our study. This highlights the importance of treatment compliance and patients being controlled, for better assessment of the relationship between treatment duration and cardiac mass.

Conclusions

This study showed that the cases had a greater systolic function than the controls, consequently increasing contractility. It also showed an increased left ventricular mass among cases leading to an altered relaxation of the left ventricle. These abnormalities were highly correlated to the late age at diagnosis and duration of treatment. This hence the necessity to introduce systematic neonatal screening for CAH to ensure early diagnosis and treatment, along with regular monitoring of heart function in children with CAH.

Abbreviations

11β-OH: 11 Beta-hydroxylase; 21-OH: 21 Hydroxylase; BMI: Body mass index; CAH: Congenital adrenal hyperplasia; LAD: Left atrial diameter; LVDd: Left ventricular diastolic diameter; LVEF: Left ventricular ejection fraction; LVFS: Left ventricular fractional shortening; LVMI: Left ventricular mass index; LVSd: Left ventricular systolic diameter; MCC/CBF: Mother and Child Center of the Chantal Biya Foundation; SV: Stroke volume; TAPSE: Tricuspid annular plane systolic excursion

Acknowledgments

1. Surrénales Cameroun's Association (SURCAM).
2. All the controls and their families.
3. BILONG Josué Armand for the statistical analysis.
4. All the medical students and nurses in the cardiology and endocrinology units of the MCC/CBF.

Funding

No funding.

Authors' contributions

Study concept and design SNU, TNJ. Literature review TNJ, SNU, KNP. Data collection and interpretation, TNJ, SNU, CD, MBR, MTF, BJ, CA, KS. Statistical analysis TNJ, SNU. Writing TNJ, SNU, MBR. Review SNU, MBR, CD, BJ, CA, KS, KNP. Study supervision: KNP. All authors read and approved the final manuscript.

Competing interest

The authors declare that they have no competing interests.

Author details

[1]Faculty of Medicine and Biomedical Sciences of Yaounde I University, P.O Box: 14855, Yaounde, Cameroon. [2]Mother and Child Centre of the Chantal Biya Foundation, Yaounde, Cameroon. [3]Yaounde General Hospital, Yaounde, Cameroon. [4]Yaounde Gyneco Obstetric and Pediatric Hospital, Yaounde, Cameroon.

References

1. Speiser PW, White PC. Congenital adrenal hyperplasia. N Engl J Med. 2003; 349(8):776–88.
2. Martin KCN. New perspectives on Mars and Venus: Unravelling the role of androgens in gender differences in cardiovascular biology and disease. Heart Lung Circ. 2007;16(3):185–92.
3. Smeets L, Legros J-J. Cœur et androgènes. /data/revues/00034266/00650002/163/ [Internet]. 2008 [cited 2016 Aug 4]; Available from: http://www.em-consulte.com/en/article/75986
4. Wierzbicka-Chmiel J, Chmiel A, Kajdaniuk D, Marek B. Vascular and cardiac function in young adults with classical congenital adrenal hyperplasia. 2015 [cited 2017 Feb 18]; Available from: http://www.endocrine-abstracts.org/ea/0037/ea0037GP.16.08.htm
5. Cornean RE, Hindmarsh PC, Brook CG. Obesity in 21-hydroxylase deficient patients. Arch Dis Child. 1998;78(3):261–3.
6. Sartorato P, Zulian E, Benedini S, Mariniello B, Schiavi F, Bilora F, et al. Cardiovascular risk factors and ultrasound evaluation of intima-media thickness at common carotids, carotid bulbs, and femoral and abdominal aorta arteries in patients with classic congenital adrenal hyperplasia due to 21-hydroxylase deficiency. J Clin Endocrinol Metab. 2007 Mar;92(3):1015–8.
7. Charmandari E, Weise M, Bornstein SR, Eisenhofer G, Keil MF, Chrousos GP, et al. Children with classic congenital adrenal hyperplasia have elevated serum leptin concentrations and insulin resistance: potential clinical implications. J Clin Endocrinol Metab. 2002;87(5):2114–20.
8. Roche EF, Charmandari E, Dattani MT, Hindmarsh PC. Blood pressure in children and adolescents with congenital adrenal hyperplasia (21-hydroxylase deficiency): a preliminary report. Clin Endocrinol. 2003;58(5):589–96.
9. Bhatia S, Muranjan MN, Lahiri KR. Left ventricular failure due to a rare variant of congenital adrenal hyperplasia. Indian J Pediatr. 2012;79(9):1241–3.
10. Metwalley KA, Farghaly HS, Sherief T. Left ventricular dysfunction and subclinical atherosclerosis in children with classic congenital adrenal hyperplasia: a single-center study from upper Egypt. Eur J Pediatr. 2016; 175(3):405–12.
11. Marra AM, Improda N, Capalbo D, Salzano A, Arcopinto M, De Paulis A, et al. Cardiovascular abnormalities and impaired exercise performance in adolescents with congenital adrenal hyperplasia. J Clin Endocrinol Metab. 2015;100(2):644–52.
12. Kampmann C, Wiethoff CM, Wenzel A, Stolz G, Betancor M, Wippermann CF, et al. Normal values of M mode echocardiographic measurements of more than 2000 healthy infants and children in Central Europe. ResearchGate. 2000;83(6):667–72.
13. Schmitz L, Koch H, Bein G, Brockmeier K. Left ventricular diastolic function in infants, children, and adolescents. Reference values and analysis of morphologic and physiologic determinants of echocardiographic Doppler flow signals during growth and maturation. J Am Coll Cardiol. 1998;32(5):1441–8.
14. Ubertini G, Bizzarri C, Grossi A, Gimigliano F, Ravà L, Fintini D, et al. Blood pressure and left ventricular characteristics in young patients with classical congenital adrenal hyperplasia due to 21-Hydroxylase deficiency. Int J Pediatr Endocrinol. 2010;2009(1):1.
15. Hanevold C, Waller J, Daniels S, Portman R, Sorof J. International pediatric hypertension Association. The effects of obesity, gender, and ethnic group on left ventricular hypertrophy and geometry in hypertensive children: a collaborative study of the international pediatric hypertension Association. Pediatrics. 2004;113(2):328–33.
16. Daniels SR. Hypertension-induced cardiac damage in children and adolescents. Blood Press Monit. 1999;4(3–4):165–70.
17. De Simone G, Daniels SR, Devereux RB, Meyer RA, Roman MJ, de Divitiis O, et al. Left ventricular mass and body size in normotensive children and adults: assessment of allometric relations and impact of overweight. J Am Coll Cardiol. 1992;20(5):1251–60.
18. Simone GD, Devereux RB, Daniels SR, Mureddu G, Roman MJ, Kimball TR, et al. Stroke volume and cardiac output in Normotensive children and adults. Circulation. 1997;95(7):1837–43.
19. Warburton DER, Nicol CW, Bredin SSD. Health benefits of physical activity: the evidence. CMAJ Can Med Assoc J. 2006 Mar 14;174(6):801.
20. Sowande OA, Adejuyigbe O. Management of ambiguous genitalia in ile ife, Nigeria: challenges and outcome. Afr J Paediatr Surg. 2009;6(1):14.
21. Rodrigues TMB, Barra CB, Santos JLS, Goulart EMA, Ferreira AVM, Silva IN, et al. Cardiovascular risk factors and increased carotid intima-media thickness in young patients with congenital adrenal hyperplasia due to 21-hydroxylase deficiency. Arch Endocrinol Metab. 2015;59(6):541–7.
22. Abdullah MA, Saeed U, Abass A, Lubna K, Weam A, Ali AS, et al. Disorders of sex development among Sudanese children: 5-year experience of a pediatric endocrinology clinic. J Pediatr Endocrinol Metab. 2012;25:1065–72.
23. Garcia PA, Schueftan DLG, Farias MLF, Beserra ICR, Schueftan DLG, Carvalho LM. Bone mineral density in children and adolescents with congenital adrenal hyperplasia. Int J Endocrinol. 2014;2014:806–95.
24. Hindmarsh PC. Management of the child with congenital adrenal hyperplasia. Best Pract Res Clin Endocrinol Metab. 2009;23(2):193–208.

25. Kliegman R, Stanton BF, St. Geme III JW, Schor NF, Behrman RE. Congenital adrenal hyperplasia and related disorders. Nelson Textbook of Pediatrics. 19th ed. USA: Elsevier; 2011. p. 1930–1938.
26. Forest MG, Tardy V, Nicolino M, David M, Morel Y. 21-Hydroxylase deficiency: an exemplary model of the contribution of molecular biology in the understanding and management of the disease. Ann Endocrinol. 2005;66(3):225–32.
27. Al Jarallah AS. Reversible cardiomyopathy caused by an uncommon form of congenital adrenal hyperplasia. Pediatr Cardiol. 2004;25(6):675–6.
28. Subbarayan A, Dattani MT, Peters CJ, Hindmarsh PC. Cardiovascular risk factors in children and adolescents with congenital adrenal hyperplasia due to 21-hydroxylase deficiency. Clin Endocrinol. 2014;80(4):471–7.
29. Reckelhoff JF, Roman RJ. Androgens and hypertension: role in both males and females? Hypertension. 2011;57(4):681–2.
30. Recklhoff JF. Gender differences in the regulation of blood pressure. Hypertens J Am Heart Assoc. 2001;37:1199–208.
31. Jones RD, Hugh Jones T, Channer KS. The influence of testosterone upon vascular reactivity. Eur J Endocrinol. 2004;151(1):29–37.
32. Cerame BI, New MI. Hormonal hypertension in children: 11beta-hydroxylase deficiency and apparent mineralocorticoid excess. J Pediatr Endocrinol Metab. 2000;13(9):1537–47.
33. Amr NH, Ahmed AY, Ibrahim YA. Carotid intima media thickness and other cardiovascular risk factors in children with congenital adrenal hyperplasia. J Endocrinol Investig. 2014;37(10):1001–8.
34. Robotham JL, Takata M, Berman M, Harasawa Y. Ejection fraction revisited. Anesthesiology. 1991;74(1):172–83.
35. Wilson C, Maas R, Estrada M. Cardiovascular Effects of Androgens. Basic and Clinical Endocrinology Up-to-Date,. Chile: Intech; 2011. p. 63–78.
36. Ho S, Nihoyannopoulos P. Anatomy, echocardiography, and normal right ventricular dimensions. Heart. 2006;92(1):2–13.
37. Thum T, Borlak J. Testosterone, cytochrome P450, and cardiac hypertrophy. Fed Am Soc Exp Biol. 2002;16(12):1537–49.

9

Chromosome microarray analysis in the investigation of children with congenital heart disease

Xiao-li Wu[†], Ru Li[†], Fang Fu, Min Pan, Jin Han, Xin Yang, Yong-ling Zhang, Fa-tao Li and Can Liao[*]

Abstract

Background: Our study was aimed to explore the clinical implication of chromosome microarray analysis (CMA) in genetically etiological diagnosis of children with congenital heart disease (CHD).

Methods: A total of 104 children with CHD with or without multiple congenital anomalies (MCA) or intellectual disabilities/developmental delay (ID/DD) but normal karyotype were investigated using Affymetrix CytoScan HD array.

Result: Pathogenic copy number variations (PCNVs) were identified in 29 children (27.9%). The detection rates in children with simple CHD and complex CHD were 31.1% (19/61) and 23.2% (10/43), respectively. The detection rates of PCNVs were 17.9% (7/39), 20% (5/25), 63.2% (12/19) and 23.8% (5/21) in isolated CHD, CHD plus MCA, CHD plus ID/DD, CHD plus MCA and ID/DD, respectively. The PCNVs rate of CHD plus ID/DD was significantly higher than that of isolated CHD. Two genomic loci including 15q11.2 deletion and 1q43-q44 deletion were considered as CHD locus. The *DVL1, SKI, STIM1, CTNNA3* and *PLN* were identified as candidate genes associated with CHD phenotypes.

Conclusion: CMA can increase the diagnostic rate and improve the etiological diagnosis in children with CHD. We suggest CMA as a first-tier test in children with CHD, especially in children with CHD plus ID/DD.

Keywords: 15q11.2 deletion, 1q43-q44 deletion, Chromosome microarray analysis, Congenital heart disease, Copy number variation, Microdeletion/microduplication

Background

Congenital heart disease (CHD) is one of the most common birth defects. The incidence of CHD in the neonate is 8-9/1000, and nearly 1.35 million CHD neonates were born every year in the whole world [1]. Despite improvement of various treatment measures, CHD is still one of the major causes of children mortality.

The causes of CHD include non-genetic factors and genetic factors. Non-genetic factors include: environmental factors, maternal exposure and infection. Chromosomal causes of CHD include chromosome aneuploidies, like trisomy 21, and copy number variations (CNVs). Chromosomal aneuploidies represent 12.5% of CHD causes [2]. The spectrum of CHD-related CNVs ranges from recurrent microdeletion and microduplication syndromes, like DiGeorge syndrome (22q11 deletion syndrome) and Williams-Beuren syndrome (7q11.23 deletion syndrome), which are associated with a distinct clinical recognizable phenotype, to rare CNVs, flanked by unique breakpoints [3–5].

The resolution of conventional karyotype analysis is limited to 5 Mb or larger genomic imbalances [6]. The drawback of fluorescence in situ hybridization (FISH) lies in its a targeted approach to detect chromosomal defects, rather than a genome-wide screening method like microarrays or MLPA [7]. Chromosome Microarray Analysis (CMA) is a routine technique in clinical molecular testing nowadays, which contains two types of arrays: oligonucleotide arrays and Single Nucleotide Polymorphism arrays (SNP arrays). Both the arrays

* Correspondence: canliao@hotmail.com
[†]Equal contributors
Prenatal Diagnostic Center, Guangzhou Women and Children's Medical Center, Guangzhou Medical University, No. 9 Jinsui Road, Guangdong, China

could detect genome-wide CNVs. Moreover, SNP arrays can detect the mosaicism, triploid, loss of heterozygosity (LOH) and uniparental disomy. In 2010, the American College of Medical Genetics issued practice guidelines for CMA, and pointed out that CMA was recommended as a first-tier test for postnatal patients with multiple congenital anomalies (MCA), intellectual disabilities/developmental delay (ID/DD) and autism spectrum disorders [8]. Recently, CMA has been successfully applied to detect CNVs in patients with CHD, which confirmed the relationship between chromosome microdeletion/microduplication and CHD [9–19].

In this study, we present the results of genome-wide high resolution SNP array analysis in 106 children with CHD in the Chinese cohort, to explore the clinical implication of CMA in genetically etiological diagnosis of CHD.

Methods

Subjects and sample

In this study, we collected children diagnosed with CHD with or without MCA or ID/DD and normal karyotype at Guangzhou Women and Children's Medical Center from January 2012 to December 2014. All the children were investigated by the complete cardiac evaluation, echocardiogram, medical history, physical examination, and/or operative reports. Considering patent ductus arteriosus (PDA) was common in children with CHD, the child with PDA was selected only if he/she was born at >37 weeks' gestational age and the PDA was unclosed after 6 weeks of life [2]. MCA included cerebral malformation, neural tube and spine defects, craniofacial and neck abnormalities, thorax abnormalities, ventral wall defect, abdomen and gastrointestinal tract defects, genitourinary malformation and skeletal dysplasia. ID/DD was diagnosed by the pediatric specialist. The peripheral blood from these children and their parents were collected. Informed consent was obtained from all the participants. The study was approved by the ethics committees of Guangzhou Women and Children's Medical Center.

According to the National Birth Defects Prevention Study [20, 21], CHD was classified into the following types: septal defect, atrioventricular septal defect (AVSD), conotruncal defects, left ventricular outflow tract obstruction (LVOTO), right ventricular outflow tract obstruction (RVOTO), LVOTO + RVOTO, single ventricle (SV), and PDA (Table 1).

Table 1 Data of pathogenic copy number variants (PCNVs) in children with congenital heart disease (CHD) and CHD classification

CHD Classification	Simple CHD			Associate CHD			Total		
	No. PCNVs	No. tested	PR (%)	No. PCNVs	No. tested	PR (%)	No. PCNVs	No. tested	PR (%)
Septal defect	9	37	24.3	1	6	16.8	10	43	23.3
ASD	5	18	27.8	0	0	0	5	18	27.8
VSD	4	19	21.1	0	0	0	4	19	21.1
VSD + ASD	0	0	0	1	6	16.8	1	6	16.8
AVSD	0	1	0	0	2	0	0	3	0
Conotruncal defects	1	3	33.3	1	13	7.8	2	16	12.5
TOF	1	3	33.3	1	2	50	2	5	40
D-TGA	0	0	0	0	11	0	0	11	0
LVOTO	2	5	40	3	9	33.3	5	14	35.7
COA	0	2	0	1	4	25	1	6	16.7
AS	2	3	66.7	0	1	0	2	4	50
IAA, A	0	0	0	2	2	100	2	2	100
COA + AS	0	0	0	0	2	0	0	2	0
RVOTO	3	3	100	2	8	25	5	11	45.5
PS/PA	3	3	100	2	8	25	5	11	45.5
LVOTO + RVOTO	0	0	0	3	4	75	3	4	75
AS + PS	0	0	0	3	4	75	3	4	75
Single Ventricle	0	0	0	0	1	0	0	1	0
PDA	4	12	33.3	0	0	0	4	12	33.3
Total	19	62	30.6	10	43	23.2	29	104	27.9

PR positive rate, *ASD* atrial septal defect, *VSD* ventricular septal defect, *AVSD* atrioventricular septal defect, *TOF* tetralogy of Fallot, *D-TGA* d-transposition of the great arteries, *COA* coarctation of the aorta, *AS* aortic stenosis, *IAA* interruption arterial arch, *PS* pulmonary stenosis, *PA* pulmonary atresia, *PDA* patent ductus arteriosus, *LVOTO* Left ventricular outflow tract obstruction, *RVOTO* Right ventricular outflow tract obstruction

According to the complexity of CHD, CHD was divided into two groups: simple CHD and complex CHD [22]. Simple CHD are defined as anatomically discrete (e.g., ventricular septal defect, VSD) or a well-recognized single entity (e.g., tetralogy of Fallot, TOF). Complex CHD are defined as combinations of different heart defects (single ventricle was included in this group).

According to whether the children with CHD have ID/DD and/or MCA, CHD was divided into two types: isolated CHD and syndromic CHD. The syndromic CHD contained CHD plus MCA, CHD plus ID/DD, and CHD plus MCA and ID/DD.

Chromosome microarray analysis

CMA was performed using Affymetrix CytoScan HD arrays according to manufacturer's instructions. The procedure included genomic DNA extraction, digestion and ligation, PCR amplification, PCR product purification, quantification and fragmentation, labeling, array hybridization, washing and scanning. Data was analyzed with Chromosome Analysis Suite software version 1.2 (Affymetrix). The reporting threshold was set at 100 kb with marker count ≥50. CNVs were interpreted as benign listed in Database of Genomic Variants (DGV) database (n > 3 studies or documented in >1% of the normal population) or no gene included (not close to known CHD genes within 1 Mb) [23]. CNVs was classified as pathogenic copy number variations (PCNVs) if these CNVs overlapped completely with the minimal critical region of a well-known microdeletion or microduplication syndrome, or if the CNV comprised a dosage-sensitive gene known to cause a similar phenotype, referring to ClinGen Dosage Sensitivity Map (http://www.ncbi.nlm.nih.gov/projects/dbvar/clingen/). Rare CNVs (<1% in normal population and without OMIM genes) that do not meet the criteria above, should be considered as variant of uncertain clinical significance (VOUS), until proven otherwise (e.g. by functional studies) [8, 23]. For interpretation of these results, our in-house database and the following public database were used: DGV (http://projects.tcag.ca/variation/), Cytogenomics Array Group CNV Database (https://www.cagdb.org), Database of Chromosomal Imbalance and Phenotype in Humans using Ensembl Resources database (DECIPHER, http://decipher.sanger.ac.uk/), Online Mendelian Inheritance in Man (OMIM, http://www.omim.org), University of California Santa Cruz (UCSC, http://genome.ucsc.edu/, hg19), ClinVar (http://www.clinvar.com/) and CHD wiki (http://homes.esat.kuleuven.be/~bioiuser/chdwiki/index.php/Main_Page). All CNVs were further confirmed by Real-Time Polymerase Chain Reaction. Parental analysis were performed to interpret VOUS.

Statistical analysis

Statistical analyses were performed using the Statistic Package for Social Science (SPSS) 13.0 statistical software package (SPSS Inc.). The PCNVs detection rates in children with simple CHD and complex CHD were compared using chi square test. Frequencies of recurrent CNVs in this study and the control cohorts were compared using fisher's exact test. P value <0.05 was statistically significant. The PCNVs detection rates in isolated CHD, CHD plus MCA, CHD plus ID/DD, and CHD plus MCA and ID/DD were pairwise compared using chi square test or fisher's exact test, p value <0.008 was statistically significant.

Results

CMA was performed in 104 children (67 males and 37 females) with CHD aged from 5 days to 8 years old. CNVs were identified in 96.2% (100/104) of the children. The size of CNVs ranged from 102 kb to 13.8 Mb. CNVs were interpreted as benign or likely benign in 69.2% (72/104) children. The detection rate for PCNVs was 27.9% (29/104), and the VOUS rate was 2.9% (3/104) after parental analysis.

Detailed CHD classification and demographic data of the children were listed in Table 1. The percentages of children with simple CHD and complex CHD were 58.7% (61/104) and 41.3% (43/104), respectively. PCNVs were identified in 31.1% (19/61) children with simple CHD and in 23.2% (10/43) children with complex CHD. Pearson Chi-square test showed that there was no significant difference between these two groups (P > 0.05). PCNVs were detected in 23.3% (10/43) of septal defect, 0 (0/3) of AVSD, 12.5% (2/16) of conotruncal defects, 35.7% (5/14) of LVOTO, 45.5% (5/11) of RVOTO, 75% (3/4) of LVOTO + RVOTO, 0 (0/1) of SV, and 33.3% (4/12) of PDA.

The detection rates of PCNVs in isolated CHD and syndromic CHD were 17.9% (7/39) and 33.8% (22/65), respectively. There was no significant difference between these two groups (P > 0.05). The detection rates for PCNVs were 20% (5/25) in CHD plus MCA, 63.2% (12/19) in CHD plus ID/DD, and 23.8% (5/21) in CHD plus MCA and ID/DD, respectively (Table 2). The PCNVs rate of CHD plus ID/DD was significantly higher than that of isolated CHD (63.2 vs 17.9%, P = 0.001) and CHD plus MCA (63.2 vs 20%, P = 0.004).

PCNVs were identified in 29 children (Table 3, including 22q11 deletion syndrome (n = 6), 22q11 duplication syndrome (n = 1), Williams-Beuren syndrome (n = 6), Angleman/Prader-Willi syndrome (n = 1), Wolf-Hirschhorn syndrome (n = 2), Schinzel-Giedion midface retraction syndrome (n = 1), 15q24 recurrent microdeletion syndrome (n = 1), 1p36 microdeletion syndrome (n = 1), Cornelia de Lange syndrome 4(n = 1), Marfan syndrome (n = 1), Opitz G/BBB syndrome (n = 1), 6q24

Table 2 Classification of children with CHD and/or other diagnoses (MCA, ID/DD)

Classification of symptoms	Simple CHD			Complex CHD			Total		
	No. pCNVs	No. tested	PR (%)	No. pCNVs	No. tested	PR (%)	No. pCNVs	No. tested	PR (%)
Isolated CHD	3	15	20.0	4	24	16.7	7	39	17.9
Syndromic CHD	16	46	34.8	6	19	31.6	22	65	33.8
CHD + MCA	4	18	22.2	1	7	14.3	5	25	20
CHD+ ID/DD	8	13	61.5	4	6	66.7	12	19	63.2
CHD + MCA+ ID/DD	4	15	26.7	1	6	16.7	5	21	23.8
Total	19	61	31.1	10	43	23.2	29	104	27.9

PR positive rate, *MCA* multiple congenital anomalies, *ID/DD* intellectual disabilities/development delay

LOH (n = 1), and CNVs overlapped with DECIPHER patient entries (n = 6).

In this study, PCNVs in 79.3% (23/29) of the children contained genes contributing to CHD (Table 3). The genes responsible for syndromic CHD included *TBX1* (22q11 deletion syndrome), *ELN* (Williams-Beuren syndrome), *EVC2* and *EVC* (Wolf-Hirschhorn syndrome), *STRA6* (15q24 recurrent microdeletion syndrome), *FBN1* (Marfan syndrome), *MID1* (Opitz G/BBB syndrome), *RAD21* (Cornelia de Lange syndrome 4) and *SETBP1* (Schinzel-Giedion midface retraction). In addition, the genes contributing to non-syndromic CHD included *CRELD1, RAF1* and *CITED2*. *DVL1* and *SKI* were identified as candidate genes for CHD in the current study.

CNVs detected in 9 children were classified as VOUS initially, further parental microarray analysis showed that CNVs in 6 children were inherited. The remaining CNVs in the other 3 children (Table 3, child 30-32) were de novo and the clinical significance was still unknown. Therefore, the VOUS rate was 2.8% in this study. The three VOUS were 11p15.4 duplication (chr11:3,923,985-4,242,111, 180 kb), 10q21.3 duplication (chr10:69,026,332-69,430,434, 400 kb) and 6q22.31 duplication (chr6:118,693,553-119,050,523, 360 kb). Three genes, *STIM1*, *CTNNA3* and *PLN* relevant with CHD, located in these fragments respectively. For the other children with benign or pathogenic CNVs, their parents rejected further parental analysis by CMA.

Discussion

In the past few years, several studies have investigated postnatal cases with syndromic CHD by array CGH (aCGH) (Table 4) [9, 11, 13, 14, 16–19]. Different arrays were used in these studies, and the PCNVs detection rate ranged from 10.9 to 25.5%. Bachman's study showed that the lowest PCNVs detection rate was 10.9% (5/46) using Roche NimbleGen 135 K arrays [18]. The highest detection rate was 25.5% (5/20) by Agilent 244 K array from Syrmou's study [19]. In our study, the total detection rate for PCNVs reached 27.9% (29/104) by CytoScan HD array, including 1,950,000 oligonucleotide probes and 750,000 SNP probes. Our results demonstrated further that denser arrays with high resolution will lead to a proportional increase in number of PCNVs [13, 24].

CMA has also been applied in children with isolated CHD previously [10–12, 15]. The PCNVs detection rates ranged from 0 to 5.3% (Table 4). Richards et al. studied 20 children with isolated CHD and 20 children with CHD plus MCA, the results showed that PCNVs detection rate in isolated CHD was 0 and that in CHD plus MCA was 25%, and the highest PCNVs detection rate was 45% in children with CHD plus neurologic defects [11]. Therefore, CMA was not recommended by Richards for children with isolated CHD. In our study, PCNVs detection rate was 17.9% (7/39) in isolated CHD. The PCNVs detection rates for CHD plus MCA, CHD plus ID/DD and CHD plus MCA and ID/DD were 20, 63.2 and 23.8%, respectively. PCNVs detection rate in CHD plus ID/DD was significantly higher than that of isolated CHD (P = 0.001) and CHD plus MCA (P = 0.004). Our data demonstrated that CMA is the most useful for genetic diagnosis in children with CHD plus ID/DD. In addition, we also recommended CMA investigation for children with isolated CHD.

In this study, PCNVs were detected in 31.1% (19/61) children with simple CHD and 23.2% (10/43) children with complex CHD by CMA. There was no significant difference between the two groups ($P > 0.05$). Detection rates in various types of CHD were different. Shaffer et al. reviewed 580 fetuses with CHD and normal karyotype by aCGH [25], and revealed the detection rates of PCNVs as follows: 16.2% (11/68) in LVOTO, 11.6% (5/43) in conotruncal defect and 10.6% (14/132) in septal defect. The above three types of CHD in fetuses were the most frequent. In our study, the PCNVs detection rates in different types of CHD in isolated or with additional anomalies were as follows in turn: 75% (3/4) in LVOTO + RVOTO, 45.5% (5/11) in RVOTO, 35.7% (5/14) in LVOTO, 33.3% (4/12) in PDA, 23.3% (10/43) in septal defect, 12.5% (2/16) in conotruncal defects. Our data demonstrate that LVOTO and/or RVOTO were most probably related to microdeletion/microduplication. Of the 29 children with PCNVs, 22 (75.9%) were complicated with MCA and/or DD/ID. High detection

Table 3 Pathogenic copy number variants and variants of unknown significance detected by Chromosome Microarray Analysis in children with CHD

Child	Age[a]	Phenotype		CNVs: Region and size	Known syndrome/Decipher number/OMIM number	Significant genes (bold fonts) /candidate genes relating to CHD[b]
		Cardiac diagnosis	MCA or ID/DD			
Pathogenic CNVs						
1	8 y	ASD	ID	Dup 11q24.2-q25 (8.5 Mb)	Decipher number 255590	None
				Del 1q43-q44 (6.2 Mb)	Decipher number 284767	None
2	7 m	PS + ASD	None	Del 22q11.21 (3.2 Mb)	22q11 deletion syndrome	***TBX1***
3	10 m	PDA	Congenital anal atresia + DD	Dup 3p26.1-p24.3 (13.8 Mb)	Decipher number 260758	***CRELD1; RAF1***
				Del 6q13-q14.1 (5.2 Mb)	Decipher number 249539	None
				Dup 17q12 (1.4 Mb)	Decipher number 278456	None
4	4 y	PDA	Leukodystrophy	Del 1p36.33-p36.31(4.8 Mb)	1p36 microdeletion syndrome	*DVL1;SKI*
5	13 m	ASD	DD	Del 15q24.1-q24.2 (3.1 Mb)	15q24 recurrent microdeletion syndrome	***STRA6***
6	5 y	PS	ID	Del 15q11.2-q13.1 (4.9 Mb)	Angelman/Prader-Willi syndrome	None
7	5 m	VSD	DD	Del 4p16.3-p16.2 (5.7 Mb)	Wolf-Hirschhorn syndrome	***EVC2; EVC***
8	2 m	ASD	Laryngeal cartilage dysplasia	Del 22q11.21 (2.4 Mb)	22q11 deletion syndrome	***TBX1***
9	2 y	VSD	ID	Del 22q11.21 (3.2 Mb)	22q11 deletion syndrome	***TBX1***
10	14 m	ASD	None	Del 22q11.21 (1.4 Mb)	22q11 deletion syndrome	***TBX1***
11	2 y	ASD	Cleft palate + ID	Dup 18q12.3 (0.64 Mb)	Schinzel-Giedion midface retraction syndrome	*SETBP1*
12	2 y	AS + PS	DD	Del 7q11.23 (1.4 Mb)	Williams-Beuren syndrome	***ELN***
13	3 y	TOF + PLSVC + Pericardial defect	Diaphragmatic hernia + ID	Dup 2q12.3 (0.42 Mb)	Decipher number 287980	None
14	1 m	IAA,A + VSD	fingers of both hands and left toe deformity	Dup Xp22.2 (0.72 Mb)	Opitz G/BBB syndrome	***MID1***
15	1 y	PS + VSD	ID	Del 22q11.21 (3.2 Mb)	22q11 deletion syndrome	***TBX1***
16	15 m	PDA	DD	Del 1p36.33 (0.35 Mb)	Decipher number 106	None
				Dup 17q25.1-q25.3 (6.4 Mb)	Decipher number 249584	None
17	18 m	ASD	Cleft palate + DD	Del 4p16.3-p16.1 (7.6 Mb)	Wolf-Hirschhorn Syndrome	***EVC2; EVC***
18	11 d	IAA, A + VSD	None	Del 7q11.23 (1.4 Mb)	Williams-Beuren syndrome	***ELN***
19	8 m	AS + PS	DD	Del 7q11.23 (1.4 Mb)	Williams-Beuren syndrome	***ELN***
20	2 y	PS	None	Dup 15q21.1 (1.58 Mb)	Marfan syndrome	***FBN1***
21	3 y	TOF	Absence of corpus callosum + cerebellar vermis hypoplasia + ID	Del 1q43-q44 (7.6 Mb)	Decipher number 249647	None
				Dup 10p15.3-p14 (6.7 Mb)	Decipher number 278831	None
22	3 y	COA + VSD + ASD	ID	LOH 6q24.1-q24.2 (5.2 Mb)	Decipher number 290225	***CITED2***
23	1 m	AS	Hemivertebra + Adduction deformity of thumb + Polydactyly + Funnel chest	Del 8q23.3-q24.11(1.24 Mb)	Cornelia de Lange syndrome 4	*RAD21*
				Dup 11p15.3-15.2 (0.75 Mb)	None	None
24	2 y	VSD	ID	Del 22q11.21 (3.2 Mb)	22q11 deletion syndrome	***TBX1***
25	2 y	PS	ID	Del 7q11.23 (1.5 Mb)	Williams-Beuren syndrome	***ELN***
26	2 m	AS	None	Del 7q11.23 (1.5 Mb)	Williams-Beuren syndrome	***ELN***
27	2 m	AS + PS	None	Del 7q11.23 (1.4 Mb)	Williams-Beuren syndrome	***ELN***
28	7 m	PDA	Cleft palate	Dup 22q11.21 (2.5 Mb)	22q11 duplication syndrome	***TBX1***
29	6 m	ASD + VSD	None	Dup 17q25.1-q25.3 (8.5 Mb)	Decipher number 254723	None
				Del 20q13.33 (1.3 Mb)	Decipher number 2615	None

Table 3 Pathogenic copy number variants and variants of unknown significance detected by Chromosome Microarray Analysis in children with CHD *(Continued)*

Variants of unknown significance						
30	1 m	CoA + Heart Enlargement	None	Dup 11p15.4 (0.18 Mb)	None	*STIM1*
31	1 m	AS + VSD	None	Dup 10q21.3 (0.4 Mb)	None	*CTNNA3*
32	1 m	D-TGA + VSD + ASD	None	Dup 6q22.31 (0.36 Mb)	None	*PLN*

ASD atrial septal defect, *PDA* patent ductus arterious, *PS* pulmonary stenosis, *VSD* ventricular septal defect, *TOF* tetralogy of Fallot, *PLSVC* persistent left superior vena cava, *AS* aortic stenosis, *IAA,A* interruption arterial arch, A type, *COA* coarctation of the aorta, *D-TGA* d-transposition of the great arteries, *DD* development delay, *ID* intellectual disabilities

[a]Age column: y, years; m, months; d, days

[b]Accordion to CHD wiki (http://homes.esat.kuleuven.be/~bioiuser/chdwiki/index.php/Main_Page)and OMIM database (http://www.omim.org)

rate in children with PDA (33.3%) was obtained in this study, and we noticed that all the 12 children with PDA were complicated with MCA and/or ID/DD. There was no PCNVs detected in children with AVSD (n = 2) and SV (n = 1), this may be due to the small sample size in our study.

Gijsbers et al. suggested that as the rising of aCGH resolution, there will be more VOUS identified [26]. In the previous studies in children with CHD by microarray, the VOUS detection rates ranged from 3.4 to 11.7% [9, 11, 16]. In this study, CNVs detected in 9 children were unknown of clinical significance. After parental microarray analysis, CNVs in 6 children were inherited, the remaining CNVs in the other 3 children (Table 3, child 30-32) were de novo and the clinical significance was still unknown. Finally, the VOUS rate was 2.9% in our study, which did not increase obviously as the resolution rise compared with previous studies. Therefore, parental analysis could assist in interpreting CNVs and reducing VOUS rate.

The clinical features of 1p36 microdeletion syndrome include microcephaly, brachycephaly, developmental delay with hypotonia, seizures and cardiac defects [27]. In our study, CMA revealed a 4.8 Mb deletion at 1p36.33-p36.31 (chr1:849,466-5,685,789) in child 4 with PDA and leukodystrophy, which contained the *SKI* and *DVL1* genes. *SKI* morphant embryos showed severe cardiac anomalies, especial complete failure in cardiac looping and malformations of the outflow tract [28]. Researchers have studied *DVL1* null mice and reported that *DVL1*-mediated planar cell polarity signal was crucially for cardiac outflow tract development [29]. Based on the above data, *SKI* and *DVL1* could be the main genes responsible for CHD phenotypes in 1p36 deletion syndrome.

A 4.9 Mb deletion at 15q11.2-q13.1 (chr15: 23,620,191- 28,540,345) was detected in child 6 (Table 3) with pulmonary stenosis plus ID. He was diagnosed as Angelman/Prader-Willi syndrome, the clinical features include ID, microcephaly, seizures, truncal ataxia, feeding difficulties in infancy and muscular hypotonia. Soemedi et al. first reported the association of 15q11.2 deletion with CHD, in their study the phenotypes contained left-side malformations, coarctation of the aorta, septal defect and TOF [30]. Geng et al. have detected

Table 4 The comparison of studies in postnatal patients with isolate/syndromic CHD

Study	Array type	No. tested	Other diagnosis	PCNVs rates	VOUS rates
Thienpont et al. 2007 [9]	1 Mb BAC	60	MCA, ID	16.7%	11.7%
Richards et al. 2008 [11]	385 K oligo arrays	20	MCA, DD/ID	25%	9.8%
		20	None	0	
Erdogan et al. 2008 [10]	1 Mb BAC or 1 × 244 K Agilent arrays	105	None	4.7%	Unknow
Greenway et al. 2009 [12]	Affymetrix SNP 6.0	114	None	5.3%	Unknow
Breckpot J et al. 2010 [13]	1 Mb array	150	MCA	17.3%	Unknow
Rauch et al. 2010 [14]	100 K Affymetrix	19	MCA	21%	Unknow
Goldmuntz et al. 2011 [16]	100 K Oligo array	58	MCA	20.7%	3.4%
Breckpot et al. 2011 [15]	Affymetrix SNP 6.0	46	None	4.3%	Unknow
Derwinska et al. 2012 [17]	180 K Oligo	150	MCA	14%	Unknow
Syrmou et al. 2013 [19]	1 × 244 K or 4 × 180 K Agilent arrays	55	MCA	25.5%	Unknow
Bachman et al. 2013 [18]	Roche NimbleGen 135 K arrays	46	MCA	10.9%	Unknow
Our study	Affymetrix CytoScan HD arrays	104	MCA, ID/DD	27.9%	2.9%

BAC bacterial artificial chromosome, *MCA* multiple congenital anomalies, *DD/ID* development delay/intellectual disabilities, *SNP* single nucleotide polymorphism

four patients with 15q11.2 deletion (size range 245-2703 kb) in 502 CHD patients, their result also showed the 15q11.2 deletion has low penetrance in CHD patients [31]. These data indicated that 15q11.2 deletion, containing the Angelman/Prader-Willi syndrome region, represents a critical CHD locus. However, further studies are need to ascertain the genes responsible for CHD.

In the present study, we identified two children with 1q43-q44 deletion. Child 1 manifested atrial septal defect (ASD) and ID. Child 21 manifested TOF and absence of corpus callosum. Our study showed significantly higher frequency of 1q43-q44 deletion (2/104) than that of the 9170 control cases (4/9170) ($P = 0.002$) [30, 32]. Therefore, 1q43-q44 should be considered as a locus associated with cardiac development. The clinical features of 1q43-44 deletion syndrome include ID, language retardation, characteristic facial features, abnormalities of the corpus callosum and seizures [33]. Summarizing the literature, patients with 1q43-q44 deletion manifesting ID/DD or structural anomaly of central nervous system (69/83, 83.1%) more frequently than CHD (19/76, 25%) ($P < 0.001$, Table 5). These data suggested 1q43-q44 deletion may have low penetrance in CHD children.

The child 11, a girl with ASD and cleft palate which had been corrected surgically. She was diagnosed with mental retardation at 2 years old by pediatric doctor. CMA test revealed chromosome 18q12.3 duplication (chr18: 41,814,626- 42,453,303). *SETBP1* gene located in the fragment which was responsible for Schinzel-Giedion midface retraction syndrome, and point mutation is the most common type. The clinical features included severe mental retardation, distinctive facial features, and multiple congenital malformations such as skeletal abnormalities and cardiac defects. A dominant-negative or gain-of-function mechanism was proposed to underlie this syndrome [34]. We sequenced the 5 exons of *SETBP1* gene, and no mutation was detected. The *SETBP1* gene duplication was in accordance with gain-of-function mechanism, and the child's manifestations were similar with the phenotypes of Schinzel-Giedion midface retraction syndrome, Therefore, *SETBP1* should be the main responsible gene for this patient.

The child 22 had coarctation of aorta, VSD, ASD (cardiac surgery was performed when he was 1 month old) and ID. Brain MRI showed normal result. CMA test revealed a 5.2 Mb LOH on chromosome 6q24.1-q24.2 (chr6:139,184,381-144,411,648). This LOH fragment included *PLAG1* and *HYMAI* genes, which were associated with imprinting disorder intrauterine growth retardation and neonatal hyperglycemia [35]. Another gene *CITED2* also located in the LOH, which has been identified associated with cardiac malformations, including atrial and ventricular septal defects, overriding aorta, double-outlet right ventricle and right-side aortic arches [36]. Therefore, this fragment was classified as PCNVs.

Of the 29 children with PCNVs, 7 (24.1%) were with 22q11 deletion ($n = 6$) or duplication ($n = 1$) syndrome, which was the most common type. The incidence of 22q11 deletion/duplication was 6.7% (7/104) in the children with CHD in the present study. These data indicate that in addition to CMA it could be more cost-effective to exclude 22q11 deletion/duplication firstly by targeted technique such as MLPA in children with CHD.

In the 3 children with VOUS, we identified CHD candidate genes such as *STIM1, CTNNA3* and *PLN. STIM1* gene mutation could cause cardiomyocyte hypertrophy [37]. *PLN* gene mutation was associated with cardiomyopathy [38]. *CTNNA3* gene mutation could cause arrhythmogenic right ventricular dysplasia, compound heterozygous deletion was related to ASD [39, 40]. However, the children's symptoms in this study were inconsistency with genotypes in the database. Further study of these genes are still needed to evaluate the clinical implication.

Conclusion

CMA has been recommended as a first-tier clinical diagnosis test in patients with DD, ID and/or MCA [8, 41]. Study from Bachman also recommended aCGH as a first-tier test in evaluation of neonates with CHD [18]. In the present study, we obtained the highest detection rate in children with CHD plus ID/DD (63.2%), while in children with isolated CHD we still obtained relatively high detection rate (17.9%). Based on the above data, we suggest CMA as a first-tier test in children with CHD, especially in children with CHD plus ID/DD.

Table 5 1q43-q44 deletion in our study compared with other studies

Phenotype	Our case	1q43 deletion[a]	1q44 deletion[b]	1q43-q44 deletion[c]	1q42-q44 deletion[d]	Total
ID/DD or CNS abnormal	2/2	22/27	24/24	15/24	6/6	69/83
Congenital heart defects	2/2	8/24	5/22	2/24	2/4	19/76

ID/DD intellectual disabilities/development delay, *CNS* central nervous system
[a]Reference to [42–45]
[b]Reference to [42–44, 46–48]
[c]Reference to [33, 49]
[d]Reference to [44]

Abbreviations

aCGH: Array CGH; AOH: Absence of heterozygosity; ASD: Atrial septal defect; AVSD: Atrioventricular septal defect; CHD: Congenital heart disease; *CITED2*: Cbp/p300-interacting transactivator, with Glu/Asp-rich carboxy-terminal domain, 2; CMA: Chromosome microarray analysis; CNVs: Copy number variations; *CRELD1*: Cysteine-rich with EGF-like domains 1; *CTNNA3*: Catenin (cadherin-associated protein), alpha 3; *CYFIP1*: Cytoplasmic FMR1 interacting protein 1; DD: Developmental delay; DECIPHER: Database of chromosomal imbalance and phenotype in humans using ensembl resources; DGV: Database of genomic variants; *DVL1*: Dishevelled segment polarity protein 1; *ELN*: Elastin; *EVC*: Ellis van Creveld syndrome; *EVC2*: Ellis van Creveld syndrome 2; *FBN1*: Fibrillin 1; *HYMAI*: Hydatidiform mole associated and imprinted (non-protein coding); ID: Intellectual disabilities; LVOTO: Left ventricular outflow tract obstruction; MCA: Multiple congenital anomalies; *MID1*: Midline 1; *NIPA1*: Non imprinted in Prader-Willi/Angelman syndrome 1; *NIPA2*: Mon imprinted in Prader-Willi/Angelman syndrome 2; OMIM: Online mendelian inheritance in man; PCNVs: Pathogenic copy number variations; PDA: Patent ductus arteriosus; *PLAG1*: Pleiomorphic adenoma gene 1; *PLN*: Phospholamban; *RAD21*: RAD21 homolog; *RAF1*: Raf-1 proto-oncogene, serine/threonine kinase; RVOTO: Right ventricular outflow tract obstruction; *SETBP1*: SET binding protein 1; *SKI*: SKI proto-oncogene; *STIM1*: Stromal interaction molecule 1; *STRA6*: Stimulated by retinoic acid 6; SV: Single ventricle; *TBX1*: T-box 1; *TTN*: Titin; *TUBGCP5*: Tubulin, gamma complex associated protein 5; UCSC: University of California Santa Cruz; VOUS: Variant of uncertain clinical significance; VSD: Ventricular septal defect

Acknowledgments

We thank all the children and their family members for their interest and cooperation.

Funding

This study was supported by Science and technology project of Guangdong Province (2014A020213015), the key project of Guangzhou Science and Information Technology Bureau (201300000086), the key project of Guangzhou Health Bureau (201102A212026) and Medical research foundation of Guangdong Province (A2013515).

Authors' contributions

XL Wu contributed to the implementation of the study, analysis and writing of this manuscript. R Li supervised the development of the manuscript and contributed to the analysis and writing. F Fu, M Pan, J H and X Yang interviewed the participants and collected and collated the data. YL Zhang and FT Li contributed to the experiment and data analysis. C Liao contributed to the study design, initiated the study, and provided comments on the manuscript. All authors read and approved the final manuscript.

Competing interests

The authors declare that they have no competing interests.

References

1. van der Linde D, Konings EE, Slager MA, Witsenburg M, Helbing WA, Takkenberg JJ, et al. Birth prevalence of congenital heart disease worldwide: a systematic review and meta-analysis. J Am Coll Cardiol. 2011;58(21):2241–7.
2. Hartman RJ, Rasmussen SA, Botto LD, Riehle-Colarusso T, Martin CL, Cragan JD, et al. The contribution of chromosomal abnormalities to congenital heart defects: a population based study. Pediatr Cardiol. 2011;32(8):1147–57.
3. Lindsay EA, Vitelli F, Su H, Morishima M, Huynh T, Pramparo T, et al. Tbx1 haploinsufficiency in the DiGeorge syndrome region causes aortic arch defects in mice. Nature. 2001;410(6824):97–101.
4. Yagi H, Furutani Y, Hamada H, Sasaki T, Asakawa S, Minoshima S, et al. Role of TBX1 in human del22q11.2 syndrome. Lancet. 2003;362(9393):1366–73.
5. Pober BR. Williams-Beuren syndrome. N Engl J Med. 2010;362(3):239–52.
6. ACOG Committee Opinion No. 446: array comparative genomic hybridization in prenatal diagnosis. Obstet Gynecol. 2009; 114(5): 1161-1163.
7. Pergament E. New molecular techniques for chromosome analysis. Baillieres Best Pract Res Clin Obstet Gynaecol. 2000;14(4):677–90.
8. Manning M, Hudgins L, Professional P, Guidelines C. Array-based technology and recommendations for utilization in medical genetics practice for detection of chromosomal abnormalities. Genet Med. 2010;12(11):742–5.
9. Thienpont B, Mertens L, de Ravel T, Eyskens B, Boshoff D, Maas N, et al. Submicroscopic chromosomal imbalances detected by array-CGH are a frequent cause of congenital heart defects in selected patients. Eur Heart J. 2007;28(22):2778–84.
10. Erdogan F, Larsen LA, Zhang L, Tumer Z, Tommerup N, Chen W, et al. High frequency of submicroscopic genomic aberrations detected by tiling path array comparative genome hybridisation in patients with isolated congenital heart disease. J Med Genet. 2008;45(11):704–9.
11. Richards AA, Santos LJ, Nichols HA, Crider BP, Elder FF, Hauser NS, et al. Cryptic chromosomal abnormalities identified in children with congenital heart disease. Pediatr Res. 2008;64(4):358–63.
12. Greenway SC, Pereira AC, Lin JC, DePalma SR, Israel SJ, Mesquita SM, et al. De novo copy number variants identify new genes and loci in isolated sporadic tetralogy of Fallot. Nat Genet. 2009;41(8):931–5.
13. Breckpot J, Thienpont B, Peeters H, de Ravel T, Singer A, Rayyan M, et al. Array comparative genomic hybridization as a diagnostic tool for syndromic heart defects. J Pediatr. 2010;156(5):810–7. 817.e811-817.e814
14. Rauch R, Hofbeck M, Zweier C, Koch A, Zink S, Trautmann U, et al. Comprehensive genotype-phenotype analysis in 230 patients with tetralogy of Fallot. J Med Genet. 2010;47(5):321–31.
15. Breckpot J, Thienpont B, Arens Y, Tranchevent LC, Vermeesch JR, Moreau Y, et al. Challenges of interpreting copy number variation in syndromic and non-syndromic congenital heart defects. Cytogenet Genome Res. 2011; 135(3-4):251–9.
16. Goldmuntz E, Paluru P, Glessner J, Hakonarson H, Biegel JA, White PS, et al. Microdeletions and microduplications in patients with congenital heart disease and multiple congenital anomalies. Congenit Heart Dis. 2011;6(6):592–602.
17. Derwinska K, Bartnik M, Wisniowiecka-Kowalnik B, Jagla M, Rudzinski A, Pietrzyk JJ, et al. Assessment of the role of copy-number variants in 150 patients with congenital heart defects. Med Wieku Rozwoj. 2012;16(3):175–82.
18. Bachman KK, Deward SJ, Chrysostomou C, Munoz R, Madan-Khetarpal S. Array CGH as a first-tier test for neonates with congenital heart disease. Cardiol Young. 2013:1–8.
19. Syrmou A, Tzetis M, Fryssira H, Kosma K, Oikonomakis V, Giannikou K, et al. Array comparative genomic hybridization as a clinical diagnostic tool in syndromic and nonsyndromic congenital heart disease. Pediatr Res. 2013; 73(6):772–6.
20. Yoon PW, Rasmussen SA, Lynberg MC, Moore CA, Anderka M, Carmichael SL, et al. The National Birth Defects Prevention Study. Public Health Rep. 2001;116(Suppl 1):32–40.
21. Rasmussen SA, Olney RS, Holmes LB, Lin AE, Keppler-Noreuil KM, Moore CA, et al. Guidelines for case classification for the National Birth Defects Prevention Study. Birth Defects Res A Clin Mol Teratol. 2003;67(3):193–201.
22. Botto LD, Lin AE, Riehle-Colarusso T, Malik S, Correa A. Seeking causes: classifying and evaluating congenital heart defects in etiologic studies. Birth Defects Res A Clin Mol Teratol. 2007;79(10):714–27.
23. Kearney HM, Thorland EC, Brown KK, Quintero-Rivera F, South ST. Working Group of the American College of medical genetics laboratory quality assurance C. American College of Medical Genetics standards and guidelines for interpretation and reporting of postnatal constitutional copy number variants. Genet Med. 2011;13(7):680–5.
24. Sagoo GS, Butterworth AS, Sanderson S, Shaw-Smith C, Higgins JP, Burton H. Array CGH in patients with learning disability (mental retardation) and congenital anomalies: updated systematic review and meta-analysis of 19 studies and 13,926 subjects. Genet Med. 2009;11(3):139–46.
25. Shaffer LG, Rosenfeld JA, Dabell MP, Coppinger J, Bandholz AM, Ellison JW, et al. Detection rates of clinically significant genomic alterations by microarray analysis for specific anomalies detected by ultrasound. Prenat Diagn. 2012;32(10):986–95.
26. Gijsbers AC, Schoumans J, Ruivenkamp CA. Interpretation of array comparative genome hybridization data: a major challenge. Cytogenet Genome Res. 2011;135(3-4):222–7.

27. Heilstedt HA, Ballif BC, Howard LA, Kashork CD, Shaffer LG. Population data suggest that deletions of 1p36 are a relatively common chromosome abnormality. Clin Genet. 2003;64(4):310–6.
28. Doyle AJ, Doyle JJ, Bessling SL, Maragh S, Lindsay ME, Schepers D, et al. Mutations in the TGF-beta repressor SKI cause Shprintzen-Goldberg syndrome with aortic aneurysm. Nat Genet. 2012;44(11):1249–54.
29. Sinha T, Wang B, Evans S, Wynshaw-Boris A, Wang J. Disheveled mediated planar cell polarity signaling is required in the second heart field lineage for outflow tract morphogenesis. Dev Biol. 2012;370(1):135–44.
30. Soemedi R, Wilson IJ, Bentham J, Darlay R, Topf A, Zelenika D, et al. Contribution of global rare copy-number variants to the risk of sporadic congenital heart disease. Am J Hum Genet. 2012;91(3):489–501.
31. Geng J, Picker J, Zheng Z, Zhang X, Wang J, Hisama F, et al. Chromosome microarray testing for patients with congenital heart defects reveals novel disease causing loci and high diagnostic yield. BMC Genomics. 2014;15(1):1127.
32. Cooper GM, Coe BP, Girirajan S, Rosenfeld JA, Vu TH, Baker C, et al. A copy number variation morbidity map of developmental delay. Nat Genet. 2011; 43(9):838–46.
33. Ballif BC, Rosenfeld JA, Traylor R, Theisen A, Bader PI, Ladda RL, et al. High-resolution array CGH defines critical regions and candidate genes for microcephaly, abnormalities of the corpus callosum, and seizure phenotypes in patients with microdeletions of 1q43q44. Hum Genet. 2012; 131(1):145–56.
34. Hoischen A, van Bon BW, Gilissen C, Arts P, van Lier B, Steehouwer M, et al. De novo mutations of SETBP1 cause Schinzel-Giedion syndrome. Nat Genet. 2010;42(6):483–5.
35. Kearney HM, Kearney JB, Conlin LK. Diagnostic implications of excessive homozygosity detected by SNP-based microarrays: consanguinity, uniparental disomy, and recessive single-gene mutations. Clin Lab Med. 2011;31(4):595–613. ix
36. Bamforth SD, Braganca J, Eloranta JJ, Murdoch JN, Marques FI, Kranc KR, et al. Cardiac malformations, adrenal agenesis, neural crest defects and exencephaly in mice lacking Cited2, a new Tfap2 co-activator. Nat Genet. 2001;29(4):469–74.
37. Henke N, Albrecht P, Pfeiffer A, Toutzaris D, Zanger K, Methner A. Stromal interaction molecule 1 (STIM1) is involved in the regulation of mitochondrial shape and bioenergetics and plays a role in oxidative stress. J Biol Chem. 2012;287(50):42042–52.
38. Schmitt JP, Kamisago M, Asahi M, Li GH, Ahmad F, Mende U, et al. Dilated cardiomyopathy and heart failure caused by a mutation in phospholamban. Science. 2003;299(5611):1410–3.
39. van Hengel J, Calore M, Bauce B, Dazzo E, Mazzotti E, De Bortoli M, et al. Mutations in the area composita protein alphaT-catenin are associated with arrhythmogenic right ventricular cardiomyopathy. Eur Heart J. 2013;34(3): 201–10.
40. Bacchelli E, Ceroni F, Pinto D, Lomartire S, Giannandrea M, D'Adamo P, et al. A CTNNA3 compound heterozygous deletion implicates a role for alphaT-catenin in susceptibility to autism spectrum disorder. J Neurodev Disord. 2014;6(1):17.
41. Miller DT, Adam MP, Aradhya S, Biesecker LG, Brothman AR, Carter NP, et al. Consensus statement: chromosomal microarray is a first-tier clinical diagnostic test for individuals with developmental disabilities or congenital anomalies. Am J Hum Genet. 2010;86(5):749–64.
42. Gentile M, Di Carlo A, Volpe P, Pansini A, Nanna P, Valenzano MC, et al. FISH and cytogenetic characterization of a terminal chromosome 1q deletion: clinical case report and phenotypic implications. Am J Med Genet A. 2003; 117A(3):251–4.
43. Hill AD, Chang BS, Hill RS, Garraway LA, Bodell A, Sellers WR, et al. A 2-Mb critical region implicated in the microcephaly associated with terminal 1q deletion syndrome. Am J Med Genet A. 2007;143A(15):1692–8.
44. Hiraki Y, Okamoto N, Ida T, Nakata Y, Kamada M, Kanemura Y, et al. Two new cases of pure 1q terminal deletion presenting with brain malformations. Am J Med Genet A. 2008;146A(10):1241–7.
45. Wagner N, Guengoer E, Mau-Holzmann UA, Maden Z, Hoopmann M, Abele H, et al. Prenatal diagnosis of a fetus with terminal deletion of chromosome 1 (q43) in first-trimester screening: is there a characteristic antenatal 1q deletion phenotype? A case report and review of the literature. Fetal Diagn Ther. 2011;29(3):253–6.
46. Roberts AE, Cox GF, Kimonis V, Lamb A, Irons M. Clinical presentation of 13 patients with subtelomeric rearrangements and a review of the literature. Am J Med Genet A. 2004;128A(4):352–63.
47. Thierry G, Beneteau C, Pichon O, Flori E, Isidor B, Popelard F, et al. Molecular characterization of 1q44 microdeletion in 11 patients reveals three candidate genes for intellectual disability and seizures. Am J Med Genet A. 2012;158A(7):1633–40.
48. Cho JH, Song ES, Kim HN, Oh BS, Choi YY. A chromosome 1q44 deletion in a 4-months-old girl; the first report in Korea. Korean J Pediatr. 2014;57(6): 292–6.
49. De Vries BB, Knight SJ, Homfray T, Smithson SF, Flint J, Winter RM. Submicroscopic subtelomeric 1qter deletions: a recognisable phenotype? J Med Genet. 2001;38(3):175–8.

Impact of preterm birth on infant mortality for newborns with congenital heart defects: The EPICARD population-based cohort study

Enora Laas[1], Nathalie Lelong[1], Pierre-Yves Ancel[1], Damien Bonnet[3], Lucile Houyel[2], Jean-François Magny[4], Thibaut Andrieu[1], François Goffinet[1,5], Babak Khoshnood[1*] and on behalf of the EPICARD study group

Abstract

Background: Congenital heart defects (CHD) and preterm birth (PTB) are major causes of infant mortality. However, limited data exist on risk of mortality associated with PTB for newborns with CHD. Our objective was to assess impact of PTB on risk of infant mortality for newborns with CHD, while taking into account the role of associated anomalies and other potentially confounding factors.

Methods: We used data on 2172 live births from a prospective population-based cohort study of CHD (the EPICARD Study) and compared neonatal, post-neonatal and overall infant mortality for infants born at <32, 32–34 and 35–36 weeks vs. those born at term (37–41 weeks).

Results: Preterm newborns had a 3.8-fold higher risk of infant death (17.9%) than term newborns (4.7%), RR 3.8, 95%CI 2.7–5.2; the risk associated with PTB was more than four-fold higher for neonatal (RR 4.3, 95% CI 2.9–6.6) and three-fold higher for post-neonatal deaths (RR 3.0, 95% CI 1.7–5.2). Survival analysis showed that newborns <35 weeks had a higher risk of mortality, which decreased but persisted after exclusion of associated anomalies and adjustment for potential confounders.

Conclusions: Preterm birth is associated with an approximately four-fold higher risk of infant mortality for newborns with CHD. This excess risk appears to be mostly limited to newborns <35 weeks of gestation and is disproportionately due to early deaths.

Keywords: Preterm birth, Congenital heart defects, Mortality

Background

Preterm birth (PTB) and congenital heart defects (CHD) are two major causes of mortality, morbidity and disability of perinatal origin [1–4]. Moreover, newborns with CHD are at a higher risk of PTB [5, 6] and both PTB and low birth weight have been shown to be risk factors for hospital mortality for newborns with CHD [7–10].

Reported infant mortality rates for newborns with CHD and preterm birth range from 20% [5] to 65% [11] with most of the deaths occurring during the first 28 days of life. There is some evidence suggesting that progress in medical and surgical management of newborns with CHD, and/or specifically those with PTB, has resulted in more favorable outcomes for infants undergoing cardiac surgery [12, 13]. However, by far most of the available literature looking at the impact of PTB on the outcomes of CHD are based on hospital series [7, 14–17] and concern essentially cases of cardiac surgery in specialized centers.

In the only previous population-based study reporting on the impact of PTB on the risk of infant mortality for newborns with CHD [5], the main focus was on the relation between risk of PTB and presence of CHD. The

* Correspondence: babak.khoshnood@inserm.fr
[1]Obstetrical, perinatal and pediatric epidemiology research team, Center for biostatistics and epidemiology, INSERM U1153, Maternité de Port-Royal, 6ème étage, 53 av. de l'Observatoire, 75014 Paris, France
Full list of author information is available at the end of the article

authors also reported descriptive data on the risk of infant mortality for CHD associated with PTB. They found that the overall infant mortality rate for newborns with CHD was 13%, whereas for the subgroup of preterm infants with CHD, risk of mortality was 20%. This study did not examine the role of associated anomalies, the degree of severity of CHD and the effects of potentially confounding factors, notably multiple pregnancies and intrauterine growth restriction (IUGR) on the risk of mortality associated with preterm birth for newborns with CHD.

Using data from a population-based cohort study of infants with CHD (the EPICARD study), we examined the association between PTB and the risk of infant mortality for newborns with CHD for: i) all CHD combined, ii) "isolated" CHD (excluding CHD associated with chromosomal or other anomalies) and iii) "isolated major CHD" (isolated CHD excluding ventricular septal defects).

Methods

Data source

EPICARD (Etude EPIdémiologique sur le devenir des enfants porteurs de CARDiopathies congénitales) is an ongoing prospective cohort follow-up study of all children with a CHD born to women in the Greater Paris area (Paris and its surrounding suburbs) between 2005 and 2008 [18].

All cases (live births, pregnancy terminations, fetal deaths) diagnosed in the prenatal period or up to one year of age in the birth cohorts between May 1st 2005 and April 31st 2008 were eligible for inclusion. Multiple sources of data including all maternity units, pediatric cardiology and cardiac surgery centers, fetal and neonatal pathology departments, neonatal and pediatric intensive units, infant units and outpatient clinics in the catchment area as well as a neighboring tertiary care center were regularly consulted to attain completeness of care registrations.

The total number of births (live births + stillbirths) in the study population base was 317,538, which included 314,022 live births. The total number of cases (live births, terminations of pregnancy for fetal anomaly and fetal deaths at >20 weeks of gestation) included in the EPICARD cohort was 2867 (Fig. 1). After excluding terminations of pregnancy for fetal anomaly (N = 466) and fetal deaths (N = 53), our initial study population comprised 2348 live births. Five (0.2%) cases had missing information on gestational age and were excluded from the analyses. We also excluded isolated atrial septal defects (N = 153, 6.5%) (ASD) in order to minimize any ascertainment bias. Preterm infant are more likely to undergo echocardiography resulting in detection of minor isolated ASD that may otherwise go undiagnosed. In addition, isolated minor ASD may be difficult to distinguish from patent foramen ovale. Finally, we excluded post term delivery (i.e. delivery after 42 weeks). After these exclusions, there were 2172 newborns in our final study population.

Cardiac anomalies associated with a known chromosomal anomaly accounted for 6.2% (N = 134), and those with anomalies of other systems, including genetic syndromes, 15.5% (N = 337) of newborns with CHD.

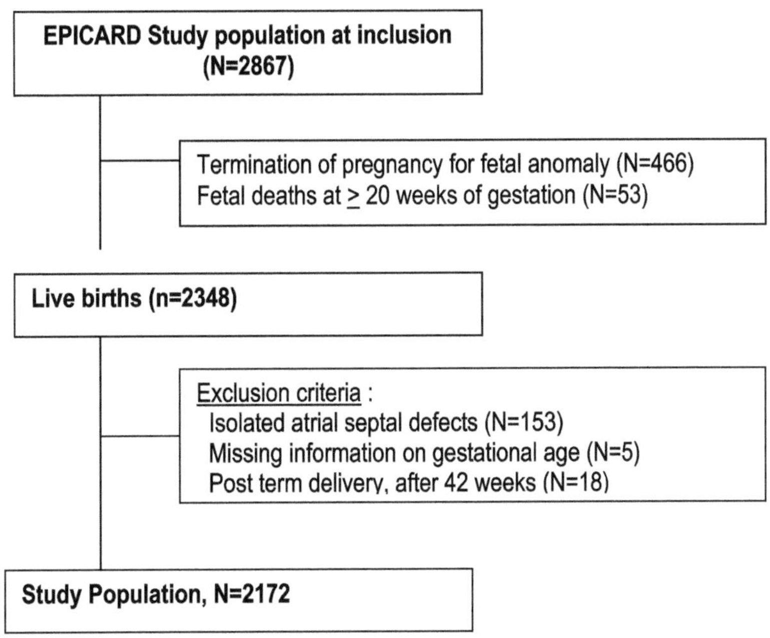

Fig. 1 Flow chart – Study Population

Statistical analysis

We compared the risk of infant mortality for newborns with preterm (gestational age < 37 weeks) vs. term (37–41 weeks) births for (i) all cases of CHD, (ii) "isolated" CHD (all cases excluding those associated with chromosomal anomalies or anomalies of other systems, including genetic syndromes; (iii) "isolated major" CHD ("isolated" CHD excluding VSD, as the latter are most frequently benign CHD that do not require any intervention).

We conducted separate analyses for timing of infant mortality for the following periods: early neonatal (< 1 week), late neonatal (7–27 days), early post-neonatal (28 days to three months) and late post-neonatal (three month to one year of age).

We calculated proportions with 95% binomial exact confidence intervals. We used poisson regression to compare the risk of death for preterm vs. term births.

In addition, for "isolated" and "isolated major" CHD, we used Kaplan-Meier survival curves to represent the risk the death over time for newborns in the following gestational age groups: 28–31 weeks, 32–34 weeks, 35–36 weeks and 37–41 weeks. Newborns with gestational age < 28 weeks were excluded as the sample size ($N = 10$) was not sufficient to examine this group separately. We used the log-rank test to determine the statistical significance of differences in the survival curves.

We used the Cox proportional hazard model to compare the risk (hazard) of death for the four gestational age groups noted above after taking into account the effects of the following potentially confounding variables: maternal age, occupation, geographic origin, diabetes mellitus, intra-uterine growth restriction (IUGR, <10th percentile) and multiple births. We tested the assumption of proportional hazards in the Cox model and found no statistically significant evidence of violation of this assumption in the Cox model. The R 2.13.2 software (R Development Core Team (2009), http://cran.r-project.org/) was used for data analysis.

Results

Study population

Table 1 shows the characteristics of the study population for preterm (< 37 weeks) and term (37–41 weeks) newborns with CHD. Overall, 13.6% (95% CI 12.2–15.1) of newborns were preterm. Median gestational age at birth was 39 weeks for term infants, and 35 weeks for preterm infants.

Mothers of preterm newborns were on average older (31.1 vs. 32.3 years $p < 0.001$), and more likely to be unemployed or from African origin. Preterm newborns were more likely to have associated chromosomal (13.2% vs. 5.1% for full term newborns) or other anomalies (24.3% vs. 14.1%) and IUGR (22.6% vs. 11.9%). Multiple pregnancies accounted for 17.9% of preterm vs. 2.4% of term newborns (all p-values <0.05). The proportion of maternal diabetes was higher (7.1% vs. 4.4%) and that of prenatal diagnosis lower (20.0% vs. 24.7%) for preterm vs. term newborns; however, these differences did not reach statistical significance (p-values 0.08 and 0.07, respectively).

The overall infant mortality rate was 6.5%. Preterm newborns had a 3.8-fold higher risk of infant death (17.9%) than term newborns (4.7%), RR 3.8, 95%CI 2.7–5.2 (Table 2). The higher risk of mortality for preterm newborns appeared to be greater in the neonatal (RR 4.3, 95% CI 2.9–6.6) than in the post-neonatal (RR 3.0, 95% CI 1.7–5.2) period. However, the confidence intervals were relatively wide and overlapping.

After excluding chromosomal and other anomalies, risk of infant mortality for preterm newborns with "isolated" CHD was 2.6-fold higher than term newborns (RR 2.6, 95% CI, 1.5–4.5). For "isolated major" CHD (i.e., CHD excluding cases associated with chromosomal or other anomalies and VSD), risk of infant mortality associated with PTB was 1.6-fold higher than for term newborns (RR 1.6; 95%CI 1.0–2.8) (Table 2).

Survival analysis

Figure 2 shows the survival curves for four gestational age groups: 28–31 weeks, 32–34 weeks, 35–36 weeks and 37–41 weeks for newborns with isolated CHD. Newborns with gestational age less than 35 weeks had significantly lower survival rates than those born at term whereas the survival curves for newborns 35–36 weeks were very similar to those born at term. Most of the differences across the survival curves were due to early deaths in the neonatal and early post-neonatal period. Differences in survival curves (Fig. 3) for isolated major CHD (isolated CHD, excluding VSD) paralleled those noted above; however the "baseline" risk of mortality was higher for all gestational age groups after exclusion of VSD.

Table 3 shows the results of the Cox proportional hazards models for estimating the hazard ratios of mortality across the four gestational age groups after taking into account the effects of potentially confounding factors including maternal age, occupation, geographic origin, diabetes mellitus, intra-uterine growth restriction (IUGR, <10th percentile) and multiple births. The adjusted hazard of mortality for children with isolated CHD was 4.0 (HR 4.0, 95%CI 1.5–10.5) and 5.4 (HR 5.4, 95%CI 2.1–13.9) higher for newborns at 28–31 weeks and 32–34 weeks of gestational age, respectively, as compared with term newborns. The hazard ratio for newborns at 35–36 weeks was not statistically significant (HR 0.9 95%CI 0.3–2.7). The adjusted hazard ratios associated with low gestational age groups for newborns with

Table 1 Maternal and fetal characteristics of the study populationn

		Term (*N* = 1876)		Preterm (*N* = 296)		p
		n	%	n	%	
Characteristics						
Fetal	Gestational age: median(range)	39 (37–41)		35 (24–36)		
	Birthweight: median(range)	3240 (1380–5550)		2080 (500–4770)		<0.001
	IUGR (< 10th percentile)	223	11.9	67	22.6	<0.001
	Multiple pregnancy	45	2.4	142	48.0	0.9
	Male	894	47.7			
	Associated anomalies					
	chromosomal	95	5.1	39	13.2	<0.001
	other systems	259	13.8	74	25	<0.001
Maternal	Age in years: mean	31.1		32.3		0.002
	< 30	710	38.1	89	30.3	<0.001
	30–34	652	35.0	103	35.0	
	35–39	376	20.2	63	21.4	
	≥ 40	124	6.7	39	13.3	
	Nulliparous	898	48.3	137	46.4	0.5
	Geographic origin					
	France	930	49.9	116	39.2	<0.001
	North african	362	19.4	65	22.0	
	African	228	12.2	57	19.2	
	Other	346	18.5	58	19.6	
	Maternal occupation					
	professional	444	25.2	49	17.6	0.01
	intermediate	354	20	46	16.6	
	administrative/public service	203	11.5	39	14.0	
	other	285	16.2	50	18.0	
	none	479	27	94	33.8	
	Diabete mellitus	82	4.4	21	7.1	0.04
	Prenatal diagnosis of CHD	375	20.0	73	24.7	0.06

isolated major CHD were 2.1 (95% CI 0.8–5.4) and 3.1 (95% CI 1.2–8.1) for newborns at 28–31 and 32–34 weeks, respectively. There was no evidence of a difference in the hazard of death between newborns at 35–36 weeks vs. term newborns (HR 0.6, 95% CI, 0.2–1.9) for newborns with "isolated major" CHD.

Discussion

Using population-based data on 2172 newborns with CHD, we found that the risk of infant mortality was about four-fold higher for preterm vs. term infants with CHD. The relative risk associated with PTB was lower (RR ~ 2.6) after cases with associated chromosomal or other anomalies were excluded and lowest in case of "isolated major" CHD ("isolated" CHD, VSD-excluded) (RR ~ 1.6). Survival analysis estimates suggested that the higher risk of mortality associated with PTB was limited to newborns with gestational age < 35 weeks and was disproportionately due to early deaths in the neonatal and early post-neonatal period. The higher risk of mortality associated with preterm births <35 weeks remained statistically significant and clinically important after exclusion of other anomalies and adjustment for potentially confounding factors.

Our estimate for the overall risk of infant mortality for preterm newborns with CHD (17.9%) are comparable to those reported by Tanner et al. in a population-based study in the British population [5]. However, in that study the authors did not examine the risk of mortality for preterm newborns in detail. In particular, the timing of mortality, the role of associated anomalies and the impact of potentially confounding factors were not analyzed.

Our estimate of the relative risk of infant mortality associated with preterm birth for newborns with CHD

Table 2 Risk on infant death in term ans preterm newborns: all cases, isolated CHD[a] and isolated majour CHD[b]

		Term		Preterm			
		%	95% CI	%	95% CI	RR	95% CI
All cases		*N* = 1876		*N* = 296			
Neonatal mortality	early <7 days	1.5	1.0–2.1	6.1	3.6–9.4	4.1	2.3–7.3
	7.3late 7-28d	1.2	0.8–1.8	5.7	3.4–9.0	4.7	2.5–8.7
	Total	2.7	2.0–3.6	11.8	8.4–16.1	4.3	2.9–6.6
Post neonatal mortality	28d-3 months	0.9	0.5–1.4	2.4	1.0–4.8	2.8	1.2–6.7
	3 m-1y	1.2	0.7–1.8	3.7	1.9–6.6	3.2	1.6–6.5
	Total	2.1	1.4–2.8	6.1	3.6–9.4	3.0	1.7–5.2
Infant mortality	<1 year	4.8	3.8–5.8	17.9	13.7–22.8	3.8	2.7–5.2
Isolated CHD[a]		*N* = 1551		*N* = 200			
Neonatal mortality	early <7 days	1.0	0.5–1.6	3.0	1.1–6.4	3.1	1.2–7.9
	7.9late 7-28d	0.8	0.5–1.4	2.5	0.8–5.7	3	1.1–8.3
	Total	1.8	1.2–2.6	5.5	2.8–9.6	3.0	1.5–6.0
Post neonatal mortality	28d-3 months	0.5	0.2–1.0	1.5	0.3–4.3	2.9	0.8–10.8
	3 m-1y	0.8	0.4–1.4	1.0	0.1–3.6	1.3	0.3–5.7
	Total	1.3	0.8–2.0	2.5	0.8–5.7	1.9	0.7–5.1
Infant mortality	<1 year	3.1	2.2–4.0	8	4.6–12.8	2.6	1.5–4.5
Isolated major CHD[b]		*N* = 542		*N* = 114			
Neonatal mortality	early <7 days	2.8	1.6–4.5	5.3	2.0–11.1	1.9	0.8–4.8
	late 7-28d	2.4	1.3–4.1	4.4	1.4–9.9	1.8	0.7–5.0
	Total	5.2	3.5–7.4	9.7	4.9–16.6	1.9	1.0–3.6
Post neonatal mortality	28d-3 months	1.5	0.6–2.9	2.6	0.6–7.5	1.8	0.5–6.6
	3 m-1y	2	1.0–3.6	1.8	0.2–6.2	0.9	0.2–3.8
	Total	3.5	2.1–5.4	4.4	1.4–9.9	1.3	0.5–3.3
Infant mortality	<1 year	8.7	6.4–11.4	14.1	8.2–21.8	1.6	1.0–2.8

[a]Isolated CHD: excluding cases with chromosomal or other anomalies
[b]Isolated major CHD: excluding cases with chromosomal or other anomalies and ventricular septal defects (VSD)

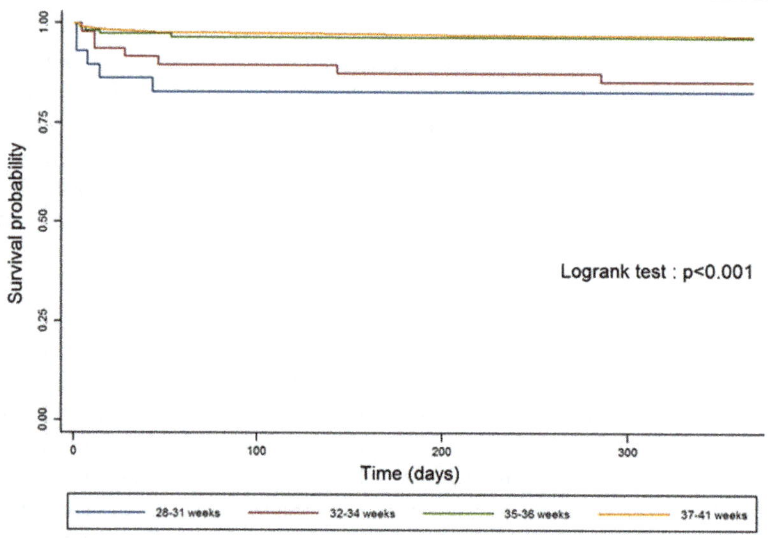

Fig. 2 Gestational-age specific Kaplan-Meier survival curves for infants with isolated CHD

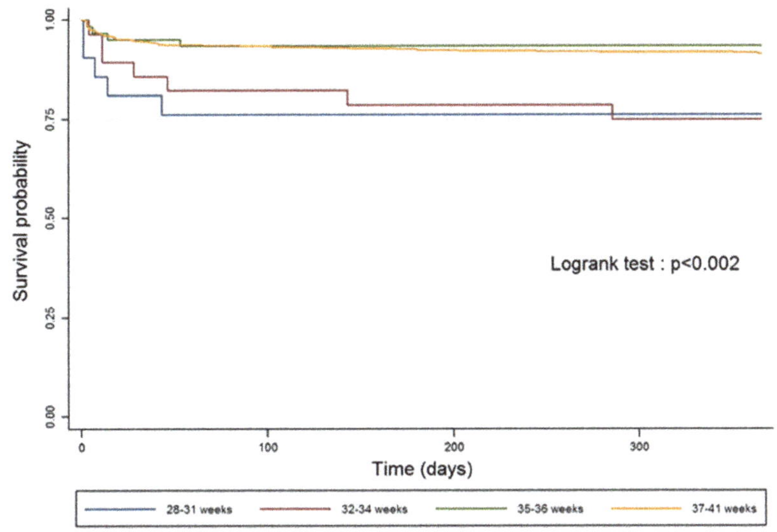

Fig. 3 Gestational-age specific Kaplan-Meier survival curves for infants with isolated *major* CHD

(RR ~ 3.8) was lower than the relative risk of mortality associated with preterm birth in the general population for several European countries and the United States; where the relative risks of infant mortality associated with preterm birth were found to be consistently greater than ten [19, 20]. This lower RR of preterm birth in newborns with CHD is of course not due to any, as it were, protective effect of CHD on the risk of mortality associated with preterm birth. Instead, this is most likely due to the fact that in newborns with CHD, particularly those with severe CHD, preterm birth may play a smaller role as a prognostic factor since the CHD pathology, in cases of moderately severe and more so severe CHD (e.g., functionally univentricular heart) can be a more important prognostic factor than the gestational age of the newborn. Indeed, we found that the relative risk associated with PTB was lower when cases of VSD, which for the most part represent benign lesions that do not require intervention, were excluded. This suggests in turn that as the severity of CHD increases, the effect of PTB, *relatively* speaking, decreases.

In addition, the effect of PTB on the risk of mortality of newborns with CHD may be in part due to differences in the spectrum of CHD associated with preterm vs. term births. A previous study [6] found that in general categories of CHD that were associated with a higher risk of PTB were also more likely to represent more severe cases of CHD.

Our study has certain limits. Even though our study population included more than 2000 cases of newborns with CHD, we were not able to examine the risk of mortality separately for extremely (< 28 weeks) PTB due to our limited sample size for this gestational age group. In addition, our study was not designed to assess the impact of different management strategies (e.g., timing of surgery [8, 12, 21–24]) for preterm vs. term newborns

Table 3 Cox proportional hazard models of the impact of preterm birth on the risk of infant death

		HR	95% CI	p[c]	HRa[d]	95%CI	p[c]
Isolated CHD[a]							
Gestational age (weeks)	28–31	6.5	2.6–16.3	<0.001	4.0	1.5–10.4	<0.001
	32–34	4.9	2.2–10.9		5.4	2.1–13.9	
	35–36	1.1	0.4–3.1		0.9	0.3–2.7	
Isolated major CHD[b]							
Gestational age (weeks)	28–31	3.3	1.3–8.4	0.003	2.1	0.8–5.4	0.045
	32–34	3.1	1.4–6.8		3.1	1.2–8.0	
	35–36	0.8	0.3–2.1		0.6	0.2–1.9	

[a]Isolated CHD: excluding cases with chromosomal or other anomalies
[b]Isolated major CHD: excluding cases with chromosomal or other anomalies and ventricular septal defects (VSD)
[c]Likelihood ratio test
[d]adjusted for maternal age, occupation, geographic origin, diabetes, intra-uterine growth restriction (IUGR) and multiple pregnancy

with CHD. We also could not examine in any detail the extent to which differences in mortality between preterm vs. term newborns with CHD may be due to differences in the spectrum of CHD or the extent to which the effect of PTB may be modified by different type of CHD.

It should be noted that while we took into account the potentially confounding effects of certain socioeconomic factors, the scope of our study was much more limited than a comprehensive analysis of the many factors associated with PTB and CHD, and in particular the potential role of socioeconomic factors such as education, income and place of residence, would require. Future studies should examine in particular the extent to which any effects of socioeconomic factors on the risk of infant mortality may be due to (mediated by) preterm birth, which is known to vary across socioeconomic groups.

Conclusion

We found that overall preterm newborns with CHD, particularly those who were born at <35 weeks of gestational age, had a substantially higher risk of mortality than those born at term (37–41). This higher risk decreased but remained statistically significant after exclusion of associated anomalies and adjustment for potentially confounding factors, including maternal sociodemographic factors, multiple pregnancies and IUGR. The *relative risk* of mortality associated with PTB was substantially lower for newborns with CHD than the comparable estimates in the general population. In terms of absolute risk differences, however, the situation was different. This is so because a given relative risk of mortality associated with preterm birth for infants with CHD "translates" into a higher absolute risk difference since the baseline risk of mortality for full-term infants with CHD is higher than full-term infants in the general population.

Future studies should examine the extent to which the higher risk of mortality associated with PTB may vary across the spectrum of CHD and assess the role of alternative clinical management strategies (e.g., age at surgery) on survival and long-term neuro-developmental outcomes of preterm newborns with CHD.

Abbreviations

ASD: Atrial septal defect; CHD: Congenital heart defect; CI: Confidence interval; EPICARD: Etude EPIdémiologique sur le devenir des enfants porteurs de CARDiopathies congénitales; HR: Hazard ratio; IUGR: Intrauterine growth restriction; OR: Odds ratio; PTB: Preterm birth; VSD: Ventricular Septal Defect

Funding

This work was supported by two grants from the French Ministry of Health (PHRC 2004 and 2008). Additional funding was provided by the AREMCAR (Association pour la Recherche et l'Etude des Maladies Cardiovasculaires) association. The funding sources had no role in the study design, data collection, data interpretation, or the writing of the manuscript.

Authors' contributions

EL participation in conceiving study with BK, conducted the statistical analyses and wrote the first draft of the manuscript. NL participated in statistical analysis and design of the study. PYA advised on the analyses in relation to his expertise in preterm birth. DB and LH advised on the analyses in relation to their expertise in CHD. TA participated in statistical analyses. FG participated in study design and the strategy for data analysis. BK conceived the study, supervised the statistical analyses and revised the first draft with EL. All authors participated in critical review of the manuscript and approved the final version submitted.

Competing interests

The authors have no competing interests to disclose.

EPICARD study group

Principal Investigators: François Goffinet, Babak Khoshnood.
Steering Committee:
Damien Bonnet (Hôpital Necker Enfants Malades, AP-HP, Centre de référence M3C, Université Paris Descartes, Paris).
Drina Candilis (Université Paris-Diderot, Paris).
Anne-Lise Delezoide (Hôpital Robert Debré, AP-HP, Service de biologie du Développement, Université Paris-Diderot, Paris).
François Goffinet (Groupe Hospitalier Cochin-Hôtel Dieu, AP-HP, Maternité Port-Royal et INSERM U1153, Equipe EPOPé, Université Paris Descartes, Paris).
Lucile Houyel (Hôpital Marie Lannelongue, Service de chirurgie des cardiopathies congénitales, Le Plessis-Robinson).
Jean-Marie Jouannic (Hôpital Trousseau, AP-HP, Centre pluridisciplinaire de diagnosticprénatal, UPMC, Paris).
Babak Khoshnood (INSERM U1153, Equipe EPOPé, Paris).
Nathalie Lelong (INSERM U1153, Equipe EPOPé, Paris).
Suzel Magnier (Hôpital Robert Debré, AP-HP, Service de cardiologie, Paris).
Jean-François Magny (Hôpital Necker Enfants Malades, AP-HP, Service de néonatologie, Paris).
Caroline Rambaud (Hôpital Raymond Poincarré, AP-HP, Service d'anatomie et cytologie pathologiques – Médecine légale, UVSQ, Garches).
Dominique Salomon (INSERM U1153, Equipe EPOPé, Paris).
Johanna Calderon (INSERM U1153, Equipe EPOPé, Paris).
Project Coordination and Data Analysis Committee:
François Goffinet, Babak Khoshnood, Nathalie Lelong, Thibaut Andrieu, Anne-Claire Thieulin, Véronique Vodovar.
Independent Data Monitoring Committee (URC Paris Centre et CIC Cochin Necker Mère Enfant): Maggy Chausson, Anissa Brinis, Laure Faure, Maryline Delattre, Jean-Marc Treluyer (Groupe Hospitalier Cochin-Hôtel Dieu, AP-HP, Université Paris Descartes, Paris).
External Scientific Committee:
Gérard Bréart, Dominique Cabrol, Alain Sérraf, Daniel Sidi, Marcel Voyer.
Participating Centers:
The Greater Paris Area (Paris and its surrounding suburbs) public (AP-HP) and private maternity units, Departments of Pediatric Cardiology and Pediatric Cardiac Surgery, pediatric cardiologists in private practice, Neonatal Intensive Care Units, Pediatric Intensive Care Units, Emergency Transfer Services (SMUR), Departments of Pathology, Sudden Death Centers, Departments of Family and Infant Protection (DFPE).

Author details
[1]Obstetrical, perinatal and pediatric epidemiology research team, Center for biostatistics and epidemiology, INSERM U1153, Maternité de Port-Royal, 6ème étage, 53 av. de l'Observatoire, 75014 Paris, France. [2]Service de chirurgie des cardiopathies congénitales, Hôpital Marie Lannelongue, 133, avenue de la Résistance, 92350 Le Plessis Robinson, France. [3]Centre de référence M3C-Necker, Université Paris Descartes, 140 rue de Sèvres, 75015 Paris, France. [4]Service de pédiatrie et réanimation néonatales CHU Necker Enfants Malades, Paris, France. [5]Maternité Port Royal, 53 avenue de l'Observatoire, 75014 Paris, France.

References

1. Dolk H, Loane M, Garne E. Congenital heart defects in Europe: prevalence and perinatal mortality, 2000 to 2005. Circulation. 2011;123(8):841–9. doi:10.1161/CIRCULATIONAHA.110.958405.
2. INSERM. Déficiences ou handicaps d'origine périnatale Dépistage et prise en charge. 2004. Available at: http://www.senat.fr/rap/r03-363/r03-inserm.pdf.
3. Lee JE, Jung K-L, Kim S-E, et al. Prenatal diagnosis of congenital heart disease: trends in pregnancy termination rate, and perinatal and 1-year infant mortalities in Korea between 1994 and 2005. J Obstet Gynaecol Res. 2010;36(3):474–8. doi:10.1111/j.1447-0756.2010.01222.x.
4. Mathews TJ, MacDorman MF. Infant mortality statistics from the 2007 period linked birth/infant death data set. Natl Vital Stat Rep. 2011;59(6):1–30.
5. Tanner K, Sabrine N, Wren C. Cardiovascular malformations among preterm infants. Pediatrics. 2005;116(6):e833–8. doi:10.1542/peds.2005-0397.
6. Laas E, Lelong N, Thieulin A-C, et al. Preterm birth and congenital heart defects: a population-based study. Pediatrics. 2012;130(4):e829–37. doi:10.1542/peds.2011-3279.
7. Dees E, Lin H, Cotton RB, Graham TP, Dodd DA. Outcome of preterm infants with congenital heart disease. J Pediatr. 2000;137(5):653–9. doi:10.1067/mpd.2000.108568.
8. Ades AM, Dominguez TE, Nicolson SC, et al. Morbidity and mortality after surgery for congenital cardiac disease in the infant born with low weight. Cardiol Young. 2010;20(1):8–17. doi:10.1017/S1047951109991909.
9. Jenkins KJ, Correa A, Feinstein JA, et al. Noninherited risk factors and congenital cardiovascular defects: current knowledge: a scientific statement from the American Heart Association Council on cardiovascular disease in the young: endorsed by the American Academy of Pediatrics. Circulation. 2007;115(23):2995–3014. doi:10.1161/CIRCULATIONAHA.106.183216.
10. Natarajan G, Anne SR, Aggarwal S. Outcomes of congenital heart disease in late preterm infants: double jeopardy? Acta Paediatr. 2011;100(8):1104–7. doi:10.1111/j.1651-2227.2011.02245.x.
11. Boldt T, Andersson S, Eronen M. Outcome of structural heart disease diagnosed in utero. Scand Cardiovasc J. 2002;36(2):73–9. doi:10.1080/140174302753675339.
12. Oppido G, Pace Napoleone C, Formigari R, et al. Outcome of cardiac surgery in low birth weight and premature infants. Eur J Cardiothorac Surg. 2004;26(1):44–53. doi:10.1016/j.ejcts.2004.04.004.
13. Wernovsky G, Rubenstein SD, Spray TL. Cardiac surgery in the low-birth weight neonate. New approaches. Clin Perinatol. 2001;28(1):249–64.
14. Andrews RE, Simpson JM, Sharland GK, Sullivan ID, Yates RWM. Outcome after preterm delivery of infants antenatally diagnosed with congenital heart disease. J Pediatr. 2006;148(2):213–6. doi:10.1016/j.jpeds.2005.10.034.
15. Cheng HH, Almodovar MC, Laussen PC, et al. Outcomes and risk factors for mortality in premature neonates with critical congenital heart disease. Pediatr Cardiol. 2011;32(8):1139–46. doi:10.1007/s00246-011-0036-3.
16. Costello JM, Polito A, Brown DW, et al. Birth before 39 weeks' gestation is associated with worse outcomes in neonates with heart disease. Pediatrics. 2010;126(2):277–84. doi:10.1542/peds.2009-3640.
17. Polito A, Piga S, Cogo PE, et al. Increased morbidity and mortality in very preterm/VLBW infants with congenital heart disease. Intensive Care Med. 2013;39(6):1104–12. doi:10.1007/s00134-013-2887-y.
18. Khoshnood B, Lelong N, Houyel L, et al. Prevalence, timing of diagnosis and mortality of newborns with congenital heart defects: a population-based study. Heart. 2012;98(22):1667–73. doi:10.1136/heartjnl-2012-302543.
19. european-perinatal-health-report.pdf. Available at: http://www.europeristat.com/images/doc/EPHR/european-perinatal-health-report.pdf. 20 Accessed Jan 2013.
20. EuroPERISTAT. 2013. Available at: http://www.europeristat.com/. Euro-Peristat project with SCPE and Eurocat. European Perinatal Health Report. The health and care of pregnant women and babies in Europe in 2010.
21. Bové T, François K, De Groote K, et al. Outcome analysis of major cardiac operations in low weight neonates. Ann Thorac Surg. 2004;78(1):181–7. doi:10.1016/j.athoracsur.2003.12.066.
22. Chang AC, Hanley FL, Lock JE, Castaneda AR, Wessel DL. Management and outcome of low birth weight neonates with congenital heart disease. J Pediatr. 1994;124(3):461–6.
23. Rossi AF, Seiden HS, Sadeghi AM, et al. The outcome of cardiac operations in infants weighing two kilograms or less. J Thorac Cardiovasc Surg. 1998;116(1):28–35.
24. Hickey EJ, Nosikova Y, Zhang H, et al. Very low-birth-weight infants with congenital cardiac lesions: is there merit in delaying intervention to permit growth and maturation? J Thorac Cardiovasc Surg. 2012;143(1):126–136, 136.e1. doi:10.1016/j.jtcvs.2011.09.008.

11

Risk factors and implications of progressive coronary dilatation in children with Kawasaki disease

Ming-Yu Liu[1], Hsin-Min Liu[1], Chia-Hui Wu[1], Chin-Hao Chang[2], Guan-Jr Huang[3], Chun-An Chen[1], Shuenn-Nan Chiu[1], Chun-Wei Lu[1], Ming-Tai Lin[1*], Luan-Yin Chang[1], Jou-Kou Wang[1] and Mei-Hwan Wu[1]

Abstract

Background: Kawasaki disease (KD) is an acute systemic vasculitis that occurs in children and may lead to cardiovascular morbidity and mortality. Progressive coronary dilatation for at least 2 months is associated with worse late coronary outcomes in patients with KD having medium or giant aneurysms. However, the risk factors and occurrence of progressive coronary dilatation in patients with KD but without medium or giant aneurysms have been insufficiently explored.

Methods: We retrospectively enrolled 169 patients with KD from a tertiary medical center in Taiwan during 2009–2013. Medical records of all patients were reviewed. Echocardiography was performed during the acute KD phase and at 3–4 weeks, 6–8 weeks, 6 months, and 12 months after KD onset. Progressive coronary dilatation was defined as the progressive enlargement of coronary arteries on three consecutive echocardiograms. Logistic regression analysis was conducted to evaluate the potential risk factors for coronary aneurysms and progressive coronary dilatation.

Results: Of a total of 169 patients with KD, 31 (18.3%) had maximal coronary Z-scores of ≥ + 2.5 during the acute KD phase, 16 (9.5%; male/female: 9/7) had coronary aneurysms at 1 month after KD onset, and 5 (3.0%) satisfied the definition of progressive coronary dilatation. Multivariate logistic regression analysis revealed that an initial maximal coronary Z-score of ≥ + 2.5 [odds ratio (OR): 5.24, 95% confidence interval (CI): 1.31–21.3, $P = 0.020$] and hypoalbuminemia (OR: 4.83, 95% CI: 1.11–20.9, $P = 0.035$) were independent risk factors for coronary aneurysms and were significantly associated with progressive coronary dilatation. However, the association between intravenous immunoglobulin unresponsiveness and the development of coronary aneurysms at 1 month after KD onset didn't reach the level of significance ($P = 0.058$).

Conclusions: In the present study, 3% (5/169) of patients with KD had progressive coronary dilatation, which was associated with persistent coronary aneurysms at 1 year after KD onset. Initial coronary dilatation and hypoalbuminemia were independently associated with the occurrence of progressive coronary dilatation. Therefore, such patients may require intensive cardiac monitoring and adjuvant therapies apart from immunoglobulin therapies.

Keywords: Kawasaki disease, Risk factors, Progressive coronary dilatation, Hypoalbuminemia

* Correspondence: mingtailin@ntu.edu.tw
[1]Department of Pediatrics, National Taiwan University Hospital and Medical College, National Taiwan University, No. 7, Chung-Shan South Road, Taipei 100, Taiwan
Full list of author information is available at the end of the article

Background

Kawasaki disease (KD) is one of the most common forms of systemic vasculitis in children [1]. Even after intravenous immunoglobulin (IVIG) treatment, coronary arterial lesions (CALs) have been observed in 5%–20% of patients with KD during the acute stage [2–4]. In Taiwan and Japan, CALs have typically been classified into three subgroups (small [<4 mm], medium [4–8 mm], and giant [≥8 mm]) based on their diameters during the acute disease phase or at 1 month after disease onset [2, 4]. Coronary artery diameter-based severity is the most significant predictor of late coronary outcomes [5]. We observed that progressive coronary dilatation for at least 2 months was associated with worse late coronary outcomes in patients with KD having medium (4–8 mm) or giant (≥8 mm) aneurysms [6]. Several studies [7, 8] have evaluated KD-associated CALs by using body surface area-normalized coronary Z-scores and have demonstrated a significant reduction in coronary Z-scores from the initial values mostly in the first 2–3 months. McCrindle and his colleagues [8] reported some risk factors associated with a greater coronary Z-scores at any time, such as younger age and lower serum albumin levels [8]. However, whether the progressive increase of coronary Z-scores occurs in all KD patients, especially those without CAL or with small aneurysms at their acute phase, remains unclear.. Therefore, in the present study, we aimed to determine (1) the maximal coronary Z-score distributions in Taiwanese patients with KD at the acute, subacute, and convalescent phases; and (2) the risk factors for coronary aneurysms and progressive coronary dilatation in Taiwanese KD patients.

Methods

This study was approved by the Institutional Review Board of National Taiwan University Hospital.

Patients

In the present study, KD was diagnosed on the basis of the clinical criteria for KD [9]. Patients with KD who were admitted to our institution between January 2009 and December 2013 and were administered IVIG (2 g/kg × 1 day or 1 g/kg × 2 days) within 10 days after fever onset were enrolled in this study. However, patients with KD who had congenital heart disease were excluded from the study. The first day of illness was considered as the first day of fever. Patients with an axillary body temperature of <37.5 °C for >24 h were considered afebrile. The aspirin dosage was reduced to 5 mg/kg/day after defervescence. Medical records of all patients were reviewed, and the manifestations, symptoms, and laboratory data (including serum albumin levels and acute-phase reactants) were obtained as described in previous studies [5, 6]. Echocardiography was performed in all children during the febrile stage and the subacute phase (3–4 and 6–8 weeks) after fever onset, and the echocardiography frequency subsequently varied depending on CAL severity.

IVIG unresponsiveness was defined as the failure to respond to the initial IVIG dosage and the presence of persistent fever for >24 h or the development of KD-associated recrudescent fever after an afebrile period [1, 4, 5]. Patients unresponsive to IVIG were administered additional IVIG doses.

Measurements

The coronary artery measurements were normalized to the body surface area using the established reference in Taiwanese children [10]. In the current study, we defined "coronary artery dilatation" as maximal Z-score > = +2.5 of any branch of coronary artery [1]. Only the coronary dilatation persisted for more than a month after disease onset were considered coronary aneurysms [5, 6]. The severity of coronary aneurysms was classified as small (+2.5 ≦ Z < +5.0), medium (+5.0 ≦ Z < 10) and giant (Z > = +10.0) [11]. CALs and the regression were diagnosed based on 2D echocardiography.

Definition of progressive coronary dilatation

Progressive coronary dilatation was defined as the progressive dilatation of coronary arteries on three consecutive echocardiograms [6]. The coronary Z-score on the second echocardiogram had to be higher than that on the first echocardiogram, and the coronary Z-score on the third echocardiogram had to be 8% higher than that on the first echocardiogram. We defined progressive coronary dilatation based on the 8% increase criterion because a previous study [10] on Taiwanese coronary Z-scores showed interobserver differences of 7.1%, 5.8%, and 5.2% for the left main coronary artery, left anterior descending coronary artery, and right coronary artery, respectively. However, in the current study, the interobserver and intraobserver differences were 6.6% and 6.1%, respectively.

Statistical analysis

Patient data are expressed as counts, percentages, medians with interquartile ranges (IQRs), and means (standard deviations). We used the independent Student *t* test and Fisher exact test for comparing continuous and categorical variables, respectively. Nonnormal variables were analyzed using the Mann–Whitney nonparametric test. A P value of <0.05 was considered statistically significant. The risk factors for coronary aneurysms derived from the univariate analysis were used in the subsequent logistic regression analysis. The logistic regression analysis was conducted to evaluate the potential risk factors for coronary aneurysms and progressive coronary dilatation. All analyses were performed using SPSS Statistics (Version 20.0. IBM Corp, Armonk, NY).

Results

Patient characteristics

Between 2009 and 2013, 175 patients with KD were admitted to our hospital. Of these 175 patients with KD, 6 (3.4%) were excluded because they received IVIG treatments beyond 10 days after fever onset. Finally, 169 patients with KD were enrolled in this study. The median age of these patients at the diagnosis of acute KD was 1.4 years (IQR: 8.1 months–2.5 years), and 99 (59%) were boys. The median duration of fever before the first course of IVIG treatment was 5 days (IQR: 4–6 days). Of the 169 KD patients, 138 (81.7%) were administered a single course of IVIG treatment (1 g/kg/day × 2 days or 2 g/kg/dose × 1 day), 20 (11.8%) received IVIG retreatment, and 11 (6.5%) did not receive IVIG treatment due to defervescence before IVIG administration. Moreover, the enrolled patients did not receive steroid therapies, and none of them died during the study period. Table 1 presents the characteristics of the patients with KD according to their maximal coronary Z-scores during the acute KD phase.

Echocardiography measurements

All enrolled patients underwent echocardiography before receiving IVIG treatment. The median maximal coronary Z-score of any coronary artery during the acute KD phase was 1.60 (IQR: +0.95 – +2.2). Table 1 shows the clinical and laboratory data of 31 and 138 patients with maximal coronary Z-scores of ≥ + 2.5 and <+2.5, respectively, during the acute KD phase. The coronary severity during the acute KD phase (before IVIG treatment) was associated with IVIG responsiveness, hypoalbuminemia, and C-reactive protein (CRP) levels. On the basis of the definition of coronary aneurysms (persistent coronary dilatation for more than 1 month after disease onset), 16 (9.5%) patients had coronary aneurysms (small, n = 14; medium, n = 2). At the end of follow-up (12 months after fever onset), four (25.0%) patients had small persistent coronary aneurysms. However, coronary aneurysms or progressive coronary dilatation was not observed in 11 patients who did not receive IVIG treatment due to defervescence within 10 days after KD onset.

Risk factors associated with the coronary aneurysms

Univariate analysis revealed three potential risk factors associated with the coronary aneurysms, including initial maximal coronary Z-score of ≥ + 2.5, IVIG unresponsiveness, and serum albumin levels [Table 2].

The median of serum albumin levels were significantly lower in the 16 KD patients with coronary aneurysms (3.4 g/dL, IQR: 2.85-3.55 g/dL) than in those without coronary aneurysms (4.0 g/dL, IQR: 3.6-4.3 g/dL; P < 0.001). When hypoalbuminemia was defined by serum albumin levels of <3.5 g/dL, it remained significantly associated with the development of coronary aneurysms (11/16 vs 25/153, P < 0.001) in this study.

Multivariate logistic regression analysis was conducted to evaluate the independent effects of an initial maximal coronary Z-score of ≥ + 2.5, hypoalbuminemia, and IVIG unresponsiveness on the development of coronary aneurysms in the 169 patients with KD. An initial maximal coronary Z-score of ≥ + 2.5 and hypoalbuminemia were independent risk factors for coronary aneurysms (odds ratio [OR] of initial maximal coronary Z-score of ≥ + 2.5: 5.24, 95% confidence interval (CI): 1.31–21.3, P = 0.020; OR of hypoalbuminemia:

Table 1 Characteristics of patients with and without coronary dilatation during their acute KD phase

	All (169)	Normal (138)	Dilatation (31)	*P* value
Male gender	99 (59%)	81 (59%)	18 (58%)	0.949
Age (yr)	1.44 (0.67; 2.56)	1.46 (0.71; 2.74)	1.12 (0.36; 2.09)	0.063
IVIG unresponsive	20 (12%)	11 (8%)	9 (29%)	0.001
Days of fever before IVIG use	5 (5; 6)	5 (4.3; 6)	5 (5; 6.3)	0.518
Albumin (g/dL)	3.9 (3.5; 4.3)	4 (3.6; 4.3)	3.5 (3.2; 4.2)	0.03
AST (U/L)	38 (29; 66.5)	37 (29; 71.5)	39.5 (25.3; 56.3)	0.379
CRP (mg/dL)	7.23 (2.22; 14.15)	6.1 (3.26; 11.93)	14.05 (6.38; 18.29)	0.009
WBC (k/μL)	13.74 (10.32; 17.56)	13.61 (10.29; 16.94)	15.36 (10.74; 19.64)	0.418
Seg (%)	62.3 (51.3; 73.6)	62.9 (53.5; 73.9)	59 (49.7; 72)	0.391
Hb (g/dL)	11.1 (10.4; 12)	11.2 (10.5; 12)	10.9 (10.4; 11.8)	0.329
PLT (k/μL)	333 (260; 412)	328 (260; 405)	343 (253; 454)	0.285

Values are expressed as medians (IQRs) and percentages (%). *IVIG* intravenous immunoglobulin, *AST* Aspartate aminotransferase, *CRP* C-reactive protein, *WBC* White blood cell, *Seg* Neutro segment WBC, *Hb* hemoglobin, *PLT* platelet

Table 2 Univariate analysis of the risk factors for coronary aneurysms

	Coronary AN (*n* = 16)	Regression (*n* = 153)	*p*-value
Male gender	9 (56%)	90 (59%)	0.842
Age (yr)	0.99 (0.33; 1.86)	1.5 (0.69; 2.7)	0.059
Initial Z-score ≥ 2.5	10 (56%)	21 (14%)	<0.001
IVIG unresponsive	8 (50%)	12 (7.8%)	<0.001
Days of fever before IVIG use	5 (5; 7)	5 (4; 6)	0.346
Albumin (g/dL)	3.4 (2.85; 3.55)	4.0 (3.6; 4.3)	<0.001
AST (U/L)	45 (25; 87)	38 (29; 60.3)	0.885
CRP (mg/dL)	12.15 (6.35; 18.18)	6.68 (3,3; 13.37)	0.058
WBC (k/μL)	17.79 (9.52; 19.19)	13..65 (10.39; 16.94)	0.426
Seg (%)	63.1 (55.7; 77.5)	61.8 (51.1; 73.5)	0.721
Hb (g/dL)	10.8 (10.4; 11.5)	11.1 (10.45; 12)	0.307
PLT (k/μL)	399 (487; 886)	333 (262; 409)	0.965

Values are expressed as medians (IQRs) and percentages (%). *IVIG* Intravenous immunoglobulin, *AST* Aspartate aminotransferase, *CRP* C-reactive protein, *WBC* White blood cell, *Seg* Neutro segment WBC, *Hb* Hemoglobin, *PLT* Platelet

4.83, 95% CI: 1.11–20.9, *P* = 0.035; OR of IVIG unresponsiveness: 4.63, 95% CI: 0.96–22.3, *P* = 0.058).

Risk factors and implications of progressive coronary dilatation

The coronary Z-scores of six patients increased from <+2.5 initially to ≥ + 2.5 at 1 month after KD onset; however, none of these patients exhibited any further increase in their coronary Z-scores on subsequent echocardiographic examinations (Fig. 1). Of the 10 patients with persistent coronary aneurysms at 1 month after KD onset, 5 showed more increased coronary Z-scores at 2 months after KD onset (Fig. 1), thus satisfying the criteria of progressive coronary dilatation on three consecutive echocardiograms. Of the five patients with progressive coronary dilatation, four had persistent coronary aneurysms even at 1 year after KD onset. Compared with the remaining 11 patients without progressive coronary dilatation, 4 patients with progressive coronary dilatation had a higher probability of persistent coronary aneurysms at 1 year after KD onset (0/11 vs 4/5, *P* = 0.003).

Of the 31 patients with KD initial coronary Z-scores of ≥ + 2.5, 5 (16.1%) had progressive coronary dilatation on three consecutive echocardiograms. However, none of the remaining 138 patients with initial coronary Z-scores of <+2.5 showed such progression (5/31 vs 0/138; $P = 2 \times 10^{-4}$). Furthermore, of the 36 KD patients with hypoalbuminemia, 5 developed progressive coronary dilatation. Moreover, the patients with normal serum albumin levels did not develop progressive coronary dilatation ($P = 3 \times 10^{-4}$). The incidence of progressive coronary dilatation did not differ significantly between the IVIG-responsive and IVIG-unresponsive patients with KD (3/138 vs 2/20, *P* = 0.11). To avoid the interaction of risk factors, multivariate logistic regression analysis was conducted to determine the risk factors for progressive coronary dilatation. The results confirmed that an initial maximal coronary Z-score of ≥ + 2.5 (OR: 10.94, 95% CI: 1.14–104.91, *P* = 0.038) and hypoalbuminemia (OR: 9.25, 95% CI: 1.001–88.93, *P* = 0.049) were independent risk factors for progressive coronary dilatation in the patients with KD. However, IVIG unresponsiveness was not significantly associated with progressive coronary dilatation (OR: 1.85, 95% CI: 0.26–13.14, *P* = 0.54)

Discussion

In this study, based on serial echocardiographic measurements, we recognized two independent clinical characteristics (initial maximal coronary Z-score of ≥ + 2.5 and hypoalbuminemia during the acute KD phase) that were significantly associated with coronary aneurysms at 1 month after KD onset as well as progressive coronary dilatation. Progressive coronary dilatation has been insufficiently explored before. McCrindle et al. [8] examined coronary artery involvement in children with KD and observed that if the maximal coronary Z-score is <+2.5 on the initial echocardiogram, it might increase above +2.5 on subsequent echocardiograms in 6% of patients, which is consistent with our study findings (6/138, 4.3%). Moreover, our recent study reported progressive coronary dilatation for at least 2 months in KD patients with medium (25.5%) or giant (48.1%) aneurysms [6]. Furthermore, the current study confirmed that progressive coronary dilatation can occur in KD patients with small aneurysms (3/14, 21.4%), though with a less probability. In 5 (31.3%) of the 16 patients with coronary aneurysms in the current study, the aneurysms enlarged on three consecutive echocardiographic examinations. Moreover, these five patients were more likely to have persistent coronary aneurysms for more than 1 year compared with those without progressive coronary dilatation (4/5 vs 0/11, *P* = 0.003). These findings support our previous observation that progressive coronary dilatation is associated with worse late coronary outcomes [6].

A recent study reported that 81% of patients with KD who eventually developed coronary aneurysms showed coronary abnormalities on their initial echocardiograms [12]. Studies have proposed the use of adjuvant therapies with agents such as atorvastatin [13], steroids [14, 15], and dalteparin [16] to ameliorate the CALs of patients with KD during the acute KD phase. Friedman et al. [17] demonstrated that the rate of coronary aneurysm regression was significantly higher in patients with KD

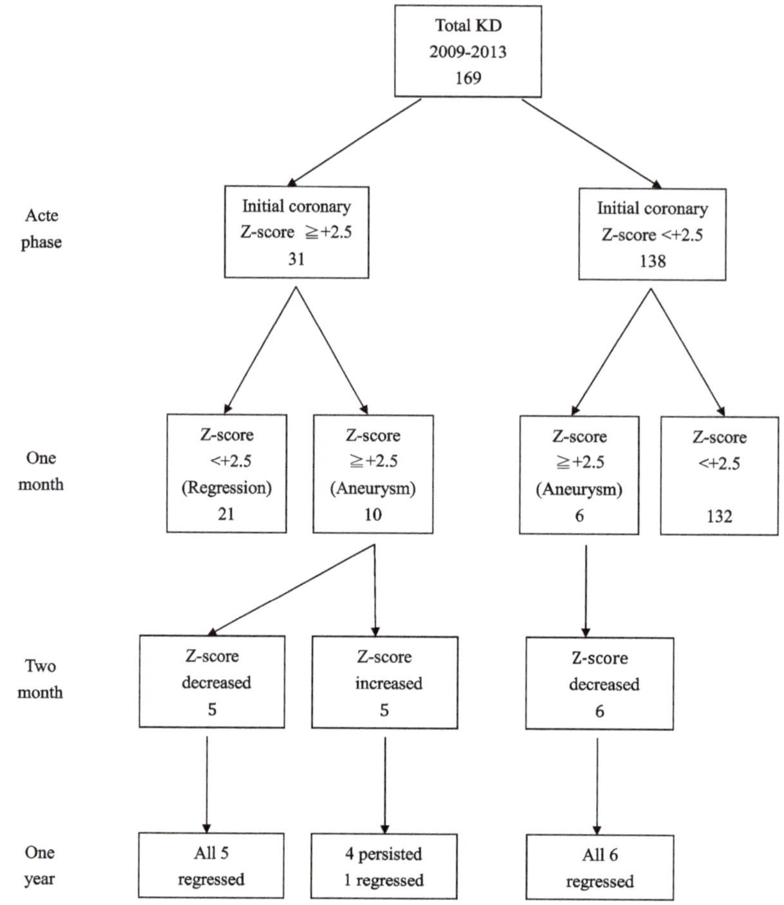

Fig. 1 Flowchart of coronary follow-up of 169 patients with KD

receiving IVIG and adjunctive medications than in those not receiving such medications (91% vs 68%, $P = 0.02$). Our present study showed that patients with KD having initial maximal coronary Z-scores of ≥ + 2.5, particularly those with hypoalbuminemia, are susceptible to progressive coronary dilatation. However, additional studies are warranted to elucidate whether IVIG and adjuvant therapies can promote the regression of coronary aneurysms and prevent their progressive dilatation in patients with KD.

Crystal et al. showed that greater coronary Z-scores over the complete study period were significantly associated with greater initial coronary Z-scores [18], which supports the findings of our studies. Previous studies have identified a few risk factors for coronary dilatation or aneurysmal formation [19–21], including late IVIG treatment, IVIG unresponsiveness, and several clinical biomarkers, such as serum albumin levels and CRP levels. In the current study, we further demonstrated hypoalbuminemia during the acute KD phase was also significantly associated with progressive coronary dilatation. In addition, of the 16 patients with coronary aneurysms at 1 month after KD onset (Fig. 1), 5 showed more increased coronary Z-scores at 2 months after KD onset. Furthermore, All of the five patients with progressive coronary dilatation had hypoalbuminemia (<3.5 g/dL, 100%), indicating that the incidence of hypoalbuminemia was higher in the aforementioned patients than in the remaining 11 patients with coronary aneurysms ($P = 0.012$). These findings may indicate that patients with KD who develop hypoalbuminemia during the acute KD phase, particularly those with coronary Z-scores of ≥ + 2.5, are susceptible to progressive coronary dilatation and may require closer cardiac monitoring and more aggressive treatments using agents such as statins [13] and steroids [14, 15].

However, the reason for the association of serum albumin levels with coronary aneurysms and progressive coronary dilatation remains unclear. Terai et al. [22] reported that IVIG-unresponsive patients with KD had higher vascular endothelial growth factor levels, which might lead to vascular leakage, decreased serum albumin levels, and pericardial effusion. Therefore, hypoalbuminemia is most likely caused by vascular inflammation and thus is associated with coronary aneurysms and progressive dilatation in patients with KD.

Previous studies have reported CRP as one of the risk factors for IVIG unresponsiveness [21] and an independent risk factor for initial coronary dilatation [23] and giant aneurysms [24] in patients with KD. However, in the current study, the CRP levels were not significantly associated with coronary aneurysms ($P = 0.058$) or progressive coronary dilatation ($P = 0.54$). Our earlier study revealed that low-grade inflammation was associated with persistent CALs in patients with KD [25]. Therefore, we investigated the association between progressive coronary dilatation and the changes in inflammatory biomarkers (CRP levels, white cell count, and neutrophil percentages) during the acute febrile and subacute phases. However, none of the changes in the three inflammatory biomarkers were associated with progressive coronary dilatation. Therefore, additional studies are warranted to elucidate the effects of CRP and other KD-associated inflammatory biomarkers, such as interleukin-4 [26] and interleukin-6 [27], on early and late CALs in patients with KD.

Limitations

Our study has several limitations. First, this study was conducted in a single tertiary medical center in Taiwan, which may have resulted in selection bias. Second, this study had a retrospective design, and a limited number of patients were enrolled. Third, information bias may have existed, because ultrasound technicians were not blinded to tentative diagnoses. Finally, we did not analyze the socioeconomic factors, febrile days on initial IVIG, and unmeasured laboratory data, such as alanine aminotransferase and bilirubin levels, which were potential confounders in the current study. Large, prospective cohort studies are necessary to reduce the influence of potential confounders.

Conclusions

Coronary artery dilatation with an initial maximal coronary Z-score of ≥ + 2.5 and hypoalbuminemia during the acute KD phase are independent risk factors for coronary artery aneurysms and progressive coronary dilatation in the subacute KD phase. These simple indicators may help clinicians in identifying high-risk KD children who may have coronary aneurysms and progressive coronary dilatation and require intensive monitoring and additional therapies.

Abbreviations

CAL: Coronary arterial lesions; CI: Confidence interval; CRP: C-reactive protein; IQR: Interquartile range; IVIG: Intravenous immunoglobulin; KD: Kawasaki disease; OR: Odds ratio

Acknowledgments

This study was supported by the Cardiac Children's Foundation, Taiwan (grant no. CCFT2013-01).

Funding

This study received funding from the Cardiac Children's Foundation, Taiwan. The funder played no role in the study design, data collection, data analysis, data interpretation, or manuscript writing.

Authors' contributions

M-Y L and HL performed data collection and interpretation and drafted the initial manuscript. CW and GH made substantial contributions to acquisition of data, especially the laboratory and echocardiographic data. C-H C provided statistical assistance. C-A C, SC, and CL managed patient care and the enrollment of eligible patients. LC revised the manuscript critically and provided instruction regarding pediatric infectious disease. JW and MW performed data interpretation. M-T L had full data access and is accountable for all aspects of the work in ensuring that questions related to the accuracy or integrity of any part of the work are appropriately investigated and resolved. All authors have read and approved the final submission.

Competing interests

The authors declare that they have no competing interests.

Author details

[1]Department of Pediatrics, National Taiwan University Hospital and Medical College, National Taiwan University, No. 7, Chung-Shan South Road, Taipei 100, Taiwan. [2]Department of Medical Research, National Taiwan University Hospital, Taipei, Taiwan. [3]Medical Information Management Office, National Taiwan University Hospital, Taipei, Taiwan.

References

1. Newburger JW, Takahashi M, Burns JC. Kawasaki disease. J Am Coll Cardiol. 2016;67:1738–49.
2. Wu MH, Chen HC, Yeh SJ, Lin MT, Huang SC, Huang SK. Prevalence and the long-term coronary risks of patients with Kawasaki disease in a general population <40 years: a national database study. Circ Cardiovasc Qual Outcomes. 2012;5:566–70.
3. Eleftheriou D, Levin M, Shingadia D, Tulloh R, Klein NJ, Brogan PA. Management of Kawasaki disease. Arch Dis Child. 2014;99:74–83.
4. JCS Joint Working Group. Guidelines for diagnosis and management of cardiovascular sequelae in Kawasaki disease (JCS 2013). Digest version Circ J. 2014;78:2521–62.
5. Lin MT, Sun LC, Wu ET, Wang JK, Lue HC, Wu MH. Acute and late coronary outcomes in 1073 patients with Kawasaki disease with and without intravenous gamma-immunoglobulin therapy. Arch Dis Child. 2015;100:542–7.
6. Chih WL, Wu PY, Sun LC, Lin MT, Wang JK, Wu MH. Progressive Coronary Dilatation Predicts Worse Outcome in Kawasaki Disease. J Pediatr. 2016;171:78–82. e1
7. de Zorzi A, Colan SD, Gauvreau K, Baker AL, Sundel RP, Newburger JW. Coronary artery dimensions may be misclassified as normal in Kawasaki disease. J Pediatr. 1998;133:254–8.
8. McCrindle BW, Li JS, Minich LL, Colan SD, Atz AM, Takahashi M, et al. Coronary artery involvement in children with Kawasaki disease: risk factors from analysis of serial normalized measurements. Circulation. 2007;116:174–9.
9. Research Committee on Kawasaki Disease. Report of Subcommittee on Standardization of Diagnostic Criteria and Reporting of Coronary Artery Lesion in Kawasaki Disease. Tokyo, Japan: Ministry of Health and Welfare; 1984.

10. Lin MT, Chang CH, Hsieh WC, Chang CE, Chang YM, Chen YC, et al. Coronary Diameters in Taiwanese Children Younger than 6 Years Old: Z-Score Regression Equations Derived from Body Surface Area. Acta Cardiol Sin. 2014;30:266–73.
11. Manlhiot C, Millar K, Golding F, McCrindle BW. Improved classification of coronary artery abnormalities based only on coronary artery z-scores after Kawasaki disease. Pediatr Cardiol. 2010;31:242–9.
12. Dominguez SR, Anderson MS, El-Adawy M, Glodé MP. Preventing coronary artery abnormalities: a need for earlier diagnosis and treatment of Kawasaki disease. Pediatr Infect Dis J. 2012;31:1217–20.
13. Tremoulet AH, Dutkowski J, Sato Y, Kanegaye JT, Ling XB, Burns JC. Novel data-mining approach identifies biomarkers for diagnosis of Kawasaki disease. Pediatr Res. 2015;78:547–53.
14. Sundel R. Clarifying the Role of Corticosteroids in Kawasaki Disease. JAMA Pediatr. 2016;170:1140–2.
15. Kobayashi T, Saji T, Otani T, Takeuchi K, Nakamura T, Arakawa H. Efficacy of immunoglobulin plus prednisolone for prevention of coronary artery abnormalities in severe Kawasaki disease (RAISE study): a randomised, open-label, blinded-endpoints trial. Lancet. 2012;379:1613–20.
16. Inamo Y, Saito K, Hasegawa M, Hayashi R, Nakamura T, Abe O. Effect of dalteparin, a low-molecular-weight heparin, as adjunctive therapy in patients with Kawasaki disease: a retrospective study. BMC Pediatr. 2014;14:27. doi:10.1186/1471-2431-14-27.
17. Friedman KG, Gauvreau K, Hamaoka-Okamoto A, Tang A, Berry E, Tremoulet AH, et al. Coronary Artery Aneurysms in Kawasaki Disease: Risk Factors for Progressive Disease and Adverse Cardiac Events in the US Population. J Am Heart Assoc. 2016;5:e003289.
18. Crystal MA, Manlhiot C, Yeung RS, Smallhorn JF, McCrindle BW. Coronary artery dilation after Kawasaki disease for children within the normal range. Int J Cardiol. 2009;136:27–32.
19. Yellen ES, Gauvreau K, Takahashi M, Burns JC, Shulman S, Baker AL, et al. Performance of 2004 American Heart Association recommendations for treatment of Kawasaki disease. Pediatrics. 2010;125:e234–41.
20. Nakamura Y, Yashiro M, Uehara R, Watanabe M, Tajimi M, Oki I, et al. Use of laboratory data to identify risk factors of giant coronary aneurysms due to Kawasaki disease. Pediatr Int. 2004;46:33–8.
21. Kobayashi T, Inoue Y, Takeuchi K, Okada Y, Tamura K, Tomomasa T, et al. Prediction of intravenous immunoglobulin unresponsiveness in patients with Kawasaki disease. Circulation. 2006;113:2606–12.
22. Terai M, Honda T, Yasukawa K, Higashi K, Hamada H, Kohno Y. Prognostic impact of vascular leakage in acute Kawasaki disease. Circulation. 2003;108:325–30.
23. Kuwabara M, Yashiro M, Kotani K, Tsuboi S, Ae R, Nakamura Y, et al. Cardiac lesions and initial laboratory data in Kawasaki disease: a nationwide survey in Japan. J Epidemiol. 2015;25:189–93.
24. Koyanagi H, Nakamura Y, Yanagawa H. Lower level of serum potassium and higher level of C-reactive protein as an independent risk factor for giant aneurysms in Kawasaki disease. Acta Paediatr. 1998;87:32–6.
25. Chen YC, Shen CT, Wang NK, Huang YL, Chiu HH, Chen CA, et al. High Sensitivity C Reactive Protein (hs-CRP) in Adolescent and Young Adult Patients with History of Kawasaki Disease. Acta Cardiol Sin. 2015;31:473–7.
26. Burns JC, Shimizu C, Shike H, Newburger JW, Sundel RP, Baker AL, et al. Family-based association analysis implicates IL-4 in susceptibility to Kawasaki disease. Genes Immun. 2005;6:438–44.
27. Fujimaru T, Ito S, Masuda H, Oana S, Kamei K, Ishiguro A, et al. Decreased levels of inflammatory cytokines in immunoglobulin-resistant Kawasaki disease after plasma exchange. Cytokine. 2014;70:156–60.

12

Neutropenia after intravenous immunoglobulin therapy is associated with coronary artery lesions in children with Kawasaki disease

Zhenquan Wang[1†], Fengfeng Weng[1†], Chen Li[2], Hongying Shi[3], Zhangke Tang[1], Huixian Qiu[1], Yue'e He[1], Rongzhou Wu[1*] and Maoping Chu[1*]

Abstract

Background: To evaluate differences in laboratory parameters, clinical presentation, and incidence of coronary artery lesions (CAL) between children with neutropenic and non-neutropenic Kawasaki disease (KD).

Methods: All consecutive KD patients that presented to the Second Affiliated Hospital and Yuying Children's Hospital of Wenzhou Medical University in Wenzhou, China between January 2005 and December 2015 were included in this study. Patients were divided into two groups (KD with neutropenia (NKD) and KD without neutropenia (NNKD)) based on whether or not they developed neutropenia during the course of treatment. We compared differences in clinical manifestations, laboratory parameters, and treatment protocols between groups. We also evaluated the relationship between neutropenia with immunoglobulin dosage and incidence of CAL.

Results: An IVIG treatment regimen of 2 g/kg*1d was associated with a lower incidence of neutropenia compared to the 1 g/kg*2d protocol. The incidence of CAL was higher in KD patients with neutropenia than in those without. Subgroup analysis showed no difference in the incidence of CAL among the different age groups between KD patients with and without neutropenia.

Conclusions: Follow up ultrasonic echocardiography should be performed in KD patients with neutropenia in order to allow for early detection of CAL and timely intervention.

Keywords: Kawasaki disease, Neutropenia, Coronary artery lesions

Background

Kawasaki disease (KD) is a systemic vasculitis of unknown etiology that occurs most commonly in infants and young children under 5 years old. The presenting features of KD include fever, bilateral nonexudative conjunctivitis, erythema of the lips and oral mucosa, changes in the extremities, rash, and cervical lymphadenopathy [1, 2]. KD has important cardiovascular sequelae which must be monitored and managed, the most common of which are coronary artery lesions (CAL). Intravenous immune globulin (IVIG) and aspirin are commonly used in the treatment of KD, and IVIG is particularly important due to its ability to relieve inflammation and reduce the incidence of coronary artery lesions [3].

Neutrophils play an important role in the pathogenesis of KD, as raised neutrophil levels during the course of disease have been shown to be related to the pathogenesis of KD and CAL [4]. In recent years, neutrophils have been found to be elevated in the acute phase of KD, despite a decrease in granulocyte counts and even a lack of granulocytes after treatment. The specific mechanism whereby raised neutrophil levels contribute to KD pathogenesis has not been clearly elucidated. Therefore, the aim of this study was to 1) investigate the effect of IVIG in patients with neutropenic KD (NKD) and non-neutropenic KD

* Correspondence: wrz71@hotmail.com; chmping@hotmail.com
†Equal contributors
[1]Children's Heart Center, the Second Affiliated Hospital and Yuying Children's Hospital, Institute of cardiovascular development and translational medicine, Wenzhou Medical University, Wenzhou, Zhejiang 325027, China
Full list of author information is available at the end of the article

(NNKD); 2) compare the effects of neutropenia on laboratory markers, clinical manifestation of disease, coronary artery lesions and non-responsiveness to IVIG; and 3) study the specificity and possible mechanism of neutropenia in KD. Finally, we aimed to investigate the relationship between neutropenia with KD treatment and prognosis.

Methods

Subjects

We performed a retrospective medical record review of all KD inpatients from January 1, 2005 to December 31, 2015 at the Second Affiliated Hospital and Yuying Children's Hospital of Wenzhou Medical University in Wenzhou, China. Additionally, follow-up information regarding CAL was extracted from outpatient medical records. Inclusion criteria were: (1) patients diagnosed in accordance with the Japanese KD diagnosis, (2) treated according to the clinical manifestations and ultrasonic echocardiography (UCG) results, and (3) patients with first presentation of KD [1]. We initially identified a total of 1667 (1111 male and 556 female). Patients were excluded if they had incomplete data. After applying these criteria, we included 1365 cases into the final analysis. Patients were divided into two groups according to the presence of neutropenia after IVIG treatment (NKD, 197 patients; and NNKD, 1168 patients). Among them, 539 patients received the 2 g/kg*1d program and 192 received the 1 g/kg*2d program, the rest of patients were not received IVIG or lack of sufficient information regarding IVIG treatment. All KD inpatients were initially treated with aspirin.

Outcomes

Outcomes of interest were the timing and dose of IVIG, use of dipyridamole, laboratory parameters, clinical manifestations, and echocardiographic results. All patients were followed up for 3 months after IVIG treatment.

Neutropenia [5]

Neutropenia is a syndrome caused by a decrease in the absolute value of peripheral blood granulocytes. Neutropenia is diagnosed based on an absolute neutrophil count less than 1.0×10^9/L in children aged 2 weeks to 1 year old, or less than 1.5×10^9/L in children aged over 1 year old. Agranulocytosis is defined as an absolute neutrophil count less than 0.5×10^9/L.

CAL [5]

The diagnosis of CAL is based on the following three criteria: 1) Coronary artery dilation: coronary artery diameter > 2.5 mm in children < 3 years old, > 3 mm in children 3–9 years old, and > 3.5 mm in children older than 9; as well as diameter of one segment of the coronary artery more than 1.5 times that of the adjacent segment; 2) Coronary artery aneurysm (CAA): ratio of the diameter of the coronary artery to the adjacent segment > 1.5, and diameter of the coronary artery > 4 mm. Small, medium, and giant CAAs are defined based on the coronary artery diameter: < 5 mm, 5–8 mm and > 8 mm, respectively. 3) Coronary artery stenosis and embolism: coronary artery diameter reduction, irregular and asymmetric tube wall or irregularity and interruption of the lumen of the continuous non echo area.

Statistical analysis

Statistical analyses were performed using SPSS version 19. Measurement data are expressed by the median and the interquartile range, and the count data is represented by the number of cases and the percentage. Continuous variables were compared using Kruskal-Wallis test and categorical variables were compared using Chi-square test. Logistic regression analysis and curve fitting were used to analyze the correlation between degree of reduction in granulocytes and CAL. All tests were considered significant under the 0.05 level.

Results

Comparison of laboratory parameters between KD patients with and without neutropenia

Table 1 shows the laboratory parameters of children in the NKD and NNKD groups. There was a statistically significant difference between groups in pre-treatment white blood cell count (WBC), absolute neutrophil count

Table 1 Laboratory parameters of children with KD

Laboratory parameters	NKD	NNKD	*P* value
CRP (mg/L)	70.1(32.90–105.0)	74.7(37.95–118.0)	0.147
WBC ($\times 10^9$/L)	14.27(11.24–19.04)	15.60(11.91–19.82)	0.028
ANC1 ($\times 10^9$/L)	0.99(0.75–1.25)	3.53(2.09–4.20)	< 0.001
ANC ($\times 10^9$/L)	8.66(5.96–12.64)	9.89(7.02–13.67)	0.002
△ANC ($\times 10^9$/L)	7.84(4.87–11.48)	6.49(3.57–10.17)	0.001
Hb (g/L)	109(102–115)	110(102–117)	0.268
ALT (U/L)	29.5(17.0–72.5)	32.0(17.8–90.0)	0.304
ESR (mm/h)	37.0(24.3–46.0)	35.0(26.0–45.0)	0.720
PLT ($\times 10^9$/L)	376(299–465)	359(294–449)	0.191
ALB (g/L)	33.0(28.9–39.1)	33.3(29.1–38.4)	0.886
BNP (pg/ml)	670(319–1543)	725(305–1934)	0.528
Na (mmol/L)	136.0(134.1–137.6)	136.1(134.2–137.7)	0.433
PT (s)	13.2(12.8–13.9)	13.6(12.9–14.3)	0.001
APTT (s)	41.0(37.6–44.8)	41.8(37.9–46.4)	0.184
TT (s)	14.8(14.2–15.4)	14.7(14.1–15.3)	0.234
FIB (g/L)	5.5(4.4–6.4)	5.9(4.9–7.0)	0.004
D-Dimer (μg/ml)	1.0(0.6–1.8)	1.4(0.8–2.3)	0.002

ANC1 absolute neutrophil count after IVIG treatment. Values are expressed as Median (interquartile range) / Number (percentage). Continuous variables were compared using Kruskal-Wallis test, categorical variables were compared using Chi-square test

(ANC), difference in absolute neutrophil count before and after treatment (△ANC), D-Dimer level, fibrinogen (FIB) level, and prothrombin time (PT). We found that (1) neutropenic KD patients had lower WBC and ANC levels in the acute phase after IVIG treatment ($P = 0.028$ and $P = 0.002$, respectively); (2) there was a greater reduction in ANC levels in the NKD group than the NNKD group ($P = 0.001$); and (3) D-Dimer, FIB and PT were lower in the NKD group than in the NNKD group ($P = 0.002$, $P = 0.004$, and P = 0.001, respectively).

Comparison of treatment protocols between KD patients with and without neutropenia

We compared differences in IVIG treatment duration, IVIG dosage, use of dipyridamole, incidence of CAL after treatment, incidence of IVIG non-responders and gender between NKD and NNKD groups. We found that (1) IVIG treatment duration differed between the two groups, being longer in the NKD than the NNKD group (P = 0.002); (2) the incidence of neutropenia in children treated with the 2 g/kg*1d scheme was lower than in those treated with 1 g/kg*2d ($P = 0.009$); (3) in patients followed up with UCG for 3 months after IVIG treatment, the incidence of CAL was higher in the NKD group than in the NNKD group ($P = 0.008$); and (4) the probability of male patients with neutropenia in the NKD was higher than that in the NNKD group, but there's no sex differences between groups ($P = 0.715$) (Table 2).

Subgroup analysis of CAL between KD patients with and without neutropenia

As mentioned above, patients followed up with UCG for 3 months after IVIG treatment, the incidence of CAL was higher in the NKD group than in the NNKD group (P = 0.008). Then we performed statistical analysis of the 3 subgroups according to the standard of CAL. As shown in Table 3, we found that the smaller the age, the greater the probability of CAL, regardless of whether there is neutropenia in children with KD. The incidence of CAL in NKD group was higher than NNKD group in children with KD less than 3 years of age, but there was no statistical difference ($P = 0..110$).

Table 2 Treatment and outcome of children with KD

Group	NKD	NNKD	*P* value
IVIG treatment duration (days)	7(6–8)	6(6–7)	0.002
IVIG dosage			0.009
2d/kg*1d	77(14.3%)	462(85.7%)	
1 g/kg*2d	43(22.4%)	149(77.6%)	
dipyridamole	39(37.5%)	224(33.3%)	0.404
CAL after treatment[a]	58(31.9%)	250(22.8%)	0.008
CAA after treatment	4(6.9%)	26(10.4%)	0.418
IVIG nonresponders	5(3.0%)	51(5.8%)	0.167
Gender			0.715
Female	63(32.0%)	389(33.3%)	
Male	134(68.0%)	779(66.7%)	

[a]CAL after treatment is defined as patients with persistent CAL after IVIG treatment. Values are expressed as Median (interquartile range) / Number (percentage). Continuous variables were compared using Kruskal-Wallis test, categorical variables were compared using Chi-square test

Comparison of the proportion of CAA in the NKD and NNKD

There are 30 patients developed CAA followed up with UCG for 3 months after IVIG treatment. The incidence of CAA in NKD was lower than NNKD, but there was no statistical difference. CAA was divided into small, medium and giant according to the size of the internal diameter, the proportion of each of the two groups was shown in Table 4. Comparison of the incidence of CAA among small and medium, medium and giant, small and giant, with no statistical significance ($P = 0.131$, $P = 0.308$ and $P = 0.656$, respectively).

Comparison of clinical manifestations between KD patients with and without neutropenia

Table 5 shows the incidence of five common clinical manifestations among children with and without neutropenic KD. There are no statistically significant differences between groups in the incidence of rash, conjunctivitis, changes in lips, and changes in extremities. However, the incidence of cervical lymphadenopathy was significantly higher in the NNKD group ($P < 0.001$).

The correlation between the degree of reduction in granulocyte count and CAL

To analyze the relationship between reduced granulocyte count and CAL, we first performed a logistic regression analysis using △ANC as the continuous variable and CAL within 3 months after treatment as the dependent variable. We found no significant correlation between the degree of reduction in granulocytes and the risk of CAL within 3 months after treatment, even after controlling for age and sex.

Secondly, we performed a logistic regression analysis using five categories of △ANC as the continuous variable and CAL within 3 months after treatment as the dependent

Table 3 Subgroup analysis of KD patients with CAL

Group	NKD	NNKD	*P* value
CAL	58(31.9%)	250(22.8%)	0.008
< 3 (years)	54(93.1%)	213(85.2%)	0.110
3–9(years)	4(6.9%)	35(14.0%)	0.143
> 9(years)	0	2(0.8%)	–

Values are expressed as Number (percentage). Categorical variables were compared using Chi-square test

Table 4 The proportion of CAA in patients with KD

Group	NKD	NNKD	*P* value
CAA	4(13.3%)	26(86.7%)	0.418
Small CAA	1(6.3%)	15(93.7%)	0.131[a]
Medium CAA	3(27.3%)	8(72.7%)	0.308[b]
Giant CAA	0	3(100%)	0.656[c]

Values are expressed as Number (percentage). Categorical variables were compared using Chi-square test. a. statistical results between small CAA and medium CAA; b. statistical results between medium CAA and giant CAA; c. statistical results between small CAA and giant CAA

variable. We found that the risk of CAL was lowest when the absolute reduction in granulocytes was between 5.653 to 7.850 (OR = 0.768; 0.507, 1.165). This was true even after controlling for age and sex (OR = 0.760; 0.499, 1.158) (Table 6).

Finally, we generated a curve using △ANC as the continuous variable and CAL within 3 months after treatment as the dependent variable (Fig. 1). Threshold effect analysis identified the break point as 6 (△ANC = 6 × 10^9/L). We found a correlation between the degree of reduction in granulocytes and CAL when the break point is greater than 6, with a higher rate of CAL in patients with a greater reduction in granulocytes ($P = 0.0323$).

Discussion

KD is a systemic vasculitis that presents as an acute febrile illness. CAL is the main complication of this disease, and its incidence can be reduced by high-dose IVIG treatment, which acts to reduce inflammation [6]. In our practice, we have found that KD patients treated with IVIG often have reduced neutrophil counts during follow up, and some even developed agranulocytosis. In this study, patients were divided into two groups for statistical analysis, and we found that the incidence of neutropenia after IVIG treatment was related to the IVIG dosage protocol. Namely, we found that the 2 g/kg*1d scheme was associated with a reduced incidence of neutropenia compared to the 1 g/kg*2d scheme. Furthermore, at the 3-month follow-up, we found that there was a statistically significant difference in the incidence of CAL between groups, which was higher in patients with NKD. Then we performed a subgroup analysis of the different age groups according to the CAL

Table 5 Clinical manifestations of KD in children

Group	NKD	NNKD	*P* value
rash	145(73.6%)	865(74.1%)	0.893
conjunctivitis	172(87.3%)	1005(86.0%)	0.634
changes in lips	177(89.8%)	1087(93.1%)	0.111
changes in extremities	139(70 .6%)	867(74.2%)	0.279
cervical lymphadenopathy	95(48.2%)	747(64.0%)	< 0.001

Values are expressed as Number (percentage). Categorical variables were compared using Chi-square test

Table 6 The independent effect of △ANC on the risk of CAL among KD patients

Exposure	Non-adjusted	Adjusted
△ANC (× 10^9/L)	1.000(0.989,1.012)0.935	1.000(0.989,1.011)0.984
△ANC(×10^9/L) (equal percentiles)		
≤ 3.015	1.0	1.0
3.016–5.652	0.879(0.585,1.320)0.534	0.873(0.578,1.319)0.519
5.653–7.850	0.768(0.507,1.165)0.214	0.760(0.499,1.158)0.202
7.851–11.474	1.042(0.700,1.552)0.839	1.021(0.682,1.528)0.919
≥ 11.475	1.091(0.734,1.621)0.667	1.138(0.762,1.702)0.527

Values are expressed as OR (95%CI) P value;
Adjusted model: age (months); gender;

criteria. It was found that the incidence of CAL in NKD group higher than NNKD group in children with KD less than 3 years of age, but there was no statistical significance. Similarly, there were no statistically significant differences in the incidence of CAL among the subgroups.

CAL is the most common complication of KD and is associated with fever duration [7–9], vascular endothelial growth factor [10, 11], B-type natriuretic peptide [12], serum albumin [13], serum sodium [14], CRP [15], platelet-neutrophil aggregates [6], and inflammatory cytokines including tumor necrosis factor-α and inter-leukin-6 [15, 16]. In this study, we found that some patients developed neutropenia after IVIG treatment. These patients were followed up with UCG at 3 months, and we identified a higher incidence of CAL in patients who developed neutropenia after treatment. The curve fitting analysis of the degree of reduction in granulocytes and CAL shows that when the breaking point is 6 (△ANC = 6 × 10^9/L); that is, the rate of CAL is higher when the degree of reduction in granulocytes is greater. Therefore, children who develop neutropenia after IVIG treatment should be followed up with regular UCG in

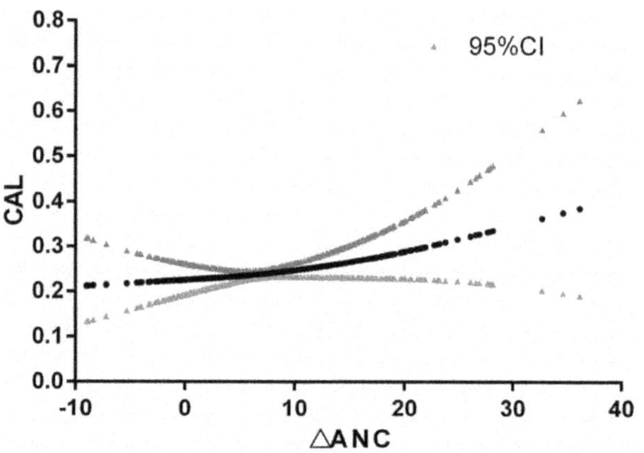

Fig. 1 Threshold effect analysis takes the break point (k) as 6. When k < 6 the OR = 0.97 (0.91, 1.03) and $p = 0.3164$; when k > 6, the OR = 1.04 (1.00, 1.07) and $p = 0.0323$

order to facilitate the early detection and treatment of CAL, and this is especially important in children with a significant reduction in granulocytes.

KD is an inflammatory disease and neutrophils are important mediators involved in the inflammatory response. Consistent with the results described in this study, Tsujimoto et al [17] found that treatment with IVIG resulted in a significant reduced in neutrophil counts. The mechanisms for this observation have not been clearly elucidated, but we propose several plausible explanations. First, in our study, 30–50 mg/kg aspirin therapy was used in children with KD on admission, drawing blood from the vein when defervescence after 3 days and aspirin did not decrease at the same time, therefore, aspirin induced neutropenia is not considered. IVIG is another effective drug for the treatment of KD, and it has been reported that IVIG can induce neutrophil apoptosis and degranulation in vitro [18]. IVIG inhibits the activated immune system, lowers the levels of inflammatory factors, and reduces the production of cytokines, thereby reducing the inhibition of neutrophil apoptosis. IVIG mainly acts through the Fas pathway and the caspase pathway. IVIG contains Fas antibody which contributes to apoptosis by activating the intracellular caspase system after binding to the Fas antigen on neutrophils and monocytes [4]. Second, KD is an autoimmune disease characterized by elevated neutrophil counts in the acute phase, with neutrophil destruction by autoantibodies during convalescence [5]. Third, the results of this study show that the level of WBC and neutrophils in children with neutropenia before IVIG treatment is lower than in those without neutropenia, and therefore it is possible that the neutropenia after treatment may be related to the basal neutrophil count at the time of disease onset.

This study is strengthened by its large sample size. However, there are certain limitations worth noting. First, our study is a single center study and therefore further multicenter studies are warranted in order to assess the generalizability of these findings. Second, the results may lack some accuracy due to the small sample of patients included in the IVIG dosage sub-analysis.

Conclusions

Neutropenia is an important complication in children with KD treated with IVIG, and is less likely among those treated with 2 g/kg*1d IVIG. The results of UCG follow-up showed that the probability of CAL was higher in patients with neutropenic KD compared to non-neutropenic KD, and in patients with a greater reduction in granulocyte counts. Therefore, children with KD should be treated with 2 g/kg*1d IVIG and monitored to prevent a large degree of reduction in granulocytes ($\triangle ANC \geq 6 \times 10^9/L$). Early diagnosis and treatment of CAL is essential to maximizing outcomes in this patient population.

Abbreviations

ALB: Albumin; ALT: Alanine transaminase; ANC: Absolute neutrophil count; APTT: Activated partial thromboplastin time; BNP: Brain natriuretic peptide; CAA: Coronary artery aneurysm; CAL: Coronary artery lesions; CRP: C-Reactive protein; ESR: erythrocyte sedimentation rate; FIB: Fibrinogen; Hb: Hemoglobin; IVIG: Intravenous immune globulin; KD: Kawasaki disease; Na: Sodium; PLT: Platelets; PT: Prothrombin time; TT: Thromboplastin time; UCG: Ultrasonic echocardiography; WBC: White blood cell

Acknowledgements

Not applicable.

Funding

None.

Authors' contributions

ZQW and FFW conceptualized and designed the study, collected the data, drafted the initial manuscript. HYS carried out the statistics. CL and ZKT made substantial contributions to the design of the paper, and its interpretation. HXQ and YEH reviewed and revised the manuscript for important intellectual content. RZW and MPC reviewed and revised the manuscript. All authors read and contributed to the present manuscript. All authors read and approved the final manuscript.

Competing interests

The authors declare that they have no competing interests.

Author details

[1]Children's Heart Center, the Second Affiliated Hospital and Yuying Children's Hospital, Institute of cardiovascular development and translational medicine, Wenzhou Medical University, Wenzhou, Zhejiang 325027, China. [2]Children's Hospital, Zhejiang University School of Medicine, Hangzhou, Zhejiang 310051, China. [3]Department of Preventive Medicine, School of Environmental Science and Public Health, Wenzhou Medical University, Wenzhou, Zhejiang 325035, China.

References

1. Research Committee of the Japanese Society of Pediatric C, Cardiac Surgery Committee for Development of Guidelines for Medical Treatment of Acute Kawasaki D. Guidelines for medical treatment of acute Kawasaki disease: report of the research Committee of the Japanese Society of pediatric cardiology and cardiac surgery (2012 revised version). Pediatr Int. 2014;56(2):135–58.
2. Newburger JW, Takahashi M, Gerber MA, Gewitz MH, Tani LY, Burns JC, Shulman ST, Bolger AF, Ferrieri P, Baltimore RS, et al. Diagnosis, treatment, and long-term management of Kawasaki disease: a statement for health professionals from the committee on rheumatic fever, Endocarditis, and Kawasaki disease, council on cardiovascular disease in the young, American Heart Association. Pediatrics. 2004;114(6):1708–33.
3. Okuma Y, Suda K, Nakaoka H, Katsube Y, Mitani Y, Yoshikane Y, Ichida F, Matsushita T, Shichino H, Shiraishi I, et al. Serum Tenascin-C as a novel predictor for risk of coronary artery lesion and resistance to intravenous immunoglobulin in Kawasaki disease- a multicenter retrospective study. Circ J. 2016;80(11):2376–81.
4. Yinhong Lu YW. Effect of intravenous immunoglobulin on neutrophil in patients with Kawasaki's disease. Zhongguo Dang Dai Er Ke Za Zhi. 2010;12(12):991–2.
5. Zhang YY, Zhou AH, Zhang YH, et al. Epidemiologic study of children admitted to hospital with Kawasaki disease in Wenzhou from 2001 to 2010. Chin J Rheumatol. 2012;16(11):763–6.

6. Ueno K, Nomura Y, Morita Y, Eguchi T, Masuda K, Kawano Y. Circulating platelet-neutrophil aggregates play a significant role in Kawasaki disease. Circ J. 2015;79(6):1349–56.
7. Beiser ASTM, Baker AL, Sundel RP, Newburger JW. A predictive instrument for coronary artery aneurysms in Kawasaki disease: US multicenter Kawasaki disease study group. Am J Cardiol. 1998;81:1116–20.
8. Ruan YYB, Zhao X. Clinical characteristics of Kawasaki syndrome and the risk factors for coronary artery lesions in China. Pediatr Infect Dis J. 2013;32:e397–402.
9. Song DYY, Ha K, Jang G, Lee J, Lee K, et al. Risk factors for Kawasaki disease-associated coronary abnormalities differ depending on age. Eur J Pediatr. 2009;168:1315–21.
10. Ohno TYT, Kariyazono H, Igarashi H, Joh-o K, Kinugawa N, et al. Serum hepatocyte growth factor combined with vascular endothelial growth factor as a predictive indicator for the occurrence of coronary artery lesions in Kawasaki disease. Eur J Pediatr. 2002;161:105–11.
11. Terai MHT, Yasukawa K, Higashi K, Hamada H, Kohno Y. Prognostic impact of vascular leakage in acute Kawasaki disease. Circulation. 2003;108:325–30.
12. Kaneko KYK, Ohashi A, Kimata T, Shimo T, Tsuji S. Prediction of the risk of coronary arterial lesions in Kawasaki disease by brain natriuretic peptide. Pediatr Cardiol. 2011;32:1106–9.
13. Printz BFSL, Newburger JW, Minich LL, Bradley T, Cohen MS, et al. Noncoronary cardiac abnormalities are associated with coronary artery dilation and with laboratory inflammatory markers in acute Kawasaki disease. J Am Coll Cardiol. 2011;57:86–92.
14. Nakamura YYM, Uehara R, Watanabe M, Tajimi M, Oki I, et al. Use of laboratory data to identify risk factors of giant coronary aneurysms due to Kawasaki disease. Pediatr Int. 2004;46:33–8.
15. Koyanagi HYH, Nakamura Y, Yashiro M. Serum C-reactive protein levels in patients with Kawasaki disease: from the results of nation-wide surveys of Kawasaki disease in Japan. Acta Paediatr. 1997;86:613–9.
16. Lin CYLC, Hwang B, Chiang BN. Cytokines predict coronary aneurysm formation in Kawasaki disease patients. Eur J Pediatr. 1993;152:309–12.
17. Tsujimoto HTS, Nakatani K, Kawamura Y, Tokutomi T, Sekine I. Intravenous immunoglobulin therapy induces neutrophil apoptosis in Kawasaki disease. Clin Immunol. 2002;103(2):161–8.
18. Ansari SSA, Khalili N, Daneshfar R, Arefi H. Neutropenia following intravenous immunoglobulin therapy in pediatric patients with idiopathic thrombocytopenic purpura. IJBC. 2014;6(2):81–5.

13

Prospective observational study on assessing the hemodynamic relevance of patent ductus arteriosus with frequency domain near-infrared spectroscopy

Christoph E. Schwarz[1*], Antonio Preusche[2], Martin Wolf[3], Christian F. Poets[4] and Axel R. Franz[5,6]

Abstract

Background: What constitutes a hemodynamically relevant patent ductus arteriosus (hrPDA) in preterm infants is unclear. Different clinical and echocardiographic parameters are used, but a gold standard definition is lacking.
Our objective was to evaluate associations between regional cerebral tissue oxygen saturation ($rcStO_2$), fraction of tissue oxygen extraction ($rcFtO_2E$) measured by frequency domain near-infrared spectroscopy (fd-NIRS) and their correlation to echocardiographic, Doppler-ultrasound, and clinical parameters in preterm infants with and without a hrPDA.

Methods: In this prospective observational study, 22 infants < 1500 g (mean [± SD]: gestational age 28.6 [±1.8] weeks, birth weight 1076 [±284] g, median (interquartile range) postnatal age at measurement 7.6 (4.6–12.9) d) with a clinical suspicion of hrPDA were analysed.
Twelve infants had left-to-right shunt through PDA, and in 6 of these the PDA was classified as hrPDA based on pre-defined clinical and echocardiographic criteria. fd-NIRS, echocardiographic and Doppler-ultrasound examinations were performed. After identification of blood hemoglobin (Hb) as confounding factor, $rcStO_2$ and $rcFtO_2E$ were corrected for this effect.

Results: Overall mean ± standard deviation (normalised to a median Hb of 13.8 mg/dl) was 57 ±5% for $rcStO_2$ and 0.39 ±0.05 for $rcFtO_2E$. Comparing no-hrPDA with hrPDA infants, there were no significant differences in mean $rcStO_2$ (58 ±5% vs. 54 ±5%; $p = .102$), but in mean $rcFtO_2E$ (0.38 ±0.05 vs. 0.43 ±0.05; $p = .038$). Echocardiographic parameter and Doppler indices did not correlate with cerebral oxygenation.

Conclusion: Oxygen transport capacity of the blood may confound NIRS data interpretation. Cerebral oxygenation determined by fd-NIRS provided additional information for PDA treatment decisions not offered by routine investigations. Whether indicating PDA therapy based on echocardiography complemented by data on cerebral oxygenation results in better outcomes should be investigated in future studies.

Keywords: Doppler-ultrasound, Cerebral oxygenation, Tissue oxygenation, Near-infrared spectroscopy, Echocardiography, Patent ductus arteriosus, Preterm infants

* Correspondence: c.schwarz@med.uni-tuebingen.de
[1]Department of Neonatology, University Children's Hospital, Calwerstr. 7, 72076 Tuebingen, Germany
Full list of author information is available at the end of the article

Background

Screening for, and therapy of, patent ductus arteriosus (PDA) in preterm infants is associated with decreased mortality and morbidity [1]. However, there is little evidence as to which parameters define a PDA that requires treatment, i.e. is hemodynamically relevant (hrPDA). Zonnenberg and de Waal summarized which echocardiographic and Doppler-ultrasound measurements, besides clinical parameters, have been used to evaluate the magnitude and clinical relevance of left-to-right shunting through a PDA [2]. Scoring Systems like the one suggested by McNamara and Sehgal include clinical and echocardiographic criteria to define hrPDA [3]. The echocardiographic part of this staging is useful to predict neonatal morbidity and may serve as a guide to clinical decision-making [4]. Resistive index (RI) in the anterior cerebral artery (ACA) was shown to be significantly higher in infants with hrPDA [5].

With frequency domain near-infrared spectroscopy (fd-NIRS) regional cerebral tissue oxygen saturation ($rcStO_2$) and (together with pulse oximetry data) tissue oxygen extraction ($rcFtO_2E$) may be monitored noninvasively. In a recent observational study using continuous wave (cw) NIRS, significant differences in cerebral oxygenation over time were observed in infants born below 32 weeks gestation within their first 6 postnatal days [6]. Such an effect, however, was not identified in other recent studies using this technique [7, 8].

To inform future studies and clinical guidelines on PDA treatment, this study aimed to evaluate the absolute cerebral oxygenation of preterm infants besides echocardiographic and Doppler-ultrasound parameters, which are frequently determined to assess the need for PDA treatment.

Methods

This prospective observational cohort study was approved by the institutional research ethics committee and written informed parental consent obtained. Inclusion criteria were gestational age (GA) <37 weeks, birth weight (bw) ≤1500 g and clinical suspicion of hrPDA such as cardiac murmur, bounding pulses, ventilator dependency, metabolic acidosis and increased oxygen requirements. Syndromal anomalies and congenital heart defects except persisting foramen ovale or atrial septal defect were exclusion criteria. Recruitment took place from June 2012 to May 2013 and September 2015 to March 2016 at the tertiary level neonatal intensive care unit of the university children's hospital, Tuebingen, Germany.

Fd-NIRS-measurements

In infants with clinical indication for echocardiography based on a clinical suspicion of PDA, fd-NIRS was measured at the time of echocardiography. The reflectance mode multi-distance fd-NIRS device OxiplexTS (ISS Inc. Champaign, Illinois, U.S.A.) measures mean intensity (DC), modulation amplitude (AC) and phase shift (PH) at 4 distances and 2 wavelengths and determines absolute values of cerebral oxy-, deoxy-, total hemoglobin concentration and $rcStO_2$. The optode was placed, as previously described [9], in a temporo-parietal position half-way between tragus and sagittal suture. The optode was held by the examiner for 5 consecutive measurements of 1 min each at either side of the head; it was repositioned between measurement runs [9]. The tissue water content was assumed to be 90% [10]. To exclude effects of tissue inhomogeneity, a quality criteria algorithm was used with r^2 >0.8 in the linear regression analyses for AC, DC and PH over the four emitter-optode distances as surrogate according to Arri et al. [11]. We decided to use this cut-off because higher cut-offs for r^2 were unable to increase precision significantly but led to loss of information. To overcome inaccuracy of single measurements [12] we used the mean of up to 10 measurements over 1 min each. Recording frequency was 1 Hz. Intra-observer repeatability was evaluated post-hoc by within-subject SD (SD_W) estimated as square root of the residual mean square by oneway-ANOVA with subject as factor according to Hyttel-Sorensen et al. [13]. The SD_W was ±7% for $rcStO_2$ and ±0.08 for $rcFtO_2E$.

Echocardiographic and Doppler-ultrasound measurements

The Parameters assessed were LA/Ao-ratio [14], diameter of the PDA at its narrowest part [15], the left-ventricular-preejection-period-to-ejection-time-ratio, calculated by including 3–4 cardiac cycles (LVPEP/LVET) [16], and the ratio of the velocity time integrals in the large vessels aorta and pulmonary artery (VTI_Ao/VTI_PA). The VTI_Ao was recorded from an apical-5-chamber-view, the VTI_PA in a parasternal short axis. We assumed that, in the absence of congenital heart defects, this ratio correlates with the ductal left-to-right shunt. After visualisation of the whole course of the PDA, its diameter was measured at its narrowest part (identified via colour-Doppler in the high left-sided parasternal "ductal" view and the suprasternal view) and measured in B-Mode to avoid the influence of gain-settings on the PDA-width. RI in celiac artery (CA) [17] and ACA [18] were measured as well. Based on our previous analyses on repeatability of echocardiographic parameters [19], mean values of repeated measurements were assessed whenever possible (i.e., in 18/22 infants, in 4 patients only single measurements were available).

All measurements were performed with a Toshiba "Aplio" using a 6.5 MHz phased array transducer (Toshiba Medical Systems, Otawara-shi, Tochigi-ken, Japan) or a Zonare ZS3 using C10–3 curved-phased array transducer (Zonare Medical Systems, Inc., Mountain View, CA,

U.S.A.). For calculation of velocity time integrals, the former device enables automatic detection while the latter device requires manual circumscription of the Doppler wave form.

Cardiorespiratory monitoring and laboratory investigations

During measurements, heart rate (HR) and peripheral arterial oxygen saturation (SpO_2) were monitored in all patients via pulse oximetry (Radical 7; Masimo Corporation, Irvine, CA, U.S.A.) and the SpO_2 was targeted at 90–95% if on supplemental oxygen and at > 89% if no supplemental oxygen was used. Averaging and recording intervals were 2 s each. As for fd-NIRS measurements, we calculated means for each 1-min measurement of these parameters. Blood hemoglobin concentration (Hb in g/dL) from clinically indicated whole blood counts was extracted from patients' charts if determined within ±12 h of NIRS-measurements or by linear interpolation of the two adjacent Hb concentrations.

Definition of hrPDA

According to the clinical standard in use in the unit, hrPDA was defined if a left-to-right shunt through a PDA was confirmed by echocardiography and at least 3 of the following 6 criteria were met:

1. LA/Ao-ratio >1.5
2. PDA diameter ≥1.5 mm/kg bodyweight
3. Need of respiratory support (mechanical Ventilation or continuous positive airway pressure with supplemental oxygen)
4. Reverse or zero end diastolic flow in ACA (=RI_ACA ≥ 1)
5. Reverse or zero end diastolic flow in CA (=RI_ CA ≥ 1)
6. LVPEP/LVET <0.32

Infants with left-to-right shunt through a PDA meeting less than 3 of the above listed criteria were classified as hiPDA (hemodynamically irrelevant) and allocated, together with infants without a PDA, to the no-hrPDA group.

Statistical analyses

$RcStO_2$ was extracted and $rcFtO_2E$ calculated from $rcStO_2$ and SpO_2 data according to Naulaers et al. [20]. Results were screened for potential confounding factors (GA, BW, age at measurement (AAM), gender, Hb, small for gestational age (SGA)) by Spearman-Rho/Pearson correlation coefficient and Fisher's exact test, as appropriate. If a statistically significant influence was identified on univariate analysis, $rcStO_2$ and $rcFtO_2E$ were normalized for the median of this confounding factor.

Patients were stratified into 2 groups: no-hrPDA and hrPDA according to echocardiographic and clinical parameters (see definition of hrPDA). Demographic, neonatal and echocardiographic parameters were tested for significant group differences using t-, Mann-Whitney-U and Fisher's exact test, oneway-ANOVA or Welch-Test, as appropriate.

$RcStO_2$ and $rcFtO_2E$ were tested for statistically significant differences with oneway-ANOVA after confirmation of normal distribution (Shapiro-Wilk) and homogeneity of variances (Levene-statistics).

A p-value below.05 was set to indicate statistical significance. Data are presented as median and interquartile range (IQR) or mean and ± standard deviation (±SD) if not noted otherwise. Where appropriate, 95% confidence intervals (CI) were added. SPSS-Statistics (Version 24.0.0.0, IBM Corporation, Armonk, NY, U.S.A.) was used for statistical analyses.

Results

Demographic and neonatal parameters

Twenty-four infants were included in the study. One infant with a BW of 1550 g was included inadvertently due to a body weight at the time of measurement of 1465 g (hiPDA). Two infants were excluded: one infant of 23 weeks GA, BW 360 g, due to fulminant sepsis a few hours after inclusion leading to its demise (hrPDA), so that cerebral oxygenation and hemodynamics could have been corrupted, the other (GA 26 weeks, BW 745 g) due to a ventricular septal defect found during his study echocardiography (hiPDA). Demographic and clinical data of the 22 preterm infants analysed in this cohort are summarized in Table 1.

Three infants in the hrPDA group had indomethacin within 24 h prior to measurements (0.1/0.2/0.4 mg/kg BW/day, respectively). Overall, 5 patients needed inotropes and 6 had medical therapy for PDA closure according to the clinical standard in use in the unit. No infant underwent surgical closure of PDA.

Echocardiographic und Doppler-ultrasound measurements

A left-to-right shunt through PDA was identified by colour-Doppler-ultrasound in 12/22 measurements. PDA-diameter at the narrowest part could rarely be measured (n = 6) due to difficulties visualizing the PDA in its complete course in B-mode. PDA staging classified 6 PDAs as hrPDA and 6 as hiPDA. All 6 parameters used to define hrPDA were relevantly different between groups. Mean VTI_Ao/VTI_PA in hrPDA vs. no-hrPDA was 1.43 ±0.56 (95% CI 0.84, 2.02) vs. 0.93 ±0.24 (95% CI 0.80,1.06), p = .085 (Table 2).

NIRS and confounding factors

The oxygen transport capacity of the blood represented by Hb concentration was identified as a confounding

Table 1 Neonatal characteristics and influence factors

Neonatal variable	hrPDA $n=6$	no-hrPDA $n=16$	p
Gestational age (weeks)	28.5 (25.9–29.4)	28.8 (28.5–29.7)	0.33
Birth weight (g)	1110 (793–1128)	1090 (879–1346)	0.43
Small for gestational age	0	2	
Male	2	11	0.18
Age at measurement (d)	4.7 (4.6–7.2)	8.1 (4.5–21.7)	0.26
Weight at measurement (g)	1118 (788–1162)	1233 (1001–1675)	0.23
Mechanical Ventilation	2	2	
CPAP	4	9	
Fraction of inspired Oxygen	0.23	0.21	0.80
Hb (g/dl)	15.0 (13.9–15.2)	12.6 (11.2–14.6)	0.08
SpO_2 (%)	94 (93–96)	95 (92–95)	0.51
HR (1/min)	163 (158–175)	161 (154–168)	0.33
meanBP (mmHg)	37 (35–40)	46 (41–49)	0.01
Inotropes	0	0	

Values are median (interquartile range) or n; CPAP: continuous positive airway pressure, Hb: hemoglobin concentration, SpO_2: pulse oximetry measured arterial oxygen saturation, HR: heart rate, meanBP: mean blood pressure

factor on $rcStO_2$ and $rcFtO_2E$ by Spearman-Rho (p = .022 and .004, respectively). Pearson correlation showed a significant influence as well (p = .023 and .003, respectively), supporting a linear relationship. We thus normalized $rcStO_2$ and $rcFtO_2E$ for Hb using the linear regression equation:

$$\text{normalized } rcStO_2 = 1,1312^*(\text{medianHb}-\text{patientHb}) + \text{measured } rcStO_2; r^2 = 0.2338$$

and

Table 2 Echocardiography/Doppler-ultrasound results

Parameter	hrPDA $n=6$	no-hrPDA $n=16$	p
Left-to-right shunt PDA	6	6	
LA/Ao	1.6 (1.4–1.8)	1.3 (1.2–1.5)	.15
PDA_diameter/kgBW	*1.6 (1.4–2.1)*	*0.6 (.6–.6)*	*ns*
RI_ACA	.86 (.83–.89)	.77 (.75–.82)	.01
RI_CA	1 (.86–1)	.77 (.71–.82)	.04
LVPEP/LVET	.26 (.21–.28)	.31 (.28–.33)	.09
VTI_Ao/VTI_PA	1.5 (.97–1.9)	.9 (.84–1.0)	.08

Values are median (interquartile range) or n; separated in hemodynamically relevant (hr) Patent ductus arteriosus (PDA) and no-hrPDA. Left atrium (LA), Aortic root (Ao), diameter of PDA, measured at its most constricted point, per kilogram of bodyweight (BW), Resistive indices (RI) in anterior cerebral artery (ACA) and celiac artery (CA), Left ventricular (LV) pre-ejection period (PEP) and ejection time (ET), Velocity time integral (VTI) and pulmonary artery (PA), bold: The ratio of VTI_Ao to VTI_PA was the only parameter not used in the definition of hrPDA, *italic*: PDA diameter/kgBW could rarely be measured (n = 6; 4 hrPDA and 2 no-hrPDA), statistical test: oneway-ANOVA or Welch-test, as appropriate

$$\text{normalized } rcFtO_2E = -0.0153^*(\text{medianHb}-\text{patientHb}) + \text{measured } rcFtO_2E; r^2 = 0.3669$$

After normalization for a median Hb value of 13.8 mg/dl, the overall mean $rcStO_2$ was 57 ±5% (95% CI: 55%, 60%) and mean $rcFtO_2E$ 0.40 ± 0.05 (95% CI 0.37, 0.41), respectively. Mean $RcStO_2$ of hrPDA vs. no-hrPDA infants was 54 ±5% (95% CI 49%, 59%) vs. 58 ±5% (95% CI 56%, 61%; p = .102). However, $rcFtO_2E$ mean was 0.43 ±0.05 (95% CI 0.38, 0.48) vs. 0.38 ±0.05 (95% CI 0.35, 0.40; p = .038) (Table 3).

None of the echocardiographic or Doppler-ultrasound parameters correlated significantly with Hb-normalized $rcStO_2$ or Hb-normalized $rcFtO_2E$.

Discussion

Using fd-NIRS and normalization for Hb, we found a significant difference in $rcFtO_2E$, but not in $rcStO_2$, between infants with vs. without hrPDA in our cohort. As neither Hb-normalized $rcStO_2$ nor $rcFtO_2E$ correlated with echocardiographic or Doppler-ultrasound parameters, fd-NIRS parameters of cerebral oxygenation may offer additional information and may help to better inform treatment decisions.

In general, a good diagnostic parameter can easily and quickly be determined, has high sensitivity and specificity and is not incriminating to measure in preterm infants. NIRS is a non-invasive technique, and lower cerebral oxygenation within the first 2 postnatal weeks has been associated with poorer neurodevelopmental long term outcome of preterm infants [21]. Suboptimal cerebral oxygenation due to a hrPDA may negatively influence brain growth at term-equivalent age [22] and, at least in animal models, $rcStO_2$ values below 40% are identified as a risk factor for an impaired neurodevelopment [23].

Data on PDA-related changes in cerebral oxygenation are still controversial, although an impact on cerebral oxygenation has been identified in several studies. In a recent prospective observational trial involving 380 infants of <32 weeks gestation studied during their first 6 days postnatal days, Dix et al. found significant differences in cerebral oxygenation over time [6]. In line with these data, $rcFtO_2E$ showed a statistically significant difference between hr- and non-hrPDA, whereas $rcStO_2$

Table 3 Cerebral Tissue Oximetry results

Parameter	hrPDA $n=6$	no-hrPDA $n=16$	p
$rcStO_2$ (%)	54 (±5)	58 (±5)	.102
$rcFtO_2E$	.43 (±.05)	.38 (±.05)	.038

Values are mean (±SD), test for significance: oneway-ANOVA, regional cerebral (rc) tissue oxygen saturation (StO_2) and fraction of tissue oxygen extraction (FtO_2E) normalized for median hemoglobin did not, but this latter observation may be due limited power due to our small sample size. Another explanation might be an effect of (small) changes in arterial oxygen saturation during measurements, which are not addressed by $rcStO_2$. Chock et al. studied 47 infants with GA below 29 weeks (21 echocardiographically stratified as hrPDA) and found no significant relationship to $rcStO_2$ [7]. In line with this, others reported data on 20 hrPDA compared with 29 non-hrPDA preterm infants (median GA 27.6 weeks, median BW 980 g) and found no significant effect on $rcStO_2$ or $rcFtO_2E$ [8]. Older observational trials found a pronounced impact of hrPDA on cerebral oxygenation in infants scheduled for surgical closure [24–28]. In the present cohort, no infants underwent surgical ligation due to a very restrictive policy on surgical PDA closure in our unit.

Contrary to previous studies using cw-NIRS devices, fd-NIRS provides absolute instead of trend values for $rcStO_2$ under the assumption of a homogenous semi-infinite tissue. Another advantage of this technique is the opportunity of extracting unprocessed optical raw data, enabling the introduction of a quality pre-analytic algorithm for using high quality data for analysis, thereby improving repeatability. A disadvantage is that this instrument is less practical for continuous bedside trend monitoring due to the use of fragile glass fibre cables as well as its non-disposable probe.

Overall mean values for $rcStO_2$ were within the (lower) normal range [29], taking into account that this "normal range" was established for the first 72 h of life, while our cohort consisted of older preterm infants. Both, device and sensor, but also the clinical suspicion of hrPDA and/or the higher postnatal age may have contributed to these slightly lower values [30].

A variety of confounding factors impacting on cerebral oxygenation as measured with NIRS are known. Growth restriction, gender and gestational age have already been identified [6, 31, 32]. We were unable to reproduce these findings, possibly due to our low sample size. Only Hb concentration was identified as a confounder so that $rcStO_2$ and $rcFtO_2E$ were normalized for median Hb before further analysis. This should be addressed in future investigations. The higher $rcFtO_2E$ observed with hrPDA supports previous suggestions to maintain higher Hb concentrations in infants with hrPDA as part of conservative management [25]. Whether this might have an effect on long term outcome has not been studied yet.

We found no significant correlation between echocardiographic or Doppler-ultrasound parameters and cerebral oxygenation. A large number of different echocardiographic and Doppler-ultrasound parameters are used to quantify left-to-right shunting through, and hemodynamic relevance of, a PDA (summarised in [2]). This is reflected in NIRS-studies on hrPDA and its effect on cerebral oxygenation by relevant differences in hrPDA definition [7, 8, 33]. This substantially complicates comparisons between studies on hrPDA. The cut-offs used here reflect local preferences and the number of parameters tested was limited to reduce examination time and hence study-driven burden on infants.

To our knowledge only Dix et al. identified a significant relation between an echocardiographic parameter (ductal diameter) and $rcStO_2$ [6]. We were only rarely able to measure PDA diameter due to our strict definition of the most constricted point at the whole course of the PDA in B-mode. In line with our results Dix et al. found no relation between LA/Ao and cerebral oxygenation.

Before embarking on this study, we assumed that the VTI_Ao/VTI_PA-ratio might be another easily determined parameter suitable for quantifying ductal left-to-right shunt under the assumption of a "normal" ratio of Ao to PA valve-area. It is also important to have in mind that it could be corrupted by inter-atrial shunting, which is commonly observed in VLBW infants (and also in 20 of the infants studied here). However, this limitation also applies to LA/Ao ratio, the most commonly used parameter. VTI_Ao/VTI_PA-ratio has a relatively low repeatability and could be corrupted by ductal jet, although it is supposed to allow discrimination between hrPDA and hiPDA [19].

Limitations of this study are its small sample size and that extremely low gestational age infants, who are most likely to develop hrPDA, were under-represented. We have been reluctant to subject the more immature and hence more vulnerable infants to the additional study-related burden.

By contrast, it is a strength of our study that fd-NIRS was used, truly generating absolute values for $rcStO_2$ and $rcFtO_2E$ and that a rigorous quality assessment of the raw data preceded further analyses. Furthermore, we identified that Hb was an important confounder of cerebral oxygenation in this context and therefore assessed Hb-normalized values of NIRS parameters.

Only 5 patients overall were ever treated for PDA – this reflects the very restrictive approach to PDA treatment present in our unit - others may be more proactive [6].

Conclusions

Oxygen transport capacity of the blood may be taken into account for NIRS data interpretation. In our cohort we found a statistically significant difference in absolute cerebral oxygenation between clinically and echocardiographically defined hrPDA compared to no-hrPDA infants. Furthermore, our data suggest that parameters of cerebral oxygenation might offer additional information for the clinical decision whether or not to treat a PDA in an individual infant. Whether indicating PDA therapy based on echocardiography complemented by data on cerebral oxygenation results in better outcomes should be investigated in future studies.

Abbreviations

AAM: Age at measurement; AC: Modulation amplitude; ACA: Anterior cerebral artery; BW: Birthweight; CA: Celiac artery; CI: Confidence interval; cw: Continuous wave; DC: Mean intensity; fd: Frequency domain; GA: Gestational age; Hb: Hemoglobin concentration; hiPDA: Hemodynamically irrelevant PDA; hrPDA: Hemodynamically relevant PDA; IQR: Interquartile range; LA/Ao: Left-atrium-to-aortic-root-ratio; LVPEP/LVET: Left-ventricular-preejection-period-to-ejection-time-ratio; NIRS: Near-infrared spectroscopy; PDA: Patent ductus arteriosus; PH: Phase shift; $rcFtO_2E$: Regional cerebral fraction of tissue oxygen extraction; $rcStO_2$: Regional cerebral tissue oxygen saturation; RI: Resistive index; SD: Standard deviation; SGA: Small for gestational age; SpO_2: Pulse oximetry measured arterial oxygen saturation; VTI_Ao: Velocity time integral ascending Aorta; VTI_PA: Velocity time integral pulmonary artery; WAM: Body weight at measurement

Acknowledgements

We like to thank the parents of our patients to take part in this study with their preterm infants, the whole stuff of the neonatal intensive care unit in Tuebingen to support this study and we like to thank the „Else Kröner-Fresenius-Stiftung "for supporting this study. We acknowledge support by Deutsche Forschungsgemeinschaft and Open Access Publishing Fund of University of Tuebingen.

Authors' contributions

CES has contributed to the design of the study, measurements, statistical analysis, has drafted and revised the manuscript. AP has contributed to the measurements, statistical analysis and writing and revision of the manuscript. MW contributed to the design of the study, measurements, statistical analysis and critically reviewed the manuscript. CFP participated in the design of the study and critically reviewed the manuscript. ARF conceived the study and participated in its design, measurements, statistical analysis, acquisition of funding and coordination and helped to draft the manuscript. All authors read and approved the final manuscript.

Competing interests

The authors have no conflict of interest to declare.

Author details

[1]Department of Neonatology, University Children's Hospital, Calwerstr. 7, 72076 Tuebingen, Germany. [2]Department of Neonatology, University Children's Hospital, Tuebingen, Germany. [3]Department of Neonatology, University Hospital Zurich, Zurich, Switzerland. [4]Department of Neonatology, University Children's Hospital, Tuebingen, Germany. [5]Department of Neonatology, University Children's Hospital, Tuebingen, Germany. [6]Center for Pediatric Clinical Studies, University Children's Hospital, Tuebingen, Germany.

References

1. Rozé JCCG, Marchand-Martin L, Gournay V, Durrmeyer X, Durox M, Storme L, Porcher R, Ancel PY, Hemodynamic EPIPAGE 2 Study Group. Association between early screening for patent ductus arteriosus and in-hospital mortality among extremely preterm infants. JAMA. 2015;313(24):2441–8.
2. Zonnenberg I, de Waal K. The definition of a haemodynamic significant duct in randomized controlled trials: a systematic literature review. Acta Paediatr. 2012;101(3):247–51.
3. McNamara PJ, Sehgal A. Towards rational management of the patent ductus arteriosus: the need for disease staging. Arch Dis Child Fetal Neonatal Edition. 2007;92(6):F424–7.
4. Schena FFG, Cappelleri A, Picciolli I, Mayer A, Mosca F, Fumagalli M. Association between hemodynamically significant patent ductus arteriosus and bronchopulmonary dysplasia. J Pediatr. 2015;166(6):1488–92.
5. Ecury-Goossen GM, Raets MM, Camfferman FA, Vos RH, van Rosmalen J, Reiss IK, Govaert P, Dudink J. Resistive indices of cerebral arteries in very preterm infants: values throughout stay in the neonatal intensive care unit and impact of patent ductus arteriosus. Pediatr Radiol. 2016;46(9):1291–300.
6. Dix L, Molenschot M, Breur J, de Vries W, Vijlbrief D, Groenendaal F, van Bel F, Lemmers P. Cerebral oxygenation and echocardiographic parameters in preterm neonates with a patent ductus arteriosus: an observational study. Arch Dis Child Fetal Neonatal Ed. 2016;101:F520–6.
7. Chock VY, Rose LA, Mante JV, Punn R. Near-infrared spectroscopy for detection of a significant patent ductus arteriosus. Pediatr Res. 2016;80(5):675–80.
8. van der Laan ME, Roofthooft MT, Fries MW, Berger RM, Schat TE, van Zoonen AG, Tanis JC, Bos AF, Kooi EM. A hemodynamically significant patent ductus arteriosus does not affect cerebral or renal tissue oxygenation in preterm infants. Neonatology. 2016;110(2):141–7.
9. Demel A, Feilke K, Schoning M, Wolf M, Poets CF, Franz AR. Healthy term and moderately preterm infants have similar cerebral oxygen saturation and cerebral blood flow volumes during early post-natal transition. Acta Paediatr. 2015;104(8):e330–6.
10. Demel A, Wolf M, Poets CF, Franz AR. Effect of different assumptions for brain water content on absolute measures of cerebral oxygenation determined by frequency-domain near-infrared spectroscopy in preterm infants: an observational study. BMC Pediatr. 2014;14:206.
11. Arri SJ, Muehlemann T, Biallas M, Bucher HU, Wolf M. Precision of cerebral oxygenation and hemoglobin concentration measurements in neonates measured by near-infrared spectroscopy. J Biomed Opt. 2011;16(4):047005.
12. Sorensen LC, Greisen G. Precision of measurement of cerebral tissue oxygenation index using near-infrared spectroscopy in preterm neonates. J Biomed Opt. 2006;11(5):054005.
13. Hyttel-Sorensen S, Hessel TW, Greisen G. Peripheral tissue oximetry: comparing three commercial near-infrared spectroscopy oximeters on the forearm. J Clin Monit Comput. 2014;28(2):149–55.
14. Green TP, Thompson TR, Johnson DE, Lock JE. Furosemide promotes patent ductus arteriosus in premature infants with the respiratory-distress syndrome. N Engl J Med. 1983;308(13):743–8.
15. Kluckow M, Evans N. Early echocardiographic prediction of symptomatic patent ductus arteriosus in preterm infants undergoing mechanical ventilation. J Pediatr. 1995;127(5):774–9.
16. Robel-Tillig E, Knupfer M, Pulzer F, Vogtmann C. Dopplersonographic findings in neonates with significant persistent ductus arteriosus. Z Geburtshilfe Neonatol. 2002;206(2):51–6.
17. Shimada S, Kasai T, Konishi M, Fujiwara T. Effects of patent ductus arteriosus on left ventricular output and organ blood flows in preterm infants with respiratory distress syndrome treated with surfactant. J Pediatr. 1994;125(2):270–7.
18. Martin CG, Snider AR, Katz SM, Peabody JL, Brady JP. Abnormal cerebral blood flow patterns in preterm infants with a large patent ductus arteriosus. J Pediatr. 1982;101(4):587–93.
19. Schwarz CE, Preusche A, Baden W, Poets CF, Franz AR. Repeatability of echocardiographic parameters to evaluate the hemodynamic relevance of patent ductus arteriosus in preterm infants: a prospective observational study. BMC Pediatr. 2016;16:18.
20. Naulaers G, Meyns B, Miserez M, Leunens V, Van Huffel S, Casaer P, Weindling M, Devlieger H. Use of tissue oxygenation index and fractional tissue oxygen extraction as non-invasive parameters for cerebral oxygenation. A validation study in piglets. Neonatology. 2007;92(2):120–6.
21. Verhagen EA, Van Braeckel KN, van der Veere CN, Groen H, Dijk PH, Hulzebos CV, Bos AF. Cerebral oxygenation is associated with neurodevelopmental outcome of preterm children at age 2 to 3 years. Dev Med Child Neurol. 2015;57(5):449–55.
22. Lemmers PM, Benders MJ, D'Ascenzo R, Zethof J, Alderliesten T, Kersbergen KJ, Isgum I, de Vries LS, Groenendaal F, van Bel F. Patent ductus arteriosus and brain volume. Pediatrics. 2016;137(4):e20153090.
23. Hou X, Ding H, Teng Y, Zhou C, Tang X, Li S, Ding H. Research on the relationship between brain anoxia at different regional oxygen saturations and brain damage using near-infrared spectroscopy. Physiol Meas. 2007; 28(10):1251–65.
24. Lemmers PM, Molenschot MC, Evens J, Toet MC, van Bel F. Is cerebral oxygen supply compromised in preterm infants undergoing surgical closure for patent ductus arteriosus? Arch Dis Child Fetal Neonatal Ed. 2010;95(6):F429–34.
25. Chock VY, Ramamoorthy C, Van Meurs KP. Cerebral oxygenation during different treatment strategies for a patent ductus arteriosus. Neonatology. 2011;100(3):233–40.

26. Zaramella P, Freato F, Quaresima V, Ferrari M, Bartocci M, Rubino M, Falcon E, Chiandetti L. Surgical closure of patent ductus arteriosus reduces the cerebral tissue oxygenation index in preterm infants: a near-infrared spectroscopy and Doppler study. Pediatr Int. 2006;48(3):305–12.
27. Huning BM, Asfour B, Konig S, Hess N, Roll C. Cerebral blood volume changes during closure by surgery of patent ductus arteriosus. Arch Dis Child Fetal Neonatal Ed. 2008;93(4):F261–4.
28. Vanderhaegen J, De Smet D, Meyns B, Van De Velde M, Van Huffel S, Naulaers G. Surgical closure of the patent ductus arteriosus and its effect on the cerebral tissue oxygenation. Acta Paediatr. 2008;97(12):1640–4.
29. Alderliesten T, Dix L, Baerts W, Caicedo A, van Huffel S, Naulaers G, Groenendaal F, van Bel F, Lemmers P. Reference values of regional cerebral oxygen saturation during the first 3 days of life in preterm neonates. Pediatr Res. 2016;79(1-1):55–64.
30. Kleiser S, Hyttel-Sorensen S, Greisen G, Wolf M. Comparison of near-infrared oximeters in a liquid optical phantom with varying Intralipid and blood content. Adv Exp Med Biol. 2016;876:413–8.
31. Cohen E, Baerts W, Alderliesten T, Derks J, Lemmers P, van Bel F. Growth restriction and gender influence cerebral oxygenation in preterm neonates. Arch Dis Child Fetal Neonatal Ed. 2016;101(2):F156–61.
32. Cohen E, Dix L, Baerts W, Alderliesten T, Lemmers P, van Bel F. Reduction in cerebral oxygenation due to patent ductus arteriosus is pronounced in small-for-gestational-age neonates. Neonatology. 2016;111(2):126–32.
33. Petrova A, Bhatt M, Mehta R. Regional tissue oxygenation in preterm born infants in association with echocardiographically significant patent ductus arteriosus. J Perinatol. 2011;31(7):460–4.

14

Gender-related differences in cardiometabolic risk factors and lifestyle behaviors in treatment-seeking adolescents with severe obesity

Lisa Ha Barstad[1], Pétur B. Júlíusson[1,2], Line Kristin Johnson[1], Jens Kristoffer Hertel[1], Samira Lekhal[1] and Jøran Hjelmesæth[1,3*]

Abstract

Background: Obesity during adolescence is associated with cardiovascular mortality in adulthood. The adverse obesity-related cardiometabolic risk profile is already observed in adolescence. We aimed to examine possible gender differences in cardiometabolic risk factors and lifestyle behaviors among adolescents with severe obesity, hypothesizing that boys would have both a higher prevalence of the metabolic syndrome as well as less healthy lifestyle behaviors than girls.

Methods: Cross-sectional study of treatment-seeking adolescents with severe obesity who attended the Morbid Obesity Centre at Vestfold Hospital Trust and who were consecutively enrolled in the Vestfold Register of Obese Children between September 2009 and September 2015. A total of 313 adolescents aged 12 to 18 years were recruited, whereof 268 subjects (49% boys) completed a food and activity frequency questionnaire and were included in the analysis.

Results: Mean (SD) age, BMI and BMI SDS were 15 (1.6) years, 38.6 (5.9) kg/m^2 and 3.5 (0.6). Levels of LDL cholesterol, fasting insulin and glucose and diastolic blood pressure (DBP) did not differ between genders. Compared to girls, boys had significantly higher triglycerides ($p = 0.037$) and systolic blood pressure (SBP) ($p = 0.003$), as well as lower HDL cholesterol ($p = 0.002$). The metabolic syndrome was present in 27% of the boys and 19% of the girls ($p = 0.140$), and the prevalence of high DBP, dyslipidemia and dysglycemia also did not differ significantly between genders. The prevalence of high SBP was higher in boys than in girls (19% vs. 9%, $p = 0.021$). Gender was associated with a number of lifestyle habits, as a larger proportions of boys had higher screen time ($p = 0.032$), more regular breakfast eating ($p = 0.023$), higher intake of sugar sweetened soda ($p = 0.036$), and lower intake of vegetables than girls ($p = 0.011$). By contrast, physical activity level and intake of fruit and berries did not differ between genders.

Conclusions: Male treatment-seeking adolescents with severe obesity had a more unfavorable set of metabolic and behavioral risk factors for cardiovascular disease than girls. Our results indicate that lifestyle behavioral markers should be thoroughly assessed in both genders, and possible gender-related differences in risk profile should be taken into account in future treatment programs.

Keywords: Severe obesity, Gender differences, Lifestyle behavior, Metabolic syndrome, Cardiovascular risk factor, Cardiovascular disease

* Correspondence: joran.hjelmeseth@siv.no
[1]Morbid Obesity Centre, Vestfold Hospital Trust, Box 2168, 3103 Tønsberg, Norway
[3]Department of Endocrinology, Morbid Obesity and Preventive Medicine, Institute of Clinical Medicine, University of Oslo, Oslo, Norway
Full list of author information is available at the end of the article

Background

Cardiovascular diseases (CVD) are the leading cause of mortality in both men and women.

Importantly, men have a 3–4-fold higher risk of an acute coronary event below age 60 than women [1], although the prevalence of ischemic heart disease in younger women is increasing [2].

During the last 30 years, the prevalence of overweight and obesity in children has increased to alarming proportions in many Western countries, with obesity currently affecting one-fifth of US adolescents aged 12 to 19 years [3, 4]. Obesity during the teen years is not only a psychosocial burden, but is also related to increased mortality in middle age from CVD and shortened life expectancy [5, 6]. The adverse cardiometabolic risk profile related to obesity is observed in early adolescence and even in early childhood [7–11], and cardiometabolic risk factors are more prevalent with the increasing degree of obesity in adolescents, particularly in boys [9, 10, 12]. Furthermore, adolescent boys tend to have larger abdominal fat deposits than girls, a condition associated with hypertension, dyslipidemia and dysglycemia [13].

A number of studies have shown that unhealthy lifestyle behaviors such as low physical activity level, high screen time, skipping breakfast, high intake of sugar-sweetened beverages (SSB) and low intake of fruits and vegetables are related to obesity and cardiometabolic risk factors in children and adolescents, and with CVD in adults [14–23]. However, the causes and consequences of obesity in adolescence differ between the genders due to biological and behavioral differences [24–26]. Thus, there is a need for a clearer focus on gender-related differences within the field of adolescent obesity. Considering that adolescent girls may be more likely to modify their diet to obtain weight control than boys [27], and boys have a more disadvantageous fat distribution after puberty, an unhealthy lifestyle could have greater impact on future CVD risk in boys. Although some cross-sectional studies of CVD risk factors in adolescents with obesity have considered boys and girls separately, few studies have examined gender-related differences specifically [7, 9, 10, 12]. In addition, to the best of our knowledge, no study has examined gender-related differences in multiple lifestyle habits and cardiometabolic risk factors among adolescents with severe obesity.

We aimed to examine possible gender differences in lifestyle behaviors and cardiometabolic risk factors in a population of treatment seeking adolescents with severe obesity. We hypothesized that compared to girls, boys would have both a higher prevalence of the metabolic syndrome and its components as well as less healthy lifestyle behaviors. Finally, we aimed to assess the possible associations between cardiometabolic risk factors and lifestyle behaviors, hypothesizing that unhealthy lifestyle habits were associated with unfavorable levels of cardiometabolic risk factors.

Methods

Treatment-seeking adolescents with severe obesity referred to a tertiary care obesity outpatient clinic (the Morbid Obesity Centre, Vestfold Hospital Trust (MOC)) in southern Norway and who were consecutively enrolled in the Vestfold Register of Obese Children from September 2009 until September 2015 were assessed for eligibility. The MOC receives patients who have severe obesity, referred by primary care practitioners. The main inclusion criterion is a BMI (body mass index) of 5 kg/m^2 or more above the obesity limits proposed by the International Obesity Task Force (IOTF 30 kg/m^2 (iso-BMI 30) + 5 kg/m^2) [28], or a BMI level below this cut-off in the presence of obesity-related comorbidity (including family history of obesity-related comorbidity, type 2 diabetes mellitus, hypertension, dyslipidemia, very rapid increase in weight, severe psychosocial problems). We have defined severe obesity as BMI ≥ iso-BMI 35 as suggested by Bervoets et al. [29]. In addition to this definition we have also included subjects with BMI ≥ iso-BMI 30 and having obesity-related conditions. Of the 313 patients included in the Vestfold Register of Obese Children during this period, 268 subjects (86%) completed the food- and activity questionnaire on their first visit to the clinic and were included in this cross-sectional study.

Food and activity frequency questionnaire

The participants' lifestyle behaviors including physical activity, screen time, breakfast eating frequency and intake of sugar-sweetened soda, fruit and vegetables were reported using a self-administered food frequency questionnaire (FFQ) including questions about physical activity. The food and activity questionnaire included questions about habitual daily consumption of specified meals and 23 food items, daily physical activity outside school and daily screen time outside school (time in front of the TV- or PC screen). For each of the questions regarding screen time, physical activity level, breakfast eating, intake of fruit, vegetables and sugar-sweetened soda there were six to eight frequency categories to choose from as shown in Additional file 1: Table S1. The questionnaire was developed by the Department of Nutrition at the University of Oslo, Norway for use in a nationwide study of diet among fourth- and eighth-grade children (9- and 13 years old) in year 2000; the UNGKOST study [30]. The food frequency part of the questionnaire in the UNGKOST study has been validated against a four-day precoded food diary also used in the same study by Lillegaard and colleagues, and they demonstrated that the FFQ can be used to distinguish between low and high consumers of various food items [31]. Furthermore, they demonstrated that self-reported data from the FFQ were more consistent with data obtained from the food diary in the UNGKOST study considering intake of drinks, fruits and vegetables compared to infrequently eaten food items such as chocolate, sweets, savory snacks and pizza [31].

In the present analysis the highest frequencies of intake of fruits, vegetables and soda intake were rarely reported, therefore the number of original response categories were reduced and recoded into 3: low, moderate or high intake of fruits and berries and vegetables and low, moderate or high intake of sugar-sweetened soda. For simplicity, the response categories for physical activity level, screen time and breakfast eating were also reduced and recoded into 3: low, moderate or high physical activity level, low, moderate or high screen-time and skipping breakfast regularly, sometimes eating breakfast or regularly eating breakfast (Additional file 1: Table S1). Low physical activity, skipping breakfast regularly, high screen time, low intake of fruits and vegetables and/or high intake of sugar-sweetened soda were considered as unhealthy lifestyle behaviors and CVD risk factors.

Anthropometric and clinical measurements

Height was measured using Heightronic Digital Stadiometer® to the nearest 0.1 cm. Weight (kg) and body fat percentage was measured using Tanita bioimpedance body composition analyzer (BC-418, 8-polar, TANITA Corp., Tokyo, Japan). Waist circumference (WC) was measured using a standardized anthropometric tape, measuring the circumference at the midpoint between the top of the iliac crest and the lower part of the lateral rib cage to the nearest 0.1 cm. Waist to height ratio (WHtR) was calculated as WC (in cm) divided by height (in cm). BMI was converted to SDS by means of the current Norwegian growth references [32].

Systolic and diastolic blood pressure (SBP and DBP) were measured using a digital oscillimetric device, Dinamap ProCare (GE Healthcare). BP measurements were taken in the sitting position using appropriate sized cuffs (the mid-upper arm circumference was measured) four times on the dominant arm, and the average between the last three measurements was calculated.

Laboratory analyses

Blood samples were obtained after an overnight fast by venipuncture in vacutainer gel tubes, and serum was separated from cells by centrifugation. Analyses of serum glucose and blood lipids were performed using dry reagent slide technology on the Vitros FS 5.1 (Ortho-Clinical Diagnostics, NY, USA). HbA1c was analyzed by high-performance liquid chromatography (HLPC) using Tosoh HLC-723 G7 (Tosoh Corporation, Tokyo, Japan). Insulin was analyzed by radioimmunossay (RIA) (Millipore Corporation, Billerica, MA, USA) until March 2012, thereafter the electrochemiluminescence immunoassay method (ECLIA) (ECLIA kit, Roche Diagnostics, Mannheim, Germany) was used. Intra- and inter-assay coefficient of variation were < 10% for all assays. Insulin resistance was estimated using the homeostasis model assessment for insulin resistance (HOMA-IR): (insulin (pmol/L) x fasting blood glucose (mmol/L)/135) [33].

Metabolic syndrome

Metabolic syndrome was identified using the definition from the International Diabetes Federation (IDF) Consensus Group Criteria: Abdominal (central) obesity (waist circumference ≥ 90th percentile for age and sex for ages < 16 years, and ≥ 94 cm for males and ≥80 cm for female for ages ≥ 16 years) and the presence of two or more of the following characteristics: 1) triglycerides ≥ 1.7 mmol/L, 2) HDL cholesterol < 1.03 mmol/L for age 10- < 16 years, and < 1.03 mmol/L in males and < 1.29 mmol/L in females for age ≥ 16 years, 3) SBP ≥ 130 mmHg or DBP ≥ 85 mmHg and 4) fasting plasma glucose ≥ 5.6 mmol/L or known type 2 diabetes [34]. Waist circumference was missing for 10 boys and 6 girls, and for these we assumed abdominal adiposity when BMI was above the International Obesity Task Force threshold for obesity [28].

Ethics

All procedures in the study were performed in accordance with the ethical standards of the institutional and/or national research committee and with the Helsinki declaration and its later amendments or comparable ethical standards. The research protocol for the Vestfold Register of Obese Children has been approved by the Regional Committees for Medical and Health Research Ethics (S-08742c 2008/19081), Norwegian Centre for Research Data (NSD) and by the Norwegian Data Inspectorate (20,789 grh/rh). The research protocol for the current study has been approved by the Regional Committees for Medical and Health Research Ethics, REK sør-øst (2016/2039). Written informed consent was obtained from all participants and the parents/guardians of participants under the age of 16 in the study.

Statistics

Continuous variables are presented as mean (SD) if normally distributed, or as median (interquartile range) if not. Categorical variables are presented as counts and percentages. Crude comparisons between variables were performed using Fisher's exact test (categorical variables), independent samples t-test and ANOVA with

Tukey's post-hoc test (continuous normally distributed data), or Mann-Whitney Wilcoxon test or Kruskal-Wallis test (for continuous skewed data such as triglycerides, fasting glucose and insulin). The standardized mean differences (Cohen's *d*) for cardiometabolic variables between the genders were calculated. The correlations between lifestyle habits (ordinal variables) and cardiometabolic markers (continuous variables) were analyzed with Spearman correlation. A probability value < 0.05 was considered statistically significant. Statistical analyses were performed with SPSS version 21 (Statistical Package for Social Science Inc., Chicago, IL, USA).

Results

Data from a total of 268 (49% boys) treatment seeking adolescents with obesity aged 12 to 18 years were included in the analyses. Mean (SD) age, BMI and BMI SDS was 15.0 (1.6) years, 38.6 (5.9) kg/m^2 and 3.5 (0.6) respectively. The boys were slightly younger than the girls (Table 1).

Cardiometabolic risk factors

The cardiometabolic characteristics presented in Table 1 demonstrate that the mean waist circumference, triglyceride levels and SBP were significantly higher in boys compared with girls. In addition, boys had lower body fat percentage and HDL cholesterol levels than girls. The standardized mean differences between genders (Cohen's *d*) are shown in Additional file 2: Table S2. Three of the participants (all boys) did not have central adiposity as defined by the IDF guidelines [34]. The prevalence of metabolic syndrome and components of the metabolic syndrome such as high DBP, dyslipidemia and dysglycemia did not differ significantly between genders (Table 2). However, the prevalence of high systolic blood pressure was higher in boys than in girls (19% vs. 9%, $p = 0.021$).

Table 1 Clinical characteristics of the study participants ($n = 268$) according to gender

	Boys ($n = 132$)	Girls ($n = 136$)	*P*-value
Age (years)	14.6 (1.7)	15.3 (1.5)	0.001
Weight (kg)	112.5 (24.8)	107.0 (18.6)	0.040
BMI (kg/m^2)	37.9 (6.1)	39.2 (5.7)	0.075
BMI SDS	3.2 (0.4)	3.8 (0.6)	< 0.001
Delta iso-BMI 30	10.0 (5.6)	10.3 (5.6)	0.647
Waist circumference (cm)	115.0 (13.3)	109.3 (11.5)	< 0.001
Waist to height ratio	0.67 (0.07)	0.66 (0.07)	0.600
Body fat (%)	42.1 (7.3)	47.2 (5.1)	< 0.001
SBP (mmHg)	119 (15)	113 (14)	0.003
DBP (mmHg)	62 (7)	61 (7)	0.418
Total cholesterol (mmol/L)	4.4 (0.9)	4.5 (0.7)	0.458
HDL cholesterol (mmol/L)	1.1 (0.2)	1.2 (0.3)	0.002
LDL cholesterol (mmol/L)	2.6 (0.7)	2.6 (0.6)	0.505
Triglycerides (mmol/L)	1.4 (1.0–2.1)	1.3 (0.9–1.7)	0.037
Fasting insulin (pmol/L)	156 (112–236)	149 (109–202)	0.209
Fasting glucose (mmol/L)	4.9 (4.7–5.1)	4.9 (4.6–5.1)	0.133
HbA1c (%)	5.4 (0.6)	5.4 (0.5)	0.516
HOMA-IR[a]	5.8 (4.1–8.9)	5.3 (3.9–7.4)	0.270

Continuous variables are shown as mean (SD) or median (interquartile range) unless otherwise indicated. [a]HOMA-IR = (insulin (pmol/L) x fasting blood glucose (mmol/L))/135

Unhealthy lifestyle behaviors

Gender was significantly associated with a number of lifestyle habits, as larger proportions of boys had higher screen time, more frequent breakfast eating, higher intake of sugar sweetened soda, and lower intake of vegetables than girls (Table 3). By contrast, physical activity level and intake of fruit and berries did not differ between boys and girls. The percentages of all adolescents reporting unhealthy lifestyle habits were 34% for low physical activity level, 55% for high screen time, 28% for not eating breakfast regularly, 25% for high intake of sugar-sweetened soda, and 18% for low intake of vegetables, fruits and berries. In a sub-analysis, those with unhealthy lifestyle behaviors (low physical activity, skipping breakfast regularly, high screen time, low intake of fruits and vegetables and/or high intake of sugar-sweetened soda) were compared with those reporting healthier lifestyle behaviors. As compared with girls, a larger proportion of boys reported high screen time ($p = 0.010$) and high intake of sugar-sweetened soda ($p = 0.041$). By contrast, the percentage of girls skipping breakfast regularly was higher than for boys ($p = 0.037$). There were no significant differences in the proportions of boys and girls with low physical activity ($p = 0.436$) or low intake of fruit ($p = 0.223$) and vegetables ($p = 0.133$). Figure 1 shows the prevalence of CVD risk factors (both cardiometabolic and lifestyle habits) according to gender.

Table 2 Participants with metabolic syndrome and risk factors according to the IDF definition [34]

	Boys, n (%)	Girls, n (%)	*P*-value
Metabolic syndrome	34 (27)	25 (19)	0.140
High triglycerides	49 (39)	36 (27)	0.064
Low HDL cholesterol	49 (39)	48 (36)	0.702
High systolic blood pressure	25 (19)	12 (9)	0.021
High diastolic blood pressure	0	0	
High fasting glucose	3 (2)	8 (6)	0.218

Fisher's exact test

Table 3 Physical activity level, screen time, breakfast eating frequency, intake of sugar-sweetened soda, fruits and vegetables

	Boys, n (%)	Girls, n (%)	*P*-value
Physical activity level			0.704
Low	46 (36)	42 (31)	
Moderate	72 (56)	82 (61)	
High	10 (8)	10 (8)	
Screen time			0.032
Low	11 (8)	15 (11)	
Moderate	38 (29)	57 (42)	
High	82 (63)	63 (47)	
Breakfast eating			0.023
Skipping regularly	21 (17)	36 (28)	
Sometimes	25 (20)	33 (25)	
Regularly	81 (64)	62 (47)	
Sugar-sweetened soda			0.036
Low	27 (22)	44 (34)	
Moderate	56 (46)	59 (46)	
High	38 (31)	25 (20)	
Fruits and berries			0.179
Low	28 (23)	18 (14)	
Moderate	62 (50)	65 (51)	
High	34 (27)	44 (35)	
Vegetables			0.011
Low	31 (24)	14 (11)	
Moderate	73 (58)	81 (63)	
High	23 (18)	34 (26)	

Fisher's exact test

Associations between cardiometabolic markers and lifestyle behaviors

The associations between lifestyle behaviors (physical activity level, breakfast eating frequency, frequency of intake of fruits, vegetables and sugar-sweetened soda) and cardiometabolic markers (total cholesterol, HDL- and LDL cholesterol, waist circumference, triglycerides, glucose, SBP and DBP) were significant only in terms of screen time and DBP, $r = 0.17$, $p = 0.005$). In the girl cohort HDL cholesterol was significantly related to breakfast intake frequency ($r = 0.21$, $p = 0.020$), whilst in boys DBP was related to screen time and fruit intake frequency ($r = 0.26$, $p = 0.002$, and $r = -0.22$, $p = 0.016$, respectively). The mean levels of HDL cholesterol, LDL cholesterol, triglycerides, SBP and DBP did not differ significantly between those with unhealthy and healthier lifestyle behaviors (Tables 4 and 5). However, fasting blood sugar was significantly higher in those with high physical activity compared with those with low physical activity (Table 4).

Discussion

In accordance with our hypothesis, we found that treatment seeking adolescent boys with obesity had a significantly worse cardiometabolic risk profile than girls, including unfavorable measures of waist circumference, blood pressure, triglycerides and HDL cholesterol. In addition, larger proportions of boys had unhealthy lifestyle behaviors such as higher screen time, higher intake of sugar-sweetened soda and lower intakes of vegetables than girls. However, in contrast with our hypothesis, the prevalence of metabolic syndrome did not differ significantly between genders, and a higher proportion of girls than boys skipped breakfast regularly. Finally, most cardiometabolic risk factors were not significantly associated with lifestyle behaviors.

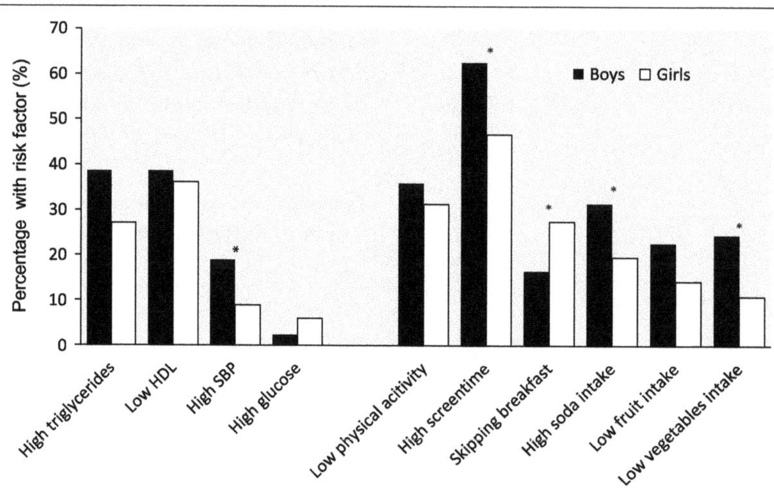

Fig. 1 Prevalence of CVD risk factors (cardiometabolic and behavioral) according to gender. $*P < 0.05$

Table 4 Cardiometabolic risk markers at different levels of breakfast eating, physical activity and screen time

Cardiometabolic risk marker	Physical activity level			Breakfast eating			Screen time		
	Low	Moderate	High	Skipping regularly	Sometimes	Regular	Low	Moderate	High
	n = 88	*n* = 154	*n* = 20	*n* = 57	*n* = 58	*n* = 143	*n* = 26	*n* = 95	*n* = 145
HDL cholesterol (mmol/L)	1.19 (0.27)	1.19 (0.26)	1.25 (0.33)	1.17 (0.24)	1.17 (0.26)	1.19 (0.28)	1.20 (0.27)	1.22 (0.27)	1.17 (0.28)
LDL cholesterol (mmol/L)	2.6 (0.6)	2.6 (0.7)	2.6 (0.7)	2.5 (0.6)	2.6 (0.7)	2.6 (0.7)	2.7 (0.7)	2.5 (0.7)	2.6 (0.7)
Triglycerides (mmol/L)	1.5 (0.8)	1.5 (0.8)	1.6 (0.9)	1.5 (0.6)	1.5 (0.7)	1.6 (0.9)	1.4 (0.6)	1.5 (0.7)	1.6 (0.8)
Fasting glucose (mmol/L)	4.9 (0.3)[a]	4.9 (0.3)	5.4 (2.0)[1]	4.9 (0.4)	4.9 (0.4)	5.0 (0.9)	4.9 (0.4)	4.9 (0.4)	4.9 (0.9)
Systolic blood pressure (mmHg)	118 (11)	115 (16)	119 (15)	116 (12)	112 (21)[a]	118 (12)[a]	111 (22)	115 (11)	118 (15)

ANOVA with post-hoc test for HDL cholesterol, LDL cholesterol and systolic blood pressure. Kruskall-Wallis test for triglycerides and fasting glucose. [a]Values within the same lifestyle category differ significantly from each other

Cardiometabolic risk factors

One out of four boys (27%) and one out of five girls (19%) had metabolic syndrome. These figures are in accordance with those from an Italian cohort of adolescents with severe obesity (30 and 19%, respectively), but lower than demonstrated in a German cohort (46 and 37%, respectively) [12]. Although in the current study the average serum triglyceride levels were higher and HDL cholesterol levels lower in boys than in girls, the percentage with high triglycerides or low HDL cholesterol did not differ significantly between genders. Furthermore, high blood pressure was diagnosed in 19% of the boys, which was significantly higher than in the girls (9%). In two other cross-sectional studies prehypertension was present in 25% of adolescents with obesity and hypertension was present in 5%, but these studies did not assess gender differences [9, 10]. However, we did not find significant differences in cardiometabolic risk factors between adolescents with unhealthy or healthier lifestyle behaviors, except for blood glucose which was higher in those with high physical activity. Thus, we could not confirm our hypothesis that unhealthy lifestyle habits were associated with more unfavorable levels of cardiometabolic risk factors in our cohort of adolescents with severe obesity.

Lifestyle behaviors

In the current study, 55, 34 and 22% of treatment seeking adolescents with severe obesity had high screen time, low physical activity and skipped breakfast regularly. These figures are considerably higher than those from a representative population of Norwegian 13-year olds taken from a national food and activity survey; the corresponding percentages were 18, 10 and 10% [30]. In the current study more boys than girls had high screen time as well as high intake of sugar-sweetened beverages. High screen time has been associated with high total cholesterol to HDL cholesterol ratio, high triglycerides and obesity in children [15, 17, 35]. In addition, Stamatakis et al. showed that screen time of 4 h or more per day in adults doubled the risk of CVD (HR:2.25 (95% CI:1.30–3.89)) [20]. A study by Shang et al. found a higher energy intake of 136 kcal and lower intake of fruits and vegetables of 0.2 servings in overweight children with high screen time in comparison with those with low screen time [36]. Data from the first National Health and Nutrition Examination Survey Epidemiologic Follow-up Study showed that adults who reported a high intake of fruits and vegetables had a 27% lower CVD mortality than those who had a low intake of fruits and vegetables [22]. Furthermore, sugar-sweetened beverages have been associated with weight gain, metabolic syndrome and type 2 diabetes [23, 37].

Furthermore, in the current study, a high proportion of boys and girls did not eat breakfast regularly, although the percentage of girls skipping breakfast regularly was higher than among boys. This is in accordance with findings of Boutelle et al. who suggest that girls may skip

Table 5 Cardiometabolic risk markers at different levels of intake of sugar-sweetened soda, fruits/berries and vegetables

Cardiometabolic risk marker	Sugar-sweetened soda			Fruits and berries			Vegetables		
	Low	Moderate	High	Low	Moderate	High	Low	Moderate	High
	n = 70	*n* = 109	*n* = 62	*n* = 45	*n* = 122	*n* = 76	*n* = 42	*n* = 150	*n* = 56
HDL cholesterol (mmol/L)	1.14 (0.27)	1.20 (0.28)	1.19 (0.25)	1.21 (0.27)	1.20 (0.28)	1.16 (0.25)	1.20 (0.31)	1.20 (0.28)	1.15 (0.23)
LDL cholesterol (mmol/L)	2.6 (0.7)	2.6 (0.7)	2.6 (0.7)	2.7 (0.6)	2.5 (0.7)	2.6 (0.8)	2.7 (0.7)	2.5 (0.7)	2.6 (0.8)
Triglycerides (mmol/L)	1.4 (0.7)	1.6 (0.9)	1.5 (0.7)	1.5 (0.6)	1.5 (0.8)	1.6 (0.8)	1.5 (0.6)	1.5 (0.8)	1.4 (0.8)
Fasting glucose (mmol/L)	5.0 (1.1)	4.9 (0.5)	4.9 (0.4)	5.0 (0.6)	4.9 (0.9)	4.9 (0.4)	4.9 (0.4)	4.9 (0.8)	4.9 (0.5)
Systolic blood pressure (mmHg)	115 (11)	116 (15)	116 (18)	111 (24)	117 (11)	116 (12)	116 (11)	116 (15)	116 (17)

ANOVA with post-hoc test for HDL cholesterol, LDL cholesterol and systolic blood pressure. Kruskall-Wallis test for triglycerides and fasting glucose

meals more often than boys as a method of losing weight [38]. Not eating breakfast regularly has been associated with increased waist circumference, high fasting insulin, high glucose and obesity in both children and adolescents [19, 39]. Skipping breakfast is associated with a poor diet quality, with low intake of whole-grain products and low micronutrient intake [18, 40].

Strengths and limitations

One strength of this study is the relatively large cohort of treatment-seeking adolescents with severe obesity. Furthermore, in the Vestfold Register of Obese Children a wide range of cardiometabolic markers with clinical relevance have been registered. There are, however, limitations to our study which need to be addressed. The questionnaire was based on self-reported data about physical activity and dietary habits. In a population classified as obese, under-reporting of unhealthy choices and over-reporting of healthy choices can be expected [41].

The apparent lack of association between lifestyle habits and cardiometabolic risk factors might be explained by either the relatively low number of participants in the extreme categories (lowest, highest), or that severe adiposity has a larger impact on cardiometabolic risk factors than lifestyle behavior.

Conclusion

Treatment-seeking adolescent boys with severe obesity had a more unfavorable cardiometabolic risk profile, higher screen time, higher intake of sugar-sweetened soda and lower intake of vegetables than girls, while a higher proportion of girls skipped breakfast regularly. In a clinical setting a thorough assessment of health-related factors including lifestyle behavioral markers should receive proper attention to be able to identify relevant treatment focus and individualize the treatment in both genders. Care providers should, however, be aware of the possibility of differences in risk profiles between boys and girls.

Abbreviations

CVD: Cardiovascular disease; FFQ: Food frequency questionnaire; IDF: International Diabetes Federation; MOC: Morbid Obese Centre, Vestfold Hospital Trust; SSB: Sugar-sweetened beverages; WC: Waist circumference; WHtR: Waist to height ratio

Acknowledgements

We would like to thank the staff (nurses, doctors and secretaries) at the Children and adolescent department of the Morbid Obesity Centre at Vestfold Hospital Trust, for gathering data for the Vestfold Register of Obese Children. Our gratitude also goes to Milada C. Småstuen for statistical advice and to Matthew McGee for proof-reading the manuscript.

Funding

This study was funded by Vestfold Hospital Trust.

Authors' contributions

LHB designed the study, carried out analysis and interpretation of the data, and drafted the initial manuscript. PBJ, LKJ and JKH contributed to drafting the manuscript and revising it critically. SL collected the data and revised the manuscript critically. JH contributed to the conception and design of the work and the interpretation of the data, as well as drafting the manuscript and revising it critically. All authors read and approved the final manuscript.

Ethics approval and consent to participate

All procedures in the study were performed in accordance with the ethical standards of the institutional and/or national research committee and with the Helsinki declaration and its later amendments or comparable ethical standards. The research protocol for the Vestfold Register of Obese Children has been approved by the Regional Committees for Medical and Health Research Ethics (S-08742c 2008/19081), Norwegian Centre for Research Data (NSD) and by the Norwegian Data Inspectorate (20,789 grh/rh). The research protocol for the current study has been approved by the Regional Committees for Medical and Health Research Ethics, REK sør-øst (2016/2039). Written informed consent was obtained from all participants and the parents/guardians of participants under the age of 16 in the study.

Competing interests

The authors declare that they have no competing interests.

Author details

[1]Morbid Obesity Centre, Vestfold Hospital Trust, Box 2168, 3103 Tønsberg, Norway. [2]Department of Clinical Science, University of Bergen, 5021 Bergen, Norway. [3]Department of Endocrinology, Morbid Obesity and Preventive Medicine, Institute of Clinical Medicine, University of Oslo, Oslo, Norway.

References

1. Group EUCCS, Regitz-Zagrosek V, Oertelt-Prigione S, Prescott E, Franconi F, Gerdts E, Foryst-Ludwig A, Maas AH, Kautzky-Willer A, Knappe-Wegner D, et al. Gender in cardiovascular diseases: impact on clinical manifestations, management, and outcomes. Eur Heart J. 2016;37(1):24–34.
2. Ostan R, Monti D, Gueresi P, Bussolotto M, Franceschi C, Baggio G. Gender, aging and longevity in humans: an update of an intriguing/neglected scenario paving the way to a gender-specific medicine. Clin Sci. 2016; 130(19):1711–25.
3. Ogden CL, Carroll MD, Lawman HG, Fryar CD, Kruszon-Moran D, Kit BK, Flegal KM. Trends in obesity prevalence among children and adolescents in the United States, 1988-1994 through 2013-2014. JAMA. 2016;315(21):2292–9.

4. Juliusson PB, Roelants M, Eide GE, Hauspie R, Waaler PE, Bjerknes R. Overweight and obesity in Norwegian children: secular trends in weight-for-height and skinfolds. Acta Paediatr (Oslo, Norway: 1992). 2007;96(9):1333–7.
5. Bjorge T, Engeland A, Tverdal A, Smith GD. Body mass index in adolescence in relation to cause-specific mortality: a follow-up of 230,000 Norwegian adolescents. American J Epidemiol. 2008;168(1):30–7.
6. Twig G, Yaniv G, Levine H, Leiba A, Goldberger N, Derazne E, Ben-Ami Shor D, Tzur D, Afek A, Shamiss A, et al. Body-mass index in 2.3 million adolescents and cardiovascular death in adulthood. N Engl J Med. 2016; 374(25):2430–40.
7. de Ferranti SD, Gauvreau K, Ludwig DS, Neufeld EJ, Newburger JW, Rifai N. Prevalence of the metabolic syndrome in American adolescents: findings from the third National Health and nutrition examination survey. Circulation. 2004;110(16):2494–7.
8. Srinivasan SR, Myers L, Berenson GS. Predictability of childhood adiposity and insulin for developing insulin resistance syndrome (syndrome X) in young adulthood: the Bogalusa heart study. Diabetes. 2002;51(1):204–9.
9. Skinner AC, Perrin EM, Moss LA, Skelton JA. Cardiometabolic risks and severity of obesity in children and young adults. N Engl J Med. 2015;373(14): 1307–17.
10. May AL, Kuklina EV, Yoon PW. Prevalence of cardiovascular disease risk factors among US adolescents, 1999-2008. Pediatrics. 2012;129(6):1035–41.
11. Martos-Moreno GA, Gil-Campos M, Bueno G, Bahillo P, Bernal S, Feliu A, Lechuga-Sancho AM, Palomo E, Ruiz R, Vela A, et al. Obesity associated metabolic impairment is evident at early ages: Spanish collaborative study. Nutr Hosp. 2014;30(4):787–93.
12. Lafortuna CL, Adorni F, Agosti F, De Col A, Sievert K, Siegfried W, Sartorio A. Prevalence of the metabolic syndrome among extremely obese adolescents in Italy and Germany. Diabetes Res Clin Pract. 2010;88(1):14–21.
13. Tchernof A, Despres JP. Pathophysiology of human visceral obesity: an update. Physiol Rev. 2013;93(1):359–404.
14. D'Addesa D, D'Addezio L, Martone D, Censi L, Scanu A, Cairella G, Spagnolo A, Menghetti E. Dietary intake and physical activity of normal weight and overweight/obese adolescents. Int J Pediatr. 2010;2010:785649.
15. Berentzen NE, Smit HA, van Rossem L, Gehring U, Kerkhof M, Postma DS, Boshuizen HC, Wijga AH. Screen time, adiposity and cardiometabolic markers: mediation by physical activity, not snacking, among 11-year-old children. Int J Obes (2005). 2014;38(10):1317–23.
16. Carlson JA, Crespo NC, Sallis JF, Patterson RE, Elder JP. Dietary-related and physical activity-related predictors of obesity in children: a 2-year prospective study. Child Obes. 2012;8(2):110–5.
17. Danielsen YS, Juliusson PB, Nordhus IH, Kleiven M, Meltzer HM, Olsson SJ, Pallesen S. The relationship between life-style and cardio-metabolic risk indicators in children: the importance of screen time. Acta Paediat (Oslo, Norway : 1992). 2011;100(2):253–9.
18. Gilardini L, Croci M, Pasqualinotto L, Caffetto K, Invitti C. Dietary habits and Cardiometabolic health in obese children. Obes Facts. 2015;8(2):101–9.
19. Smith KJ, Gall SL, McNaughton SA, Blizzard L, Dwyer T, Venn AJ. Skipping breakfast: longitudinal associations with cardiometabolic risk factors in the childhood determinants of adult health study. Am J Clin Nutr. 2010;92(6): 1316–25.
20. Stamatakis E, Hamer M, Dunstan DW. Screen-based entertainment time, all-cause mortality, and cardiovascular events: population-based study with ongoing mortality and hospital events follow-up. J Am Coll Cardiol. 2011; 57(3):292–9.
21. Lee IM, Shiroma EJ, Lobelo F, Puska P, Blair SN, Katzmarzyk PT, Lancet Physical Activity Series Working G. Effect of physical inactivity on major non-communicable diseases worldwide: an analysis of burden of disease and life expectancy. Lancet (London, England). 2012;380(9838):219–29.
22. Bazzano LA, He J, Ogden LG, Loria CM, Vupputuri S, Myers L, Whelton PK. Fruit and vegetable intake and risk of cardiovascular disease in US adults: the first National Health and nutrition examination survey epidemiologic follow-up study. Am J Clin Nutr. 2002;76(1):93–9.
23. Malik VS, Popkin BM, Bray GA, Despres JP, Willett WC, Hu FB. Sugar-sweetened beverages and risk of metabolic syndrome and type 2 diabetes: a meta-analysis. Diabetes Care. 2010;33(11):2477–83.
24. Govindan M, Gurm R, Mohan S, Kline-Rogers E, Corriveau N, Goldberg C, Durussel-Weston J, Eagle KA, Jackson EA. University of Michigan Health S: gender differences in physiologic markers and health behaviors associated with childhood obesity. Pediatrics. 2013;132(3):468–74.
25. Sweeting HN. Gendered dimensions of obesity in childhood and adolescence. Nutr J. 2008;7:1.
26. Campbell MK. Biological, environmental, and social influences on childhood obesity. Pediatr Res. 2016;79(1–2):205–11.
27. Neumark-Sztainer D, Rock CL, Thornquist MD, Cheskin LJ, Neuhouser ML, Barnett MJ. Weight-control behaviors among adults and adolescents: associations with dietary intake. Prev Med. 2000;30(5):381–91.
28. Cole TJ, Bellizzi MC, Flegal KM, Dietz WH. Establishing a standard definition for child overweight and obesity worldwide: international survey. BMJ. 2000; 320(7244):1240–3.
29. Bervoets L, Massa G. Defining morbid obesity in children based on BMI 40 at age 18 using the extended international (IOTF) cut-offs. Pediatr Obes. 2014;9(5):e94–8.
30. Andersen LF, Lillegaard IT, Overby N, Lytle L, Klepp KI, Johansson L. Overweight and obesity among Norwegian schoolchildren: changes from 1993 to 2000. Scand J Public Health. 2005;33(2):99–106.
31. Lillegaard IT, Overby NC, Andersen LF. Evaluation of a short food frequency questionnaire used among Norwegian children. Food Nutr Res. 2012;56. doi: https://doi.org/10.3402/fnr.v56i0.6399.
32. Juliusson PB, Roelants M, Nordal E, Furevik L, Eide GE, Moster D, Hauspie R, Bjerknes R. Growth references for 0-19 year-old Norwegian children for length/height, weight, body mass index and head circumference. Ann Hum Biol. 2013;40(3):220–7.
33. Matthews DR, Hosker JP, Rudenski AS, Naylor BA, Treacher DF, Turner RC. Homeostasis model assessment: insulin resistance and beta-cell function from fasting plasma glucose and insulin concentrations in man. Diabetologia. 1985;28(7):412–9.
34. Alberti KG, Zimmet P, Shaw J. The metabolic syndrome–a new worldwide definition. Lancet (London, England). 2005;366(9491):1059–62.
35. Grontved A, Ried-Larsen M, Moller NC, Kristensen PL, Wedderkopp N, Froberg K, Hu FB, Ekelund U, Andersen LB. Youth screen-time behaviour is associated with cardiovascular risk in young adulthood: the European youth heart study. Eur J Prev Cardiol. 2014;21(1):49–56.
36. Shang L, Wang J, O'Loughlin J, Tremblay A, Mathieu ME, Henderson M, Gray-Donald K. Screen time is associated with dietary intake in overweight Canadian children. Prev Med Rep. 2015;2:265–9.
37. Malik VS, Pan A, Willett WC, Hu FB. Sugar-sweetened beverages and weight gain in children and adults: a systematic review and meta-analysis. Am J Clin Nutr. 2013;98(4):1084–102.
38. Boutelle K, Neumark-Sztainer D, Story M, Resnick M. Weight control behaviors among obese, overweight, and nonoverweight adolescents. J Pediatr Psychol. 2002;27(6):531–40.
39. Freitas Junior IF, Christofaro DG, Codogno JS, Monteiro PA, Silveira LS, Fernandes RA. The association between skipping breakfast and biochemical variables in sedentary obese children and adolescents. J Pediatr. 2012;161(5): 871–4.
40. Leech RM, Worsley A, Timperio A, McNaughton SA. Understanding meal patterns: definitions, methodology and impact on nutrient intake and diet quality. Nutr Res Rev. 2015;28(1):1–21.
41. Collins CE, Watson J, Burrows T. Measuring dietary intake in children and adolescents in the context of overweight and obesity. Int J Obes (2005). 2010;34(7):1103–15.

15

Biomarkers of endothelial dysfunction predict sepsis mortality in young infants

Julie Korol Wright[1], Kyla Hayford[2], Vanessa Tran[2], Gulam Muhammed Al Kibria[3], Abdullah Baqui[4], Ali Manajjir[5], Arif Mahmud[4], Nazma Begum[4], Mashuk Siddiquee[6], Kevin C. Kain[1,2†] and Azadeh Farzin[4,7*†]

Abstract

Background: Reducing death due to neonatal sepsis is a global health priority, however there are limited tools to facilitate early recognition and treatment. We hypothesized that measuring circulating biomarkers of endothelial function and integrity (i.e. Angiopoietin-Tie2 axis) would identify young infants with sepsis and predict their clinical outcome.

Methods: We conducted a matched case-control (1:3) study of 98 young infants aged 0–59 days of life presenting to a referral hospital in Bangladesh with suspected sepsis. Plasma levels of Ang-1, Ang-2, sICAM-1, and sVCAM-1 concentrations were measured at admission. The primary outcome was mortality ($n = 18$); the secondary outcome was bacteremia ($n = 10$).

Results: Ang-2 concentrations at presentation were higher among infants who subsequently died of sepsis compared to survivors (aOR 2.50, $p = 0.024$). Compared to surviving control infants, the Ang-2:Ang-1 ratio was higher among infants who died (aOR 2.29, $p = 0.016$) and in infants with bacteremia (aOR 5.72, $p = 0.041$), and there was an increased odds of death across Ang-2:Ang-1 ratio tertiles (aOR 4.82, $p = 0.013$).

Conclusions: This study provides new evidence linking the Angiopoietin-Tie2 pathway with mortality and bacteremia in young infants with suspected sepsis. If validated in additional studies, markers of the angiopoietin-Tie2 axis may have clinical utility in risk stratification of infants with suspected sepsis.

Keywords: Neonatal Sepsis, Endothelial activation, Angiopoietins, Biomarkers

Background

Globally, sepsis and its sequelae are leading causes of childhood morbidity and mortality. Among neonates, sepsis is a major contributor to an estimated 2.6 million annual deaths and accounts for approximately 3 % of all disability adjusted life years [1, 2]. Early recognition and initiation of antimicrobial therapy are essential to reduce the morbidity and mortality of neonatal sepsis. However, early signs of sepsis are subtle and we currently lack diagnostic tools to enable rapid triage and management of at-risk infants, especially in low-resource settings where 99% of the world's neonatal deaths occur [3, 4].

Septic shock represents a final common pathway for a variety of life-threatening infections and culminates in multiple organ failure and death. While the pathobiology of septic shock is complex and incompletely understood, dysregulated systemic inflammatory responses and endothelial dysfunction are believed to play key roles [5–7]. These altered host responses are associated with decreased systemic vascular resistance, loss of endothelial integrity, and microvascular leak, which compromise tissue perfusion and organ function [8].

The Angiopoietin proteins are a family of endothelium-derived angiogenic factors that have potent effects on the vascular endothelium. Angiopoietins interact with their

* Correspondence: azadehfarzin57@gmail.com
†Equal contributors
[4]International Centre for Maternal and Newborn Health, Department of International Health, Bloomberg School of Public Health, Johns Hopkins University, Baltimore, MD, USA
[7]Division of Neonatology, Department of Pediatrics, Johns Hopkins University School of Medicine, Baltimore, MD, USA
Full list of author information is available at the end of the article

cognate tyrosine kinase receptor, Tie2, expressed on the luminal endothelium. When bound by Angiopoietin-1 (Ang-1), Tie2 signaling promotes endothelial quiescence by enhancing cell survival, maintaining stable adherens junctions through the inhibition of nuclear factor kappa-light-chain-enhancer of activated B cells (NFkB), and downregulating pro-inflammatory cell adhesion molecules including intercellular adhesion molecule-1 (ICAM-1) and vascular cell adhesion molecule-1 (VCAM-1) [9–11]. Endothelial injury stemming from a range of insults including inflammation and hypoxia, stimulates exocytosis of endothelial Weibel-Palade bodies and the release of Angiopoietin-2 (Ang-2) [9, 12]. Ang-2 generally functions as a competitive antagonist for Ang-1 binding to Tie2. Under the influence of Ang-2, activated endothelial cells increase the surface expression of cellular adhesion molecules including ICAM-1 and VCAM-1, and undergo alterations in endothelial cell-cell junctions resulting in microvascular leak [9, 13, 14].

During embryonic, fetal, and early postnatal development, the Angiopoietin-Tie2 axis regulates angiogenesis by directing blood vessel formation, remodeling, and stabilization [15] (reviewed in [16]). Beyond this developmental window the angiopoietin family of ligands continues to regulate important endothelial phenotypes. Multiple disease states are characterized by endothelial activation and microvascular leak including septic shock [17], the hemolytic uremic syndrome [18], toxic shock syndrome [19], malaria [20–24], dengue [25], and acute lung injury / acute respiratory distress syndrome [26–28]. Each of these life-threatening conditions also manifest alterations in Ang-2:Ang-1 plasma concentrations favoring Ang-2 antagonism of Tie2 signaling (reviewed in [29, 30]).

A growing body of evidence has delineated the role and temporal kinetics of Angiopoietin-Tie2 related endothelial activation in septic shock, multiorgan dysfunction, and death (reviewed in [29, 31]). Circulating levels of soluble ICAM-1 (sICAM-1) have been associated with mortality in ICU patients [32, 33], adult systemic inflammatory response syndrome (SIRS) and sepsis severity [33–35], and bacteremia [36]. However among neonates, this association is less consistent with some studies reporting no association between sICAM-1 and sepsis [37, 38], while others demonstrate a positive association [39–42], even in the early stages of sepsis [43]. Soluble-VCAM-1 (sVCAM-1) has been shown in some adult studies to be associated with sepsis [32, 34], whereas in neonates circulating sVCAM-1 was not associated with sepsis but rather only with bacteremia [43]. Taken together, these studies suggest that the Angiopoietin-Tie2 axis may have pleiotropic effects within the immature vascular endothelium of the neonate.

The Tie2 ligands, Ang-1 and Ang-2, have been studied for potential diagnostic and prognostic utility in sepsis. Among adult patients with severe sepsis admitted to the ICU, survivors had higher circulating Ang-1 levels and lower Ang-2 levels than non-survivors [7]. When plasma angiopoietin levels were assessed in adult patients with sepsis on presentation to the Emergency Department, admission Ang-2 levels were predictive of sepsis severity including septic shock and death [17]. Similar findings are documented in the pediatric literature, where Ang-2 levels were associated with sepsis and correlate with disease severity [28, 44–46]. However, none of these studies included neonates or young infants. Globally, and especially in resource-poor settings, children under two months of age bear a high burden of sepsis-related morbidity and mortality [47].

In this matched case-control study conducted at a pediatric referral facility in Bangladesh, young infants under the age of two months who were admitted to hospital with presumed sepsis were enrolled and circulating levels of Ang-2, Ang-1, sICAM-1, and sVCAM-1 were assessed from admission blood samples. We hypothesized that elevated levels of circulating Ang-2 at admission would correlate with clinical outcomes. The primary outcome was mortality and the secondary outcome was bacteremia. These angiogenic biomarkers were selected for study based on their mechanistic role in the pathophysiology of sepsis, and their potential to be predictive of outcome in this vulnerable population.

Methods

Study population

This matched case-control study was nested in an observational cohort study investigating the prognostic potential of circulating angiogenic and inflammatory biomarkers for identifying young infants at triage who are at risk of severe sepsis and death. The study was conducted at the Sylhet MAG Osmani Medical College Hospital (SOMCH), in Sylhet, Bangladesh between July 16, 2013 and December 31, 2014.

Enrollment criteria

Children aged 0–59 days of life with suspected sepsis were recruited upon presentation to the SOMCH Pediatrics ward. Clinical suspicion of sepsis was based upon the assessment of the treating physician, and the patients' parents/guardians were approached for study enrollment upon meeting the inclusion criteria. Inclusion criteria were based on the World Health Organization (WHO) Integrated Management of Childhood Illness (IMCI) algorithm [48] and included: 1) history of difficulty feeding, 2) history of convulsions, 3) movement only when stimulated, 4) respiratory rate of 60 breaths per minute or more, 5) severe chest indrawing, 6) temperature greater than 37.5 °C or less than 35.5 °C.

Infants were excluded if there was suspicion of a congenital disorder involving a major organ system, any suspected chromosomal abnormalities, or if their presentation was attributed to an acquired structural illnesses (eg. pneumothorax or necrotizing enterocolitis), intrapartum-related complications, or morbidities of prematurity and low birthweight. Infants were also excluded if no research specimen was collected or if there was inadequate follow up of the infant. Due to a low rate of positive blood cultures in enrolled infants, there was an interim amendment to the study protocol to exclude infants with antibiotic exposure within 24 h of presentation.

Clinical management

All infants received standard clinical care during the study and were visited daily by the study physician while inpatients. Families who left against the treating physician's recommendation and prior to clinical improvement were contacted after discharge using the provided mobile phone number. In cases where the family left prior to improvement and could not be reached in person or via phone follow up, the infants were categorized as insufficient follow up and excluded, as described above. Standard clinical care included supportive measures such as intravenous fluids, oxygen administration in cases of cyanosis, gavage enteral feeds, thermal support using infant incubators, and the provision of empiric antibiotics on clinical suspicion of sepsis. Common antibiotic regimens for the management of presumed sepsis included intravenous ampicillin and gentamicin, ampicillin and cefotaxime, or ceftazidime and amikacin. All infants enrolled in the study had blood cultures performed.

Blood sample collection and processing for biomarker analysis and blood culture

Upon enrollment into the study, venipuncture was performed for collection of the research specimen and blood culture, which was provided at no cost for all enrolled participants. SOMCH is a tertiary care centre for a population with significant resource limitations and therefore many children presented with severe illness at the time of diagnosis. For ethical reasons, we ensured that specimen collection for blood culture and research purposes did not delay administration of the first dose of antibiotics. The timing of blood collection in relation to antibiotic administration was recorded as part of research data collection.

For blood cultures, 2.0 mL of venous blood was collected into Lysis-Direct Plating (LDP) tubes on admission. Alternatively, in 29 cases where LDP tubes were not available, eight samples were collected into BACTEC bottles, and 21 blood samples were inoculated into Tryptic Soy Broth for incubation. The protocol for the isolation and detection of bacteria was adapted from Saha et al. [49].

For the research specimen, 1–2 mL of venous blood was collected into an EDTA blood collection tube and transferred to the laboratory within two hours in a 4 °C container. Specimens were centrifuged for 10 min at 2500 rpm to separate plasma, which was collected into sterile cryovials and stored at -20 °C prior to being batch transferred in liquid nitrogen to the central laboratory in Dhaka for storage at -70 °C. The frozen plasma samples were transferred to Toronto, Canada for analysis.

Biomarker testing

Plasma concentrations of Ang-1, Ang-2, sICAM-1, and sVCAM-1 were measured in duplicate by Enzyme Linked Immunosorbent Assay (ELISA) (DuoSets, R&D Systems, Minneapolis, MN) as described in [22]. Laboratory technicians were blinded to patient outcome. Sample dilutions were optimized for the detection of each protein using a dilution curve obtained using a selection of case and control plasma samples. The final ELISA plates were read by spectrophotometry at 405 nm with a correction of 570 nm. Concentrations were extrapolated from a 4-parameter non-linear regression curve using Gen5 software (v1.02.8). The range of detection for each biomarker was as follows: Ang-1 (1.562–100 ng/mL), Ang-2 (1.875–120 ng/mL), sICAM-1 (62.50–4000 ng/mL), sVCAM-1 (312.5–20,000 ng/mL). Results below the lower limit of detection were adjusted according to the formula: 1/2 * lower limit of detection for the biomarker in the diluted sample. Results above the upper limit of detection were assigned the value of the upper limit of detection in the diluted sample.

Outcome definitions

The primary outcome of this study was death during the index admission; infants who were discharged home in anticipation of an imminent death were also included in this primary outcome. The primary controls, termed 'Survivors', were young infants in the study cohort without bacteremia who were observed for at least 48 h at the hospital with evidence of clinical improvement prior to discharge, or confirmation of improvement provided by the family after discharge. Controls were retrospectively selected at a 3:1 ratio matched on birth weight (±500 g) and age at admission by category (0–2, 3–6, 7–13, 14–27, or > 27 days of life) as these were potentially confounding variables.

The secondary outcomes for this study were 1) culture-confirmed bacteremia, and 2) a combined outcome of death or bacteremia. Controls for secondary outcomes were matched using the same criteria as the primary analysis and termed 'Non-Bacteremia' and 'Controls', respectively.

Data analysis

Demographic characteristics, location and type of delivery, antibiotic exposure and clinical findings at admission were compared for those infants with the primary or secondary outcomes and their controls using bivariate conditional logistic regression for continuous variables and exact McNemar's test for binary variables to account for matching. No informative missingness was observed for independent variables. Two missing values for temperature and lethargy were randomly imputed and sensitivity analyses were conducted. Non-normally distributed continuous variables were natural log transformed. Multivariate conditional logistic regression models were generated to estimate the association of log-transformed biomarker levels at admission for the primary outcome and secondary outcomes. Because there are no clinically informative cutoffs among young infants for these biomarkers, biomarker distribution were divided into tertiles and analysed for an association with the Death outcome. Adjusted odds ratios (aOR) and 95% confidence intervals (CI) are reported. Final model selection was based on variables selected a priori (sex) and variables that balance parsimony with model fit. There were no changes in inferences in the sensitivity analyses. Analyses were performed in Stata 14 (Stata Corporation, College Station, TX).

Results

Patient characteristics

Four hundred and twenty three infants admitted with sepsis met eligibility criteria for the parent study and of these, parental/guardian consent for enrollment was given for 420. Mortality among this cohort was 10.4% (44/420) and the rate of culture-confirmed bacteremia was 3.1% (13/420). Of the mortality cases, 9.1% (4/44) had culture-confirmed bacteremia.

In total, angiogenic biomarkers were assessed in 98 infant plasma samples from the parent study cohort using a matched case-control design (Fig. 1). There were 18 primary outcomes (death) and 10 infants with culture-confirmed bacteremia, of which three died. Thus 25

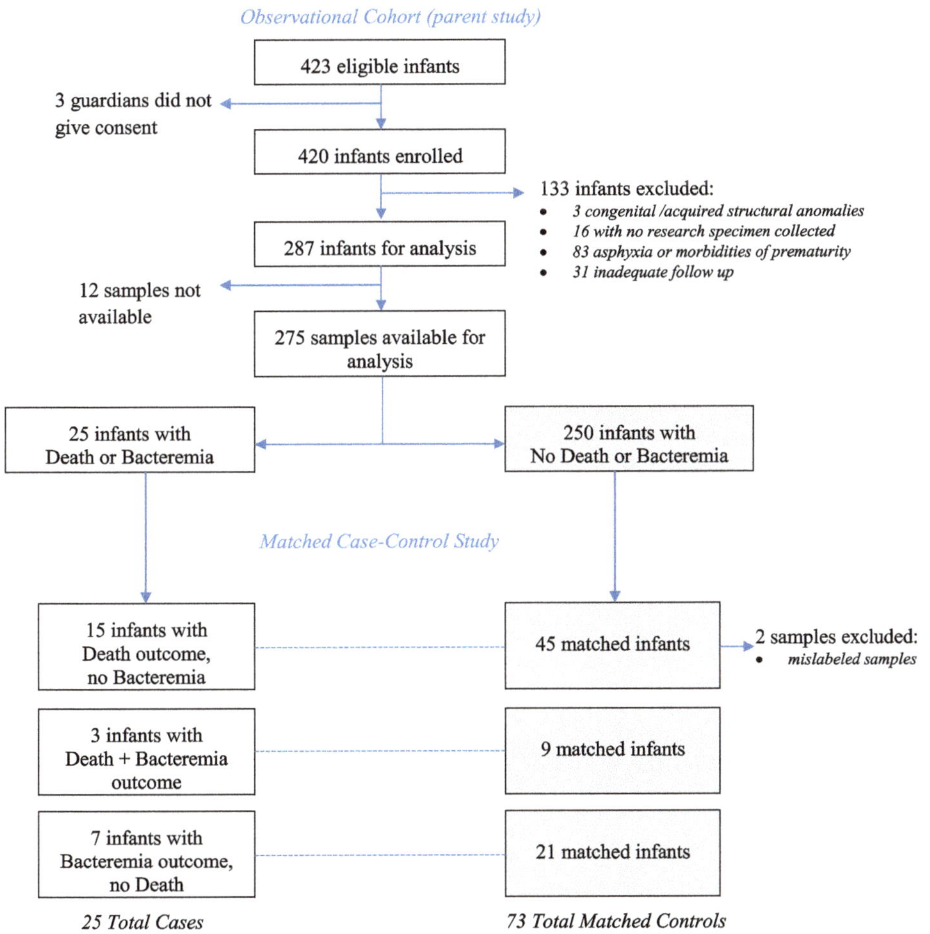

Fig. 1 Study Flow Diagram. Infants in the matched case-control analysis included all infants from the Observational Cohort Study with an outcome of death ($n = 18$) or culture-confirmed bacteremia ($n = 10$) plus control infants who were randomly selected at a 3:1 ratio after matching on birthweight and age at admission

infants fit the Combined Outcome group (death or bacteremia). Controls were selected from among the infants without bacteremia who survived to discharge at a 3:1 ratio for each outcome: 52 controls for the primary outcome, termed 'Survivors' (two samples were initially misclassified and excluded); and 30 controls for the Bacteremia group, termed 'non-Bacteremia'. For the Combined Outcome group, there were a total of 73 combined controls, termed 'Controls'.

The median age at admission was 14.5 days of life [interquartile range (IQR): 7, 27], and the median admission weight was 2.5 kg [IQR: 2.2, 3.0]. Males comprised 62% of the study population. All outcome groups had a significantly higher proportion of males compared with their respective controls (Table 1). Thirty-two per cent of infants had been born in a hospital and 10% had been delivered by Caesarean section. Between the Death and Survivor groups there were no statistically significant differences in these delivery characteristics; however, the rate of Caesarean section was significantly lower among the Bacteremia group and the Combined Outcome group compared to their controls ($p = 0.039$ and $p = 0.014$, respectively Table 1).

There were no significant differences in baseline clinical parameters at admission (temperature, respiratory rate, or lethargy) between any of the outcome groups and their respective controls (Table 1). The median time from admission to death was 19.5 h [IQR: 9, 40 h]. Forty-four per cent of infants in this study cohort received antibiotics within seven days prior to venipuncture for blood culture sample collection. Overall, prior antibiotic exposure was significantly associated with the Control group ($p = 0.013$) (Table 1). There was no statistically significant difference in the probability of positive culture result based on blood culture method in both the unmatched parent-study cohort ($n = 420$) and the matched case-control study population ($n = 98$). Among the 10 bacterial isolates from blood cultures, seven were gram positive organisms and three were gram negative (Additional file 1: Table S1). Due to the variety of organisms and low overall rate of bacteremia, correlations between pathogens and mortality or biomarker levels were not conducted.

Increased concentrations of circulating Ang-2, Ang-2:Ang-1 ratio, and sICAM-1 at admission are associated with infant mortality

Median plasma Ang-2 concentration at presentation was significantly higher among infants with suspected sepsis who subsequently died compared to those who survived (5.4 ng/mL [IQR: 3.1, 10.1] vs 3.3 ng/mL [IQR: 2.1, 4.1], aOR 2.50, $p = 0.024$) (Fig. 2; Table 2). The relative odds of death increased with each tertile increase of plasma Ang-2 concentration, and the trend approached

Table 1 Demographic and Clinical Characteristics of Enrolled Infants

	Deaths (n = 18)	Survivors (n = 52)	*p-value* [a,b]	Bacteremia (n = 10)	Non-Bacteremia (n = 30)	*p-value* [a,b]	Combined Outcome (n = 25)	Control (n = 73)	*p-value* [a,b]
Demographic characteristics									
Age, median in days [IQR]	16.5 [9, 24]	17 [10, 27]	*0.552*	11 [4, 24]	10.5 [3, 16]	*0.951*	16 [8, 24]	14 [7, 27]	*0.482*
Weight, median in kg [IQR]	2.1 [1.9, 3.0]	2.4 [2.0, 2.8]	*0.059*	2.7 [2.5, 3.1]	2.7 [2.3, 3.0]	*0.455*	2.5 [2.0, 3.0]	2.5 [2.2, 3.0]	*0.294*
Male, % (#)	**67 (12)**	**58 (30)**	**< 0.001**	**90 (9)**	**55 (16)**	**< 0.001**	**72 (18)**	**59 (43)**	**< 0.001**
Birth characteristics									
Born in hospital, % (#)	22(4)	31 (16)	0.715	20 (2)	37 (11)	0.648	24 (6)	34 (25)	0.451
Delivery by Caesarian section, % (#)	6 (1)	16 (9)	0.169	**0 (0)**	**7 (2)**	**0.039**	**4 (1)**	**13 (9)**	**0.014**
Clinical findings at admission									
Temperature, ° C [IQR]	36.7 [36.2, 37.8]	37.6 [36.7, 37.8]	0.062	37.5 [37.1, 38.6]	37.7 [37.3, 38.2]	0.435	37.2 [36.4, 37.8]	37.7 [36.9, 38.1]	0.147
Lethargy, % (#)	38.9 (7)	18.0 (9)	0.824	20.0 (2)	13.3 (4)	0.388	32 (8)	15 (11)	0.345
Respiratory rate, breaths per minute [IQR]	66 [42,75]	57 [48.5, 69.5]	0.729	64.5 [56, 78]	62 [53, 66]	0.476	66 [52, 75]	61 [49, 68]	0.481
Antibiotics prior to blood culture, % (#)	50 (9)	38 (20)	0.215	40 (4)	50 (15)	0.078	**40 (10)**	**45 (33)**	**0.013**

Ang-1 angiopoietin-1, *Ang-2* angiopoietin-2, *Ang2:1* ratio of Ang-2 to Ang-1, *sICAM* soluble intercellular adhesion molecule-1, *sVCAM* soluble vascular adhesion molecule-1, *IQR* inter-quartile range

[a]Test for differences between groups not reported for variables that were used to match cases and controls (age and weight)

[b]Continuous variables compared using bivariate conditional logistic regression. Binary variables compared using exact McNemar's test

Comparisons with *p*-values less than or equal to 0.05 marked in bold

statistical significance (p-trend = 0.061) (Table 3). There was no statistically significant difference in median plasma Ang-1 levels among infants who died versus those who survived (11.7 ng/mL [IQR: 4.7, 21.5] vs 15.8 ng/mL [IQR: 10.5, 25.0], aOR 0.51, $p = 0.119$) (Fig. 2; Table 2). All models with the primary outcome were adjusted for prior antibiotic exposure, lethargy, and sex.

Because Ang-1 and Ang-2 can have competitive effects that contribute to microvascular permeability, the ratio of the circulating levels of these two ligands was examined. The median Ang-2:1 ratio was 0.48 [IQR: 0.25, 0.87] among infants who died compared to 0.21 [IQR: 0.10, 0.31] among survivors (aOR 2.29, $p = 0.016$) (Fig. 2 and Table 2). Young infants whose Ang-2:Ang-1 ratio at admission was in the top tertile had 4.82-fold increased odds of death compared with infants in the bottom tertile (p-trend = 0.013) (Table 3).

Higher circulating Ang-2 levels are often associated with increased levels of sICAM-1 and sVCAM-1, reflective of endothelial activation. We examined the association between these downstream targets of Ang-2 signaling and infant sepsis outcomes. Median circulating sICAM-1 concentrations at admission were higher among the septic infants who subsequently died compared with those who survived (276.0 ng/mL [IQR: 160.9, 484.7] vs 197.2 ng/mL [IQR: 150.1, 346.8], aOR 14.11, $p = 0.023$) (Fig. 2, Table 2). When sICAM-1 was categorized into tertiles, the odds of death increased between the first and last tertiles but the trend was not statistically significant ($p = 0.116$) (Table 3). Soluble VCAM-1 concentrations were not associated with the mortality outcome (Fig. 2, Tables 2 and 3).

The Ang-2:Ang-1 ratio is associated with bacteremia

Among the study cohort, 10 infants had microbiologically confirmed bacterial bloodstream infections, of which three died. Ang-2 concentrations trended higher in bacteremic infants than in non-bacteraemic infants (median 4.1 ng/mL vs 3.4 ng/mL, aOR 6.12, $p = 0.072$). When combined with Ang-1, the ratio of Ang-2:Ang-1 was significantly associated with bacteremia (aOR 5.72, $p = 0.041$) (Fig. 2, Table 2). Soluble-ICAM-1 concentrations trended towards higher concentrations among bacteremic infants than their controls (265.1 ng/mL vs 161.0 ng/mL, aOR 26.72, $p = 0.062$), but the small sample size limits analytical power. There was no difference in Ang-1 or sVCAM-1 concentrations among bacteremic infants compared with their controls.

Increased circulating markers of endothelial activation at admission are associated with clinical outcomes among young infants

When the primary and secondary outcome groups were combined, the plasma Ang-2 concentration was significantly associated with the Combined Outcome group (aOR 3.20, $p = 0.006$), as was the Ang-2:Ang-1 ratio (aOR 2.56, $p = 0.004$). Soluble ICAM-1 was also significantly higher among these cases compared with the controls (262.0 ng/mL [IQR: 146.3, 409.1] vs 179.9 ng/mL [IQR: 144.0, 272.6], aOR 10.25, $p = 0.005$). Plasma Ang-1 levels displayed a trend towards lower values among the Combined Outcome group compared to the Controls group (11.2 ng/mL [IQR: 5.7, 20.4] vs 15.2 ng/mL [IQR: 8.9, 25.0], aOR 0.54, $p = 0.089$). Soluble-VCAM-1 was not associated with the Combined Outcome (Table 2).

Discussion

Sepsis remains a significant cause of global infant and child mortality [1]. Early administration of antimicrobial therapy and supportive care can improve outcomes, however early recognition is challenging due to the subtle presentation of sepsis in the newborn. Despite numerous clinical scoring tools to help identify infants at risk for septicemia and death, clinical evaluation of sepsis severity and prognostication remains imprecise [48, 50] and ancillary laboratory investigations are costly and frequently not available in the settings where most neonatal deaths occur. In agreement with previous studies, we found the prognostic utility of typical clinical indicators of infection such as temperature, heart rate, respiratory rate, and lethargy, to be limited with no significant differences observed between infants who died of sepsis compared to those who survived (Table 1). In cases of adult sepsis, determining the levels of immune and endothelial dysfunction at clinical presentation appears to have utility in triage and prognostication but this has not been well studied in the context of neonatal sepsis.

In this study we tested the hypothesis that circulating markers of endothelial dysfunction would identify young infants with life-threatening infections when they first present to a health care facility. We showed an association between biomarkers of endothelial activation and mortality among young infants aged ≤59 days with suspected sepsis at presentation to a pediatric referral centre in a resource-poor setting. Young infants who subsequently died of sepsis had increased circulating concentrations of Ang-2 and the Ang-2:1 ratio at presentation compared with age- and birthweight-matched infants who survived. Plasma levels of sICAM-1, a downstream target of the Angiopoietin-Tie2 pathway, was also significantly associated with mortality. A similar trend was observed among infants with culture-proven bacteremia, but the low rate of bacteremia in this cohort (due in part to pre-hospital antibiotic use) limited analytic power. An increased ratio of circulating Ang-2:Ang-1 was significantly associated with bacteremia,

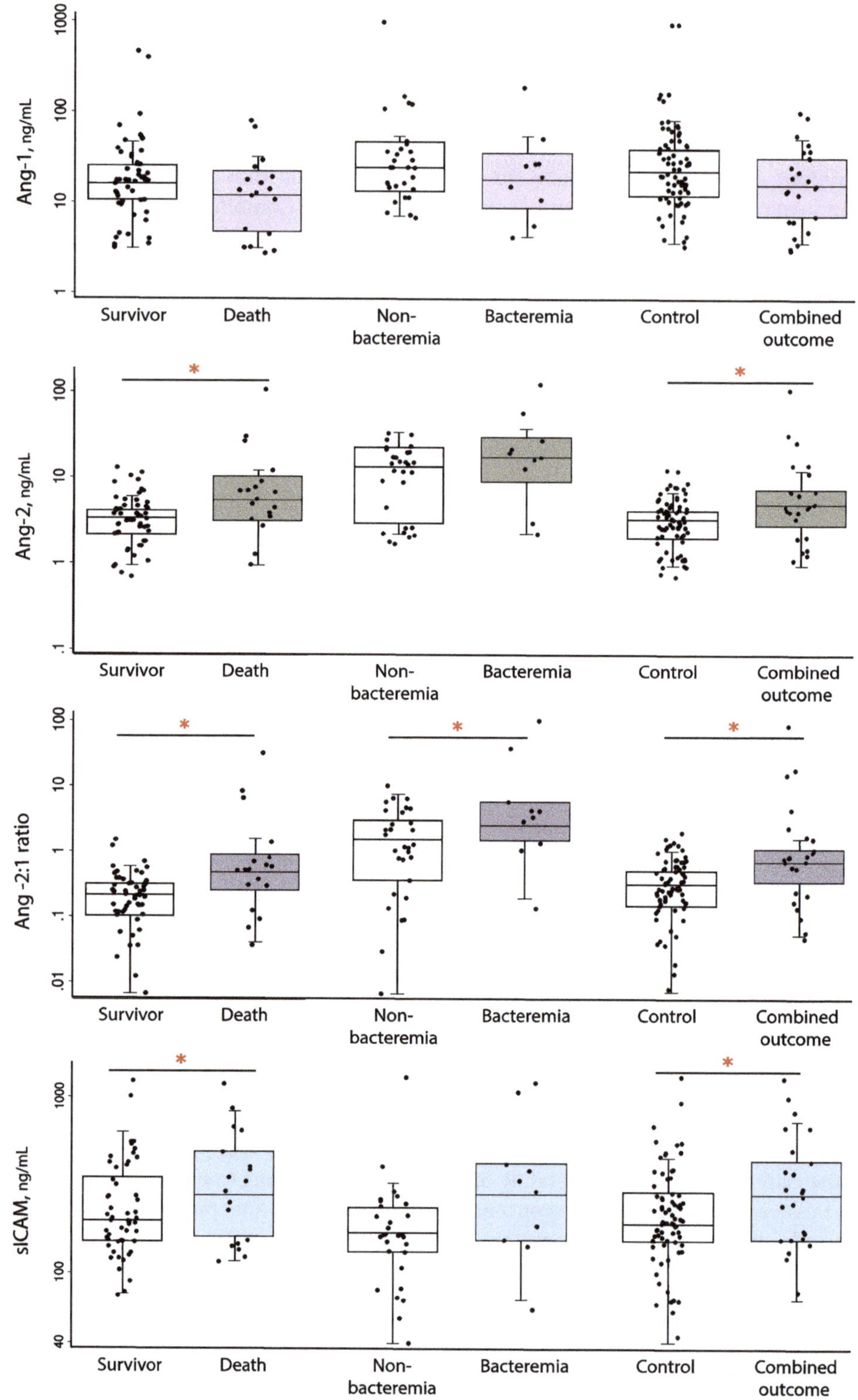

Fig. 2 Distribution of angiogenic biomarkers by mortality, bacteremia, and combined outcomes. Circulating levels of Ang-2, sICAM-1 and the Ang-2:1 ratio at admission were associated with increased risk of death and the combined outcome of death and bacteremia. Only the Ang-2:1 ratio was significantly associated with bacteremia. Ang-1 levels at admission were not associated with any of the clinical outcomes. * indicates $p < 0.05$ based on conditional logistic regression adjusting for relevant confounding variables: sex and lethargy for mortality outcome, sex for bacteremia outcome, and sex, lethargy and temperature for combined case outcome

Table 2 Median values of angiogenic biomarkers and odds of death or bacteremia

Biomarker	Death (n = 18) median [IQR]	Survivor (n = 52) median [IQR]	aOR (95% CI)	*p -value**	Bacteremia (n = 10) median [IQR]	Non-bacteremia (n = 30) median [IQR]	aOR (95% CI)	*p -value**	Combined Outcome (n = 25) median [IQR]	Control (n = 73) median [IQR]	aOR (95% CI)	*p -value**
Ang-1 (ng/mL)	11.7 [4.7, 21.5]	15.8 [10.5, 25.0]	0.51 (0.22, 1.19)	0.119	11.2 [6.0, 20.4]	14.7 [8.7, 26.2]	0.49 (0.17, 1.44)	0.194	11.2 [5.7, 20.4]	*15.2 [8.9, 25.0]*	*0.54 (0.26, 1.10)*	*0.089*
Ang-2 (ng/mL)	**5.4 [3.1, 10.1]**	**3.3 [2.1, 4.1]**	**2.50 (1.13, 5.54)**	**0.024**	*4.1 [2.6, 6.1]*	*3.4 [1.2, 5.0]*	*6.12 (0.85, 44.00)*	*0.072*	**4.9 [2.8, 7.1]**	**3.3 [2.0, 4.1]**	**3.20 (1.40, 7.34)**	**0.006**
Ang 2:1 ratio	**0.48 [0.25, 0.87]**	**0.21 [0.10, 0.31]**	**2.29 (1.16, 4.46)**	**0.016**	**0.28 [0.20, 0.46]**	**0.20 [0.01, 0.31]**	**5.72 (1.07, 30.50)**	**0.041**	**0.28 [0.20, 0.46]**	**0.21 [0.01, 0.31]**	**2.56 (1.35, 4.87)**	**0.004**
sICAM (ng/mL)	**276.0 [160.9, 484.7]**	**197.2 [150.1, 346.8]**	**14.11 (1.4, 137.83)**	**0.023**	*265.1 [146.3, 398.8]*	*161.0 [125.0, 222.9]*	*26.72 (0.84, 846.9)*	*0.062*	**262.0 [146.3, 409.1]**	**179.9 [144.0, 272.6]**	**10.25 (2.04, 51.34)**	**0.005**
sVCAM (ng/mL)	1236.6 [950.8, 1544.3]	1154.5 [884.6, 1071.0]	2.38 (0.56, 10.04)	0.239	1166.6 [795.2, 1410.3]	1149.9 [861.1, 1552.7]	1.66 (0.26, 10.67)	0.594	1289.7 [950.8, 1541.1]	1168.0 [886.2, 1647.3]	2.77 (0.80, 9.56)	0.149

aOR adjusted odds ratio, *CI* confidence interval, *Ang-1* angiopoietin-1, *Ang-2* angiopoietin-2, *Ang2:1* ratio of Ang-2 to Ang-1, *sICAM* soluble intercellular adhesion molecule-1, *sVCAM* soluble vascular adhesion molecule 1, *IQR* inter-quartile range

**P*-value for conditional logistic regression for sex, lethargy and prior antibiotic exposure for Death outcome; sex and prior antibiotic exposure for Bacteremia outcome; sex, lethargy, temperature and prior antibiotic exposure for combined outcome. Biomarkers were log transformed

Comparisons with p-value less than or equal to 0.05 marked in bold, and less than or equal to 0.10 marked in italics

Table 3 Angiogenic biomarkers tertiles and relative odds of death

Biomarker	N	Tertile 1 aOR	Tertile 2 aOR (95% CI)	Tertile 3 aOR (95% CI)	p-value for trend
Ang-1	70	1.00 (ref)	0.37 (0.09, 1.52)	0.39 (0.09, 1.62)	0.301
Ang-2	*70*	*1.00 (ref)*	*1.39 (0.26, 7.36)*	*5.27 (1.15, 24.07)*	*0.061*
Ang 2:1 ratio	**70**	**1.00 (ref)**	**0.57 (0.09, 3.54)**	**4.82 (1.22, 19.03)**	**0.013**
sICAM	70	1.00 (ref)	0.50 (0.09, 2.75)	2.43 (0.60, 9.90)	0.116
sVCAM	70	1.00 (ref)	0.95 (0.22, 4.11)	1.40 (0.36, 5.45)	0.834

aOR adjusted odds ratio, *CI* confidence interval, *Ang-1* angiopoietin-1, *Ang-2* angiopoietin-2, *Ang2:1* ratio of Ang-2 to Ang-1, *sICAM* soluble intercellular adhesion molecule-1, *sVCAM* soluble vascular adhesion molecule-1. P-value for trend using conditional logistic regression adjusted for sex, lethargy and prior antibiotic exposure
Comparisons with *p*-value less than or equal to 0.05 marked in bold and 0.05–0.10 marked in italics

and both Ang-2 and sICAM-1 displayed positive trends with this outcome despite the small number of cases.

Circulating Angiopoietins are associated with clinical outcomes of sepsis in young infants

This study adds to a growing body of evidence implicating microvascular endothelial injury in the pathophysiology of severe sepsis. Widespread activation of the endothelium triggers endothelial cell dissociation and microvascular leak resulting in hemodynamic collapse and the multi-organ failure associated with septic shock [9, 10, 13]. The Angiopoietin-Tie2 axis is emerging as a critical regulator of the microvascular response to infection [29] and may provide novel targets for intervention to improve outcomes [51, 52].

Studies of sepsis from North American academic hospitals have profiled protein markers of endothelial activation in both the adult and pediatric populations. Among adults, circulating levels of angiopoietins obtained on transfer to the ICU have shown increased circulating concentrations of Ang-2 and decreased levels of Ang-1 in patients who succumbed to sepsis [7, 53]. Mikacenic et al. also found that these endothelial biomarkers correlated with sepsis severity independently of the degree of inflammatory response. Similarly, among adults initially presenting to the Emergency Department with sepsis, Ang-2 levels correlated with sepsis severity and death [17]. Studies involving both young (10 months to 32 months) and older (9 years to 13 years) children with sepsis found that circulating concentrations of Ang-2 at the time of transfer to the Pediatric ICU correlated with sepsis severity and death [44, 45]. Outside of North America, a study conducted in Blantyre, Malawi involving 293 septic children aged two months to 16 years again found mortality to be associated with increased levels of Ang-2 and decreased levels of Ang-1 in plasma samples collected on admission to hospital [46].

This study provides new evidence for a role of the Angiopoietin-Tie2 axis in septic infants less than two months of age. Similar to patterns observed in adults and older children, the circulating concentrations of angiopoietins were associated with clinically significant endpoints of sepsis. Increased levels of Ang-2 were associated with mortality and trended with bacteremia outcomes, but our study was not powered for the latter outcome. Ang-1 levels did not vary with mortality or bacteremia outcomes, consistent with previous pediatric studies [44]. Overall, these findings suggest that despite the immaturity of the vascular endothelium in neonates and young infants, the initiating mechanisms of sepsis and vascular leak are regulated by similar pathways as those now well-characterized in older populations. The angiopoietin-Tie2 pathway may therefore serve as both a clinically important diagnostic marker and a therapeutic target for future interventions aimed to mitigate the effects of sepsis and microvascular leak in this vulnerable neonatal population [52].

Soluble-ICAM-1 is associated with clinical outcomes of sepsis in young infants

The activation of the vascular endothelium by Ang-2 results in an increase in endothelial surface expression of endothelial-leukocyte adhesion molecules including ICAM-1 and VCAM-1 [9]. After the initiation of leukocyte rolling along an activated endothelium, ICAM-1 and VCAM-1 facilitate the firm adhesion of leukocytes with endothelial cells allowing for transendothelial migration and inflammation of surrounding tissues that may ultimately contribute to end organ damage [54–57]. The shedding of sICAM-1 and sVCAM-1 from the endothelial surface is brought about by the activity of proteolytic proteins called sheddases and may represent the initial down-regulation phase of the sepsis response [58]. Levels of these circulating adhesion molecules may be indicative of the degree of endothelial activation as well as a host mechanism to limit the sepsis response by binding leukocytes in circulation and preventing their adherence and diapedesis across the endothelial barrier. The functional significance of the soluble adhesion proteins in newborn sepsis requires further study within larger cohorts.

Several studies among adults have established positive associations between circulating levels of sICAM-1 and SIRS, sepsis and sepsis severity including hemodynamic shock, multi-organ failure, and death [32–36, 54, 59–61];

findings from the neonatal and newborn populations have been less consistent. Berner et al. and Dollner et al. did not find an association between sICAM among septic infants [37, 38]. In contrast, studies by Hansen et al., Apostolu et al., and Figueras et al. found increased levels of sICAM-1 among septic infants compared with controls [40, 43, 62], and Edgar et al. demonstrated that sICAM-1 levels predicted infection in newborns [41, 42]. Interestingly even in non-septic newborns, levels of circulating sICAM-1 have been shown to increase over the first week of life; by 30 days of life, plasma concentrations can exceed those of healthy adults [63]. In our study, circulating sICAM-1 concentration in young infants on presentation to a pediatric hospital was positively associated with mortality and culture-proven bacteremia after matching on age. Within this small subset of bacteremic infants (n = 10, ages all less than 30 days), those who succumbed to sepsis (n = 3) had higher circulating levels of sICAM-1 than those who survived (n = 7) (median values 398.0 ng/mL vs 182.5 ng/mL, respectively).

Among adults, the association between sVCAM-1 and sepsis severity has been variable with some studies demonstrating a positive association between sVCAM-1 and sepsis outcomes [34, 53], while others showed no association with sepsis severity or mortality [36]. Soluble-VCAM-1 levels have not been as extensively studied in newborns. One reported study showed that sVCAM-1 levels only increased among septic infants with culture-proven bacteremia, as opposed to the septic, culture-negative comparators [43]. In our study, sVCAM-1 levels were not significantly associated with either mortality or bacteremia.

The discrepant associations between soluble adhesion molecules and sepsis, and the heterogeneity between the adult and newborn populations, suggests potential developmental changes in the pathophysiology of sepsis. In a review by Zonneveld et al., circulating endothelial adhesion molecule concentrations among healthy and septic individuals were studied across neonatal, child and adult age groups. Overall, the concentrations of soluble adhesion molecules, including sICAM-1 and sVCAM-1, increased during sepsis but both the relative and absolute extent of increase were markedly lower among neonates compared with the older age groups. The authors posit that the failure to robustly upregulate circulating sICAM-1 may be reflective of either an immature, hyporesponsive immune response, or age-related differences in the production of sheddases [58]. The functional significance of the soluble adhesion proteins in newborn sepsis requires further study.

Study limitations

This study was conducted in a resource-poor setting where tools for clinical assessment are limited and laboratory indicators of sepsis severity were not available. Medical management of the septic newborns was left to the discretion of the treating physician and this is a potential source of bias. Notably, among the parent-study cohort of septic infants from which our study sample was derived, the rate of bacteremia was 3.1%, less than expected; moreover, the pathogens typically isolated from newborns in Bangladesh, including *Staphylococcus aureus* and gram negative organisms [64, 65], were not predominant in this cohort (Additional file 1: Table S1). Importantly, 44% of our study cohort had antibiotic exposure prior to blood sampling for culture and 45% of those with negative blood cultures received antibiotics prior to sampling. Thus the rate of bacteremia identified by blood culture may underestimate the true prevalence of bacteremia in this cohort, and the reported organisms may not have identified all of the causative pathogens. Finally, due to changes in specimen storage in Bangladesh, samples collected from the first 71 enrolled infants were not available for analysis. Additional prospective studies will be required to validate the findings of this study.

Conclusions

Sepsis and its sequelae remain leading causes of infant morbidity and mortality, particularly in resource-poor settings where rates are highest, and the availability of intensive supportive care are the lowest. Our results demonstrate that circulating markers of endothelial dysfunction at the time that infants present for medical attention have the potential to risk stratify those in most need of aggressive medical support. If these findings are externally validated by additional prospective studies, point-of-care tests incorporating these markers may enable rapid triage of critically ill neonates at risk of death from sepsis.

Abbreviations

Ang-1: Angiopoietin-1; Ang-2: Angiopoietin-2; aOR: adjusted odds ratio; ELISA: Enzyme-Linked Immunosorbent Assay; ICAM-1: Intercellular adhesion molecule-1; NFkB: Nuclear Factor kappa-light-chain-enhancer of activated B cells; sICAM: Soluble Intercellular adhesion molecule-1; SIRS: Systemic inflammatory response syndrome; SOMCH: Sylhet MAG Osmani Medical College Hospital; sVCAM: Soluble Vascular cell adhesion molecule-1; VCAM-1: Vascular cell adhesion molecule-1; WHO: World Health Organization

Acknowledgements

The authors would like to acknowledge the contributions of Dr. Andrea Conroy to the experimental protocols and assistance conducting the experiments. They would also like to acknowledge all the members of the PROJAHNMO team, the physicians and nurses of the Department of Pediatrics at the Sylhet M.A.G. Osmani Medical College Hospital who participated in study.

Funding

This work was supported by the Canadian Institutes of Health Research (CIHR) grants MOP-13721, MOP-115160, MOP-136813, and a CIHR Foundation grant FDN-148439 (K.C.K.), the Canada Research Chair Program (K.C.K.), the

Johns Hopkins (KL2) Mentored Career Development Award (A.F), National Institute of Child Health and Human Development (NICHD; K08 HD 073315), The Dr. Sydney H. Kane, Emma B. Kane, David M. Kane and Family Endowment Fund (A.F), and The Sheila S. and Lawrence C. Pakula, M.D. Endowment for Neonatal Research (A.F). None of the funders were involved in the study design, data analysis, manuscript preparation, or decision to disseminate and publish the study findings.

Authors' contributions

Conceived and designed the experiments: JKW KH VT KCK; Performed the experiments: JKW VT; Contributed reagents/materials and data analysis tools: KCK; Experimental data (biomarker) analysis: JKW KH VT KCK; Developed the clinical study design: GMK, AB, AM1, AM2, MS AF; Patient recruitment SOMCH: GMK AB, AM1, AM2, AF; Patient sample and/or data collection, and clinical data analysis: GMK AB, AM1. AM2, NB MS AF; Statistical analysis: KH; Wrote the paper: JKW KH KCK AF. All authors read and approved the final manuscript.

Competing interests

K.C.K. is listed as an inventor on patents related to the use of angiopoietin markers, entitled "Angiopoietin-1 and -2 biomarkers for infectious diseases that compromise endothelial integrity" (application no. WO2009059404) and "Biomarkers for early determination of a critical or life threatening response to illness and monitoring response to treatment" (application no. CA2769433). For the remaining authors, no competing interests were declared.

Author details

[1]Tropical Disease Unit, Division of Infectious Diseases, Department of Medicine, University of Toronto, Toronto, ON, Canada. [2]Sandra Rotman Centre for Global Health, University Health Network-Toronto General Hospital, Department of Medicine, University of Toronto, Toronto, ON, Canada. [3]Department of International Health, Bloomberg School of Public Health, Johns Hopkins University, Baltimore, MD, USA. [4]International Centre for Maternal and Newborn Health, Department of International Health, Bloomberg School of Public Health, Johns Hopkins University, Baltimore, MD, USA. [5]Department of Pediatrics, Sylhet MAG Osmani Medical College Hospital, Sylhet, Bangladesh. [6]Dhaka Shishu (Children's) Hospital, Sher-E-Bangla Nagar, Dhaka, Bangladesh. [7]Division of Neonatology, Department of Pediatrics, Johns Hopkins University School of Medicine, Baltimore, MD, USA.

References

1. GBD 2015 Child Mortality Collaborators. Global, regional, national, and selected subnational levels of stillbirths, neonatal, infant, and under-5 mortality, 1980-2015: a systematic analysis for the global burden of disease study 2015. Lancet. 2016;388:1725–74.
2. Seale AC, Blencowe H, Manu AA, Nair H, Bahl R, Qazi SA, et al. Estimates of possible severe bacterial infection in neonates in sub-Saharan Africa, South Asia, and Latin America for 2012: a systematic review and meta-analysis. Lancet Infect Dis. 2014;14:731–41.
3. Lawn JE, Cousens S, Zupan J. Lancet Neonatal Survival Steering Team 4 million neonatal deaths: when? Where? Why? Lancet. 2005;365:891–900.
4. Edmond K, Zaidi A. New approaches to preventing, diagnosing, and treating neonatal sepsis. PLoS Med. 2010;7:e1000213.
5. Delano MJ, Ward PA. Sepsis-induced immune dysfunction: can immune therapies reduce mortality? J Clin Invest. 2016;126:23–31.
6. Lee WL, Slutsky AS. Sepsis and endothelial permeability. N Engl J Med. 2010; 363:689–91.
7. Ricciuto DR, Santos dos CC, Hawkes M, Toltl LJ, Conroy AL, Rajwans N, et al. Angiopoietin-1 and angiopoietin-2 as clinically informative prognostic biomarkers of morbidity and mortality in severe sepsis. Crit Care Med 2011; 39:702–710.
8. Lee WL, Liles WC. Endothelial activation, dysfunction and permeability during severe infections. Curr Opin Hematol. 2011;18:191–6.
9. Fiedler U, Reiss Y, Scharpfenecker M, Grunow V, Koidl S, Thurston G, et al. Angiopoietin-2 sensitizes endothelial cells to TNF-alpha and has a crucial role in the induction of inflammation. Nat Med. 2006;12:235–9.
10. Brindle NPJ, Saharinen P, Alitalo K. Signaling and functions of angiopoietin-1 in vascular protection. Circ Res. 2006;98:1014–23.
11. Kim I, Moon SO, Park SK, Chae SW, Koh GY. Angiopoietin-1 reduces VEGF-stimulated leukocyte adhesion to endothelial cells by reducing ICAM-1, VCAM-1, and E-selectin expression. Circ Res. 2001;89:477–9.
12. Fiedler U, Augustin HG. Angiopoietins: a link between angiogenesis and inflammation. Trends Immunol. 2006;27:552–8.
13. Scharpfenecker M, Fiedler U, Reiss Y, Augustin HG. The Tie-2 ligand angiopoietin-2 destabilizes quiescent endothelium through an internal autocrine loop mechanism. J Cell Sci. 2005;118:771–80.
14. Paulus P, Jennewein C, Zacharowski K. Biomarkers of endothelial dysfunction: can they help us deciphering systemic inflammation and sepsis? Biomarkers. 2011;16(Suppl 1):S11–21.
15. Maisonpierre PC, Suri C, Jones PF, Bartunkova S, Wiegand SJ, Radziejewski C, et al. Angiopoietin-2, a natural antagonist for Tie2 that disrupts in vivo angiogenesis. Science. 1997;277:55–60.
16. Jones N, Iljin K, Dumont DJ, Alitalo K. Tie receptors: new modulators of angiogenic and lymphangiogenic responses. Nat Rev Mol Cell Biol. 2001;2: 257–67.
17. David S, Mukherjee A, Ghosh CC, Yano M, Khankin EV, Wenger JB, et al. Angiopoietin-2 may contribute to multiple organ dysfunction and death in sepsis*. Crit Care Med. 2012;40:3034–41.
18. Page AV, Tarr PI, Watkins SL, Rajwans N, Petruzziello-Pellegrini TN, Marsden PA, et al. Dysregulation of angiopoietin 1 and 2 in Escherichia coli O157:H7 infection and the hemolytic-uremic syndrome. J Infect Dis. 2013;208:929–33.
19. Page AV, Kotb M, McGeer A, Low DE, Kain KC, Liles WC. Systemic dysregulation of angiopoietin-1/2 in streptococcal toxic shock syndrome. Clin Infect Dis. 2011;52:e157–61.
20. Lovegrove FE, Tangpukdee N, Opoka RO, Lafferty EI, Rajwans N, Hawkes M, et al. Serum angiopoietin-1 and -2 levels discriminate cerebral malaria from uncomplicated malaria and predict clinical outcome in African children. PLoS One. 2009;4:e4912.
21. Conroy AL, Lafferty EI, Lovegrove FE, Krudsood S, Tangpukdee N, Liles WC, et al. Whole blood angiopoietin-1 and -2 levels discriminate cerebral and severe (non-cerebral) malaria from uncomplicated malaria. Malar J. 2009;8:295.
22. Conroy AL, Phiri H, Hawkes M, Glover S, Mallewa M, Seydel KB, et al. Endothelium-based biomarkers are associated with cerebral malaria in Malawian children: a retrospective case-control study. PLoS One. 2010;5: e15291.
23. Silver KL, Zhong K, Leke RGF, Taylor DW, Kain KC. Dysregulation of angiopoietins is associated with placental malaria and low birth weight. PLoS One. 2010;5:e9481.
24. Conroy AL, Glover SJ, Hawkes M, Erdman LK, Seydel KB, Taylor TE, et al. Angiopoietin-2 levels are associated with retinopathy and predict mortality in Malawian children with cerebral malaria: a retrospective case-control study*. Crit Care Med. 2012;40:952–9.
25. Michels M, van der Ven AJAM, Djamiatun K, Fijnheer R, de Groot PG, Griffioen AW, et al. Imbalance of angiopoietin-1 and angiopoetin-2 in severe dengue and relationship with thrombocytopenia, endothelial activation, and vascular stability. Am J Trop Med Hyg. 2012;87:943–6.
26. Agrawal A, Matthay MA, Kangelaris KN, Stein J, Chu JC, Imp BM, et al. Plasma angiopoietin-2 predicts the onset of acute lung injury in critically ill patients. Am J Respir Crit Care Med. 2013;187:736–42.
27. Hoeboer SH, Groeneveld ABJ, van der Heijden M, Oudemans-van Straaten HM. Serial inflammatory biomarkers of the severity, course and outcome of late onset acute respiratory distress syndrome in critically ill patients with or at risk for the syndrome after new-onset fever. Biomark Med. 2015;9:605–16.
28. Zinter MS, Spicer A, Orwoll BO, Alkhouli M, Dvorak CC, Calfee CS, et al. Plasma angiopoietin-2 outperforms other markers of endothelial injury in prognosticating pediatric ARDS mortality. Am J Physiol Lung Cell Mol Physiol. 2016;310:L224–31.
29. Page AV, Liles WC. Biomarkers of endothelial activation/dysfunction in infectious diseases. Virulence. 2013;4:507–16.
30. Koh GY. Orchestral actions of angiopoietin-1 in vascular regeneration. Trends Mol Med. 2013;19:31–9.

31. Siner JM. A tale of two ligands: angiopoietins, the endothelium, and outcomes. Crit Care. 2013;17:1007.
32. Boldt J, Wollbrück M, Kuhn D, Linke LC, Hempelmann G. Do plasma levels of circulating soluble adhesion molecules differ between surviving and nonsurviving critically ill patients? Chest. 1995;107:787–92.
33. Sessler CN, Windsor AC, Schwartz M, Watson L, Fisher BJ, Sugerman HJ, et al. Circulating ICAM-1 is increased in septic shock. Am J Respir Crit Care Med. 1995;151:1420–7.
34. Cowley HC, Heney D, Gearing AJ, Hemingway I, Webster NR. Increased circulating adhesion molecule concentrations in patients with the systemic inflammatory response syndrome: a prospective cohort study. Crit Care Med. 1994;22:651–7.
35. Kayal S, Jaïs JP, Aguini N, Chaudière J, Labrousse J. Elevated circulating E-selectin, intercellular adhesion molecule 1, and von Willebrand factor in patients with severe infection. Am J Respir Crit Care Med. 1998;157:776–84.
36. Kung C-T, Hsiao S-Y, Su C-M, Tsai T-C, Cheng H-H, Tsai N-W, et al. Serum adhesion molecules as predictors of bacteremia in adult severe sepsis patients at the emergency department. Clin Chim Acta. 2013;421:116–20.
37. Berner R, Niemeyer CM, Leititis JU, Funke A, Schwab C, Rau U, et al. Plasma levels and gene expression of granulocyte colony-stimulating factor, tumor necrosis factor-alpha, interleukin (IL)-1beta, IL-6, IL-8, and soluble intercellular adhesion molecule-1 in neonatal early onset sepsis. Pediatr Res. 1998;44:469–77.
38. Døllner H, Vatten L, Austgulen R. Early diagnostic markers for neonatal sepsis: comparing C-reactive protein, interleukin-6, soluble tumour necrosis factor receptors and soluble adhesion molecules. J Clin Epidemiol. 2001;54:1251–7.
39. Hansen TM, Singh H, Tahir TA, Brindle NPJ. Effects of angiopoietins-1 and -2 on the receptor tyrosine kinase Tie2 are differentially regulated at the endothelial cell surface. Cell Signal. 2010;22:527–32.
40. Apostolou M, Dimitriou H, Kaleyias J, Perdikogianni C, Stiakaki E, Costalos C, et al. Levels of soluble ICAM-1 in premature and full-term neonates with infection. Mediat Inflamm. 2002;11:95–8.
41. Edgar JD, Wilson DC, SA MM, Crockard AD, Halliday MI, Gardiner KR, et al. Predictive value of soluble immunological mediators in neonatal infection. Clin Sci. 1994;87:165–71.
42. Edgar D, Gabriel V, Craig A, Wheeler D, Thomas M, Grant J. A low serum sICAM-1 level may assist in the exclusion of neonatal infection. Biol Neonate. 2002;81:105–8.
43. Figueras-Aloy J, Gómez-López L, Rodríguez-Miguélez J-M, Salvia-Roiges MD, Jordán-García I, Ferrer-Codina I, et al. Serum soluble ICAM-1, VCAM-1, L-selectin, and P-selectin levels as markers of infection and their relation to clinical severity in neonatal sepsis. Am J Perinatol. 2007;24:331–8.
44. Giuliano JS, Lahni PM, Harmon K, Wong HR, Doughty LA, Carcillo JA, et al. Admission angiopoietin levels in children with septic shock. Shock. 2007;28:650–4.
45. Giuliano JS, Tran K, Li F-Y, Shabanova V, Tala JA, Bhandari V. The temporal kinetics of circulating angiopoietin levels in children with sepsis. Pediatr Crit Care Med. 2014;15:e1–8.
46. Mankhambo LA, Banda DL, IPD Study Group, Jeffers G, White SA, Balmer P, et al. The role of angiogenic factors in predicting clinical outcome in severe bacterial infection in Malawian children. Crit Care. 2010;14:R91.
47. Liu L, Johnson HL, Cousens S, Perin J, Scott S, Lawn JE, et al. Global, regional, and national causes of child mortality: an updated systematic analysis for 2010 with time trends since 2000. Lancet. 2012;379:2151–61.
48. Young Infants Clinical Signs Study Group. Clinical signs that predict severe illness in children under age 2 months: a multicentre study. Lancet. 2008; 371:135–42.
49. Saha SK, Khan WA, Saha S. Blood cultures from Bangladeshi children with septicaemia: an evaluation of conventional, lysis-direct plating and lysis-centrifugation methods. Trans R Soc Trop Med Hyg. 1992;86:554–6.
50. Dorling JS, Field DJ, Manktelow B. Neonatal disease severity scoring systems. Arch Dis Child Fetal Neonatal Ed. 2005;90:F11–6.
51. Ghosh CC, David S, Zhang R, Berghelli A, Milam K, Higgins SJ, et al. Gene control of tyrosine kinase TIE2 and vascular manifestations of infections. Proc Natl Acad Sci U S A. 2016;113:2472–7.
52. Higgins SJ, Purcell LA, Silver KL, Tran V, Crowley V, Hawkes M, et al. Dysregulation of angiopoietin-1 plays a mechanistic role in the pathogenesis of cerebral malaria. Sci Transl Med. 2016;8:358ra128.
53. Mikacenic C, Hahn WO, Price BL, Harju-Baker S, Katz R, Kain KC, et al. Biomarkers of endothelial activation are associated with poor outcome in critical illness. PLoS One. 2015;10:e0141251.
54. Gearing AJ, Newman W. Circulating adhesion molecules in disease. Immunol Today. 1993;14:506–12.
55. Parrillo JE. Pathogenetic mechanisms of septic shock. N Engl J Med. 1993; 328:1471–7.
56. Leeuwenberg JF, von EJ A, Jeunhomme TM, Buurman WA. IFN-gamma regulates the expression of the adhesion molecule ELAM-1 and IL-6 production by human endothelial cells in vitro. J Immunol. 1990;145:2110–4.
57. Alon R, Feigelson S. From rolling to arrest on blood vessels: leukocyte tap dancing on endothelial integrin ligands and chemokines at sub-second contacts. Semin Immunol. 2002;14:93–104.
58. Zonneveld R, Martinelli R, Shapiro NI, Kuijpers TW, Plötz FB, Carman CV. Soluble adhesion molecules as markers for sepsis and the potential pathophysiological discrepancy in neonates, children and adults. Crit Care. 2014;18:204.
59. Cummings CJ, Sessler CN, Beall LD, Fisher BJ, Best AM, Fowler AA. Soluble E-selectin levels in sepsis and critical illness. Correlation with infection and hemodynamic dysfunction. Am J Respir Crit Care Med. 1997;156:431–7.
60. Endo S, Inada K, Kasai T, Takakuwa T, Yamada Y, Koike S, et al. Levels of soluble adhesion molecules and cytokines in patients with septic multiple organ failure. J Inflamm. 1995;46:212–9.
61. Zaki ME-S, el-Sayed H. Evaluation of microbiologic and hematologic parameters and E-selectin as early predictors for outcome of neonatal sepsis. Arch Pathol Lab Med. 2009;133:1291–6.
62. Hansen AB, Verder H, Staun-Olsen P. Soluble intercellular adhesion molecule and C-reactive protein as early markers of infection in newborns. J Perinat Med. 2000;28:97–103.
63. Phocas I, Sarandakou A, Giannaki G, Malamitsi-Puchner A, Rizos D, Zourlas PA. Soluble intercellular adhesion molecule-1 in newborn infants. Eur J Pediatr. 1998;157:153–6.
64. Hamer DH, Darmstadt GL, Carlin JB, Zaidi AKM, Yeboah-Antwi K, Saha SK, et al. Etiology of bacteremia in young infants in six countries. Pediatr Infect Dis J. 2015;34:e1–8.
65. Choi Y, Saha SK, Ahmed ASMNU, Law PA, Chowdhury MAKA, Islam M, et al. Routine skin cultures in predicting sepsis pathogens among hospitalized preterm neonates in Bangladesh. Neonatology. 2008;94:123–31.

16

Selected risk factors for atherosclerosis in children and their parents with positive family history of premature cardiovascular diseases

Elzbieta Pac-Kozuchowska[1], Paulina Krawiec[1] and Ewelina Grywalska[2*]

Abstract

Background: The aim of the study was to evaluate serum parameters of lipid metabolism, homocysteine, soluble adhesion molecules and common carotid artery wall thickness in children from families with early symptoms of atherosclerosis.

Methods: The first stage included 137 pairs of mothers and newborns, and the second 18 children from the same group (age 18-30 months) and their parents (age 21-46 years) with a history of premature coronary artery disease (CAD), as well as 12 age- and sex-matched controls.

Results: During the first stage, inverse correlations were found between birthweight, cord blood concentrations of triglycerides (TG), VLDL cholesterol and apolipoprotein B (Apo B). Serum concentrations of total cholesterol (TC), apolipoprotein A1 (Apo A1), LDL and HDL cholesterol and were significantly higher in female than in male newborns. During the second stage, children from families with a history for premature CAD were shown to present with significantly higher serum concentrations of TG, VLDL cholesterol and lipoprotein A (Lp(a)) than the controls. Furthermore, their TC correlated positively with vascular cell adhesion molecule-1 ($Rs=0.717$, $p<0.05$) and intracellular adhesion molecule-1 (sICAM-1) levels ($Rs=0.833$, $p<0.05$). Moreover, positive correlations were found between maternal carotid intima media thickness (IMT) and TC ($Rs=0.831$, $p<0.01$), as well as between paternal IMT and Apo B ($Rs=0.692$, $p<0.05$), TG and sICAM-1 ($Rs=0.912$, $p<0.01$), TG and sE-selectin ($Rs=0.678$, $p<0.05$).

Conclusions: Serum Lp(a) may serve as a maker of cardiovascular risk in children and adolescents.

Keywords: Atherosclerosis, Cardiovascular risk, Lipid profile

Background

Although cardiovascular diseases based on atherosclerosis, like ischemic heart disease or stroke, manifest in adulthood, there is a compelling evidence that the process of atherosclerosis begins in childhood and progresses to measureable vascular changes in adulthood [1, 2].

The pathogenesis of atherosclerosis has undergone many changes over the last decades. The traditional viewpoint established atherosclerosis as a localized cholesterol storage disease with flow-limiting arterial stenosis [3]. We currently understand atherosclerosis as a chronic inflammatory process of arterial wall resulting from interplay of lipid metabolism imbalance, maladaptive immune response and genetic alterations [3–5].

Traditionally cardiovascular modifiable risk factors included cigarette smoking, hypercholesterolemia, hypertension and diabetes [6–8]. Approximately 20% of cardiovascular events occur in the absence of above mentioned conventional risk factors [9].

Intense investigations on novel risk factors are conducted to define cardiovascular risk in individuals without traditional risk factors. Recent studies have shown several important non-traditional risk factors for atherosclerosis including hs-CRP, homocysteine, small dense

* Correspondence: ewelina.grywalska@gmail.com
[2]Department of Clinical Immunology and Immunotherapy, Medical University of Lublin, Chodzki 4a Street, 20-093 Lublin, Poland
Full list of author information is available at the end of the article

low density lipoprotein particles (small dense LDL), oxidized low density lipoprotein (oxy-LDL), apolipoprotein A1 and B (Apo A1 and Apo B), lipoprotein a (Lp(a)), fibrinogen and triglyceride-rich lipoprotein remnants [10].

Non- modifiable atherosclerosis risk factors include age, gender and family history of premature cardiovascular diseases (CVD). The growing body of evidence indicates that the family history of premature coronary artery disease (CAD) is an independent risk factor for CVD and significant predictor for CAD [11–14]. According to The Third Report of the Expert Panel on Detection, Evaluation, and Treatment of the High Blood Cholesterol in Adults (ATP III) family history of premature CAD, specify as myocardial infarction or sudden death before 55 years of age in father or other male first-degree relative, or before 65 years of age in mother or other female first-degree relative) was found as the major risk factor of CAD [15]. Accumulation of family history of premature CVD with obesity, hypertension and diabetes is often accompanied. Thus, lifestyle intervention including dietary modification, increased physical activity, weight control and smoking cessation may be more efficient when undertaken by the entire family than the individual due to built-in support mechanism of the family [16].

The aim of the study was to evaluate the parameters of lipid metabolism, i.e. triglycerides (TG), total cholesterol (TC) and its fractions: HDL, LDL and VLDL cholesterol, apolipoprotein A1 and B (Apo A1 and Apo B), lipoprotein(a) (Lp(a)), homocysteine, soluble adhesion molecules (sICAM-1, sVCAM-1 and sE-selectin) in the blood serum and the thickness of common carotid artery wall (IMT) in children from families in which early symptoms of atherosclerosis.

Methods

The study was performed in two stages. During the first stage, the study group was composed of 137 pairs of mothers and their newborns (74 girls and 63 boys). To the study group we recruited healthy newborns, from pregnancies free of complications, born at term by spontaneous vaginal delivery with Apgar score 8-10 points at first minute after birth. The family history of cardiovascular diseases (ischemic heart disease, stroke) and risk factors for atherosclerosis like obesity, hypertension, type 2 diabetes mellitus and hypercholesterolemia was undertaken from mothers. There were selected 41 of 137 families (29.9%) with risk factors for atherosclerosis.

In all 137 pairs of mothers and newborns we assessed nutritional status and serum concentrations of TG, TC, HDL, LDL, VLDL, Apo A1, Apo B and Lp(a).

The prospective evaluation of all newborns and their parents was planned in 18 to 30 months after birth. The information about the next stage of the study was sent to all 137 families participated in the first stage of the study. However, only 41 families volunteered to the second stage of the study. In that group we selected 29 families with risk factors for atherosclerosis and 18 with positive history for premature CAD. We presumed that parents who participated in second stage of the study were aware of the cardiovascular disease danger.

Ultimately, in the second stage of the study we included 18 children (8 girls and 10 boys) aged 18 to 30 months and their parents (aged 21-46 years) with positive history for premature coronary artery disease. The control group consisted of 12 age- and sex-matched children without a family history of CAD. In all children and their parents we assessed serum concentrations of TG, TC, HDL, LDL, VLDL, Apo A1, Apo B, Lp(a), homocysteine (Hcy), intracellular adhesion molecule-1 (sICAM-1), vascular cell adhesion molecule-1 (sVCAM-1) and sE-selectin.

The blood samples were taken fasting from the cord blood in newborns and from the ulnar vein in children and their parents. The serum the concentration of TG, TC and HDL was determined by the Cormay reagents and the Cobas Mira S analyzer. The concentration of Apo A1, Apo B and Lp(a) was determined by immunoturbidimetric method (Roche and Human). The concentration of homocysteine was determined by ELISA method using Axis Homocysteine EIA Package Insert by Axis-Shield AS. The concentrations of sICAM-1, sVCAM-1 and sE-selectin were determined by ELISA method, with the application of kits human sICAM-1 BMS201, human sVCAM-1 BMS232, human sE-selectin BMS205 (Bender Med Systems Diagnostics GmbH). The concentration of LDL and VLDL was defined by using the formula by Friedewald [17].

To identify early atherosclerotic changes common carotid intima and media combined layers thickness (IMT) was measured with an ATL 3500 ultrasound system with a 12 MHz linear transducer. The IMT was evaluated both on the right and left side, no significant differences were noticed thus the mean IMT value was calculated. A schematic diagram of the study design is presented at Fig. 1.

The statistical analysis of the results was made with application of Statistica 5.1 PL software. The distribution of studied data sets were checked up by Shapiro-Wilk test. The distribution of the examined parameters was skewed, thus Mann Whitney U test was applied for the analysis of the differences between two groups or Kruskal-Wallis ANOVA and multiple comparisons of mean ranks (as post-hoc analysis) for the analysis of differences between more than two groups. The Spearman R correlation test was used to assess the relationships between the parameters tested. The p values of $p<0.05$ were considered statistically significant.

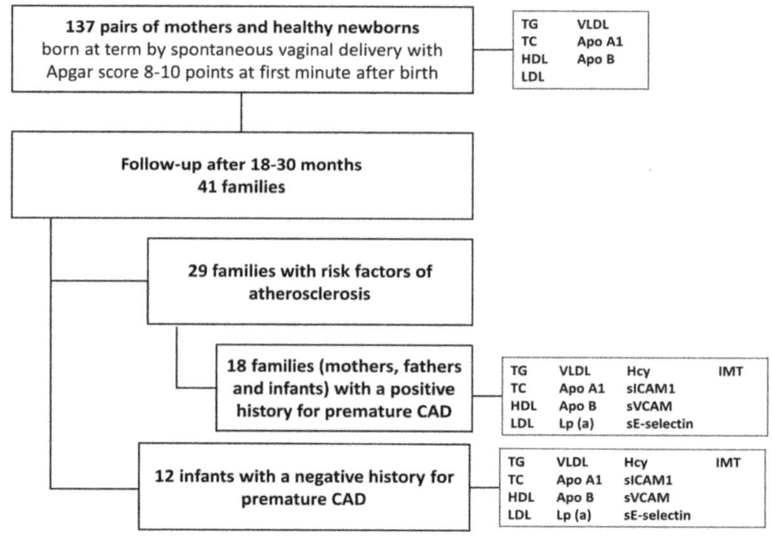

Fig. 1 Schematic diagram of the study design

The written informed consent to this research study was obtained from parents. The paper has been approved by Medical University Bioethical Committee (number KE-0254/74/2009).

Results

During the first stage of the study, we recruited 137 pairs of healthy mothers and their newborns. Newborns included 74 girls (54%) and 63 boys (45%), with the mean birth weight 3268.0±529.4 g and mean body length 54.4±3.1cm. The mean gestational age was 39.1±1.5 weeks.

Table 1 presents the lipid profile and apolipoprotein concentration in newborns and their mothers.

The results, as shown in Table 2, indicated no significant differences in newborns' lipids parameters according to family history for cardiovascular diseases.

In the second stage of the study volunteered 18 families with positive family history for premature CAD.

Table 1 Lipid and apolipoprotein concentrations (means ± SD) in newborns' cord blood and mothers' serum

Parameter	Newborns	Mothers
TG (mg/dl)	58.75±66.72	221.99±89.58
TC (mg/dl)	65.05±21.39	263.58±58.01
HDL (mg/dl)	19.63±8.40	64.23±15.86
%HDL	30.74±9.27	25.20±7.48
LDL (mg/dl)	34.12±14.08	155.14±49.44
VLDL (mg/dl)	11.46±9.93	48.83±17.83
Apo A1 (mg/dl)	86.50±18.60	232.02±39.07
Apo B (mg/dl)	37.90±17.70	149.00±41.03

The results, as shown in Table 3, showed significantly higher serum concentration of TG, VLDL and Lp(a) in children aged 18 to 30 months from families with positive history for premature CAD compared to controls. Table 4 compares the serum lipid profile, Apo A1, Apo B, sVCAM-1, sICAM-1, Hcy and sE-selectin concentration and IMT in mothers and fathers of subjects.

In children with a positive family history for premature CAD were found positive correlations between TC and sVCAM-1 (Rs=0.717, p<0.05), and TC and sICAM-1 (Rs=0.833, p<0.05). In mothers we stated significant positive correlation between IMT and TC concentration (Rs=0.831, p<0.01). In fathers there were positive correlations between IMT and Apo B (Rs=0.692, p<0.05), TG and sICAM-1 (Rs=0.912, p<0.01), TG and sE-selectin (Rs=0.678, p<0.05).

Lipid profile and concentration of apolipoproteins in newborns' cord blood according to their birth weight is presented in Table 5. A significant correlation was found between body mass at birth and cord blood concentration of TG, VLDL and Apo B. Newborns with the lowest

Table 2 Lipid and apolipoprotein concentrations (means ± SD) in newborns' cord blood according to family history of CVD

Parameter	Positive history (n=41)	Negative history (n=96)	p
TG (mg/dl)	54.73±45.10	60.47±73.67	ns
TC (mg/dl)	63.39±16.67	65.76±22.98	ns
LDL (mg/dl)	33.15±11.49	34.54±14.96	ns
VLDL (mg/dl)	11.31±8.97	11.52±10.26	ns
HDL (mg/dl)	19.25±6.49	19.79±9.04	ns
Apo A1 (mg/dl)	87.80±16.78	90.28±19.18	ns
Apo B (mg/dl)	36.85±15.25	38.41±18.65	ns

ns – non-significant

Table 3 Comparison of selected risk factors in 18- to 30-month±-old children with a positive history for premature CAD and controls (means ± SD); 2nd stage of the study

Parameter	Positive history (n=18)	Negative history (n=12)	p
TG (mg/dl)	105.44±69.04	83.03±29.26	<0.05
TC (mg/dl)	165.56±30.99	167.83±33.15	ns
HDL (mg/dl)	55.46±14.28	47.35±11.92	ns
LDL (mg/dl)	88.96±37.14	103,87±32.30	ns
VLDL (mg/dl)	21.09±13.81	16.62±5.85	<0.05
Apo A1 (mg/dl)	154.22±18.73	147.33±19.90	ns
Apo B (mg/dl)	73.11±18.82	77.58±17.59	ns
Lp (a) (mg/dl)	18.27±26.11	5.89±3.65	<0.05
Hcy (μmol/L)	12.20±2.46	10.67±2.41	ns
sVCAM-1 (ng/ml)	1616.11±561.92	1516.13±501.75	ns
sICAM-1 (ng/ml)	391.15±95.28	384.31±57.96	ns
sE-selectin (ng/ml)	58.37±17.17	72.57±38.16	ns
IMT (mm)	0.43±0.04	0.39±0.06	ns

ns – non-significant

birth weight (2250-2500g), had the highest concentration of these parameters. In female newborns concentration of TC, LDL, HDL and Apo A1 was significantly higher than in male newborns ($p<0.05$). There were no correlation between sex and concentration of TG, VLDL and Apo B.

The mean maternal age was 26±3 years. In the study group, 64 (46.7%) women were in first pregnancy, 31 (22.6%) in their second pregnancy, 22 (16.1%) in third pregnancy and 20 (14.6%) in fourth or next pregnancy. There were also no significant differences between newborns lipids parameters and pregnancy order or gestational age. The body mass index (BMI) before pregnancy ranged between 20 and 24.9 kg/m^2 in 62.8% of mothers.

Table 4 Selected risk factors for atherosclerosis in parents (means ± SD); 2nd stage of the study

Parameter	Mothers (n=18)	Fathers (n=18)
TG (mg/dl)	74.56±25.59	160.00±84.40
TC (mg/dl)	177.89±34.28	180.56±23.82
HDL (mg/dl)	67.77±19.94	51.07±15.26
LDL (mg/dl)	95,21±26.80	97.49±33.00
VLDL (mg/dl)	14.91±5.12	32.00±16.88
Apo A1 (mg/dl)	189.56±33.71	162.89±15.73
Apo B (mg/dl)	70.00±16.24	106.89±43.78
Lp (a) (mg/dl)	29.60±34.48	15.43±14.47
Hcy (μmol/L)	11.63±4.19	15.07±4.26
sVCAM-1 (ng/ml)	952.98±249.80	930.41±492.07
sICAM-1 (ng/ml)	294.50±62.13	363.93±134.46
sE-selectin (ng/ml)	29.28±19.44	34.08±37.51
IMT (mm)	0.59±0.2	0.61±0.10

BMI lower than 19.9kg/m^2 was reported by 22 women (16.1%), another 22 (16.1%) had BMI between 25 to 29.9 kg/m^2 and 7 (5.1%) women were obese (BMI over 30 kg/m^2). Table 6 presents newborns' cord blood lipids parameters according to mothers BMI before pregnancy.

Discussion

The most current American Academy of Pediatrics (AAP) guidelines for cardiovascular health recommend to fasting lipid profile in children at increased risk for CVD for the first time between 2 and 10 years of age. In risk groups are children with: 1) a positive family history of dyslipidemia or premature (≤55 years of age for men and ≤65 years of age for women) CVD or dyslipidemia, 2) unknown family history, 3) other CVD risk factors, such as overweight (BMI ≥ 85th percentile, <95th percentile), obesity (BMI ≥95th percentile), hypertension (blood pressure ≥ 95th percentile), cigarette smoking, or diabetes mellitus [18].

The National Cholesterol Education Program (NCEP) Expert Panel on Blood Cholesterol Levels in Children and Adolescents specify positive family history in biological parents and grandparents for CVD as myocardial infarction, angina pectoris, peripheral or cerebral vascular disease, sudden death, coronary artery bypass-surgery or balloon angioplasty before age 55 [19]. It should be noted that in children CVD risk we evaluate medical history of first and second-degree relatives.

The most remarkable result of our study is significant increase of TG and VLDL serum concentration in children aged 1.5-2.5 years with a family history of premature CAD compared to controls. However we did not

Table 5 Lipid and apolipoprotein concentrations (means ± SD) in newborns' cord blood according to birth weight

Parameter	Birth weight (g)	Newborns (n)	Concentration	p
TG (mg/dl)	2250-2500	12	91.83±75.00	<0.05
	2501-3000	36	44.97±22.70	1:2
	3001-3500	44	62.39±94.38	1:3
	3501-4000	36	62.14±53.33	1:5
	4001-4500	9	38.44±6.48	4:5
TC (mg/dl)	2250-2500	12	70.67±3.44	ns
	2501-3000	36	63.36±27.27	
	3001-3500	44	66.29±18.94	
	3501-4000	36	63.14±18.98	
	4001-4500	9	65.89±20.73	
LDL (mg/dl)	2250-2500	12	34.41±10.30	ns
	2501-3000	36	33.45±17.94	
	3001-3500	44	35.84±13.19	
	3501-4000	36	32.39±11.61	
	4001-4500	9	34.96±12.19	
VLDL (mg/dl)	2250-2500	12	18.37±15.00	p<0.05
	2501-3000	36	9.00±4.58	1:5
	3001-3500	44	11.30±10.57	3:5
	3501-4000	36	12.75±10.58	4:5
	4001-4500	9	7.69±1.30	
HDL (mg/dl)	2250-2500	12	17.89±8.90	ns
	2501-3000	36	21.16±7.96	
	3001-3500	44	19.44±7.19	
	3501-4000	36	17.99±9.05	
	4001-4500	9	23.24±9.42	
Apo A1 (mg/dl)	2250-2500	12	89.17±10.02	ns
	2501-3000	36	90.14±20.41	
	3001-3500	44	90.25±18.80	
	3501-4000	36	89.11±14.35	
	4001-4500	9	85.89±29.25	
Apo B (mg/dl)	2250-2500	12	47.25±18.01	<0.05
	2501-3000	36	33.97±14.88	1:2
	3001-3500	44	35.48±12.82	
	3501-4000	36	41.47±22.27	
	4001-4500	9	39.33±20.24	

ns – non-significant

Table 6 Lipid and apolipoprotein concentrations (means ± SD) in newborns' cord blood according to maternal pre-pregnancy BMI

Parameter	BMI (kg/m^2)	Newborns (n)	M ±SD	p
TG (mg/dl)	<19.9	22	43.19±20.73	ns
	20-24.9	86	57.36±49.61	
	25-29.9	22	82.73±128.70	
	>30	7	47.14±13,80	
TC (mg/dl)	<19.9	22	59.00±17.37	ns
	20-24.9	86	65.57.22.27	
	25-29.9	22	71.09±21.53	
	>30	7	58.71±11.03	
LDL (mg/dl)	<19.9	22	31.78±13.91	ns
	20-24.9	86	34.32±14.11	
	25-29.9	22	37.16±14.62	
	>30	7	29.53±7.49	
VLDL (mg/dl)	<19.9	22	8.89±4.20	<0.05
	20-24.9	86	11.80±9.97	1:2
	25-29.9	22	13.32±13.73	
	>30	7	9.43±2.76	
HDL (mg/dl)	<19.9	22	18.90±5.18	ns
	20-24.9	86	19.55±9.46	
	25-29.9	22	20.61±7.16	
	>30	7	19.76±4.55	
Apo AI (mg/dl)	<19.9	22	87.05±10.80	<0.05
	20-24.9	86	88.30±20.08	1:3
	25-29.9	22	97.77±18.69	2:3
	>30	7	86.71±6.56	3:4
Apo B (mg/dl)	<19.9	22	31.55±6.73	<0.05
	20-24.9	86	39.64±20.51	1:2
	25-29.9	22	38.95±13.68	1:3
	>30	7	34.00±7.63	

ns – non-significant

find any differences in lipid profile in newborns with a positive family history of premature CAD and controls.

Kelishadi et al. reported a significantly higher levels of TG, TC and LDL, and lower levels of HDL in children of parents with premature CAD [20]. Romaldini et al. showed hypercholesterolemia in 27.5% and hypertriglyceridemia in 12.8% of children of high-risk families [21]. In young adults aged 19 -30 years with parental premature CAD only TC concentration was significantly higher than in controls [22]. Marcovecchio et al. reported significant differences regarding TG and HDL between adolescents with a history of parental dyslipidemia and non-risk controls [23]. Mendes et al. revealed higher values of TC and lower of HDL in offspring of young adults with CAD than in controls [24]. It should be noted that our study was conducted only in children aged 1.5-2.5 years and most of mentioned studies were performed among older children and adolescents. Lipids and lipoproteins concentrations are the lowest during intrauterine life and at birth, and then increase until 2 years of age. Human lipid levels became quite constant up to adolescence [25]. Moreover, to understand some of these differences the ethnic and racial disparities should be also taken into consideration.

Elevated Lp(a) levels have been identified as independent risk factor for CAD that promotes atherogenesis and thrombogenesis [10, 26]. Several studies in children have found a positive association between Lp(a) level and positive family history of CVD [27–29]. This concept has been challenged by Tonstad et al. demonstrating that Lp(a) was marginally lower in the children with a history of premature cardiovascular death in male relatives ($p = 0.033$) [30]. In our study children, but not newborns, from kindreds with a history of premature CAD were also distinguished from controls by significantly higher Lp(a) levels. Since Lp(a) level is fully expressed in the first year of life, has a genetic adjustment, does not vary with age and, is almost unaltered by environmental factors, it should be widely applied to identification children at increased risk of CVD [28].

IMT is a well-established non-invasive marker of cardiovascular risk in adults. It has been showed that IMT >0.9 mm is related to significant atherosclerotic risk in adults [31]. In our study, the mean values of IMT in mothers and fathers did not exceed that cut-off level. Litwin et al. summarize growing body of evidence for increased IMT in children and adolescents with cardiovascular risk factors like obesity, hypertension or hyperlipidemia. It has been also reported that children with parental history of premature myocardial infarction have increased IMT independently of traditional atherosclerotic risk factors [32, 33]. However, it should be highlighted that age is the most important determinant of IMT, and increased IMT mostly was not seen in children under 10 years of age [31]. That fact may explain the lack of differences in IMT between children with a family history of premature CAD and controls in our study. Thus, efforts should be focused on enhance IMT measurements.

Several limitations to this study need to be acknowledged. The final sample size is quite small and there is no control group composed of adults. Moreover, no correction for multiple testing is a limitation. In the second stage of the study we do not evaluate impact of environmental cardiovascular risk factors like diet or physical activity on lipids parameters and IMT. It is suggested that the association of these factors is investigated in future studies. Further investigation, among the same subjects, to determine current cardiovascular risk is strongly recommended.

Conclusions

The present study make several noteworthy contributions to atherosclerosis research. Measurement of serum Lp(a) level may be apply to identification cardiovascular risk in children and adolescents. IMT is not a reliable measure of atherosclerosis in the youngest children. Early detection of cardiovascular risk in children with a family history of premature cardiovascular diseases should result in prevention intervention in the entire family.

Abbreviations

AAP: American Academy of Pediatrics; Apo A1: apolipoprotein A1; Apo B: apolipoprotein B; BMI: body mass index; CAD: coronary artery disease; CVD: cardiovascular disease; Hcy: homocysteine (Hcy); HDL: high density lipoprotein; hs-CRP: high-sensitivity C-reactive protein; IMT: intima-media thickness; LDL: low density lipoprotein; Lp(a): lipoprotein a; NCEP: National Cholesterol Education Program; NHLBI: National Heart, Lung, and Blood Institute; oxy-LDL: oxidized low density lipoprotein; sICAM-1: soluble intercellular adhesion molecule-1; sVCAM-1: soluble vascular cell adhesion molecule-1; TC: total cholesterol; TG: triglycerides; VLDL: very low density lipoprotein

Acknowledgements

Not applicable.

Funding

None.

Authors' contributions

EPK and PK designed the study and conducted the collection of data. EPK, PK and EG contributed to the data analysis and interpretation. EPK, PK and EG analyzed the data and drafted the manuscript. EPK, PK and EG proofread the manuscript. All authors read and approved the final manuscript.

Authors' information

Not applicable.

Competing interests

The authors declare that they have no competing interests.

Author details

[1]Department of Paediatrics and Gastroenterology, Medical University of Lublin, Gebali 6 Street, 20-093 Lublin, Poland. [2]Department of Clinical Immunology and Immunotherapy, Medical University of Lublin, Chodzki 4a Street, 20-093 Lublin, Poland.

References

1. Berenson BS. Cardiovascular risk begins in childhood: A time for action. Am J Prev Med. 2009;37(1S):S1–2.
2. Gidding SS, McMahan CA, McGill HC, Colangelo LA, Schreiner PJ, Williams OD, et al. Prediction of coronary artery calcium in young adults using the Pathobiological Determinants of Atherosclerosis in Youth (PDAY) risk score: the CARDIA study. Arch Intern Med. 2006;166:2271–6.
3. Libby P, Theroux P. Pathophysiology of coronary artery disease. Circulation. 2005;111:3481–8.
4. Weber C, Noels H. Atherosclerosis: current pathogenesis and therapeutic options. Nat Med. 2011;17:1410–22.
5. Singh RB, Mengi SA. Xu YJ, Arneja AS, Dhalla NS. Pathogenesis of atherosclerosis: A multifactorial process. Exp Clin Cardiol. 2002;7:40–53.
6. Libby P. Changing concepts of atherogenesis. J Intern Med. 2000;247: 349–58.
7. Dawber TR, Kannel WB. The Framingham Study: an epidemiological approach to coronary heart. Circulation. 1966;34:553–5.
8. Kannel WB, McGee D, Gordon T. A general cardiovascular risk profile: The Framingham Study. Am J Cardiol. 1976;38:46–51.
9. Khot UN, Khot MB, Bajzer CT, Sapp SK, Ohman EM, Brener SJ, et al. Prevalence of conventional risk factors in patients with coronary heart disease. JAMA. 2003;290:898–904.

10. Fruchart D, Nierman MC, Stroes ESG, Kastelein JJP, Duriez P. New risk factors for atherosclerosis and patient risk assessment. Circulation. 2004; 109:15–9.
11. Pourebrahim R, Fakhrzadeh H, Bandarian F, Tabatabie O, Noori M, Djalilpour F, et al. Household cardiovascular screening of high-risk families: A school-based study. Eur J Cardiovasc Prev Rehabil. 2006;13:229–35.
12. Assimes TL. Family history of heart disease: The re-emergence of a traditional risk factor. J Am Coll Cardiol. 2011;57:628–9.
13. Ripatti S, Tikkanen E, Orho-Melander M, Havulinna AS, Silandere K, Sharma A, et al. A multilocus genetic risk score for coronary heart disease: Case-control and prospective cohort analyses. Lancet. 2010;376:1393–400.
14. Jaquith BC, Harris MA, Penprase B. Cardiovascular disease risk in children and adolescents. J Pediatr Nurs. 2013;28:258–66.
15. National Cholesterol Education Program (NCEP) Expert Panel on Detection, Evaluation, and Treatment of High Blood Cholesterol in Adults (Adult Treatment Panel III). The Third Report of the Expert Panel on Detection, Evaluation, and Treatment of High Blood Cholesterol in Adults (Adult Treatment Panel III). Third Report of the National Cholesterol Education Program (NCEP) Expert Panel on Detection, Evaluation, and Treatment of High Blood Cholesterol in Adults (Adult Treatment Panel III) final report. Circulation. 2002;106: 3143-3421.
16. Hunt SC, Gwinn M, Adams TD. Family history assessment: strategies for prevention of cardiovascular disease. Am J Prev Med. 2003;24:136–42.
17. Friedewald WT, Levy RI, Fredrickson DS. Estimation of the concentration of low-density lipoprotein cholesterol in plasma, without use of the preparative ultracentrifuge. Clin Chem. 1972;18:499–502.
18. Daniels SR, Greer FR. The Committee on Nutrition. Lipid screening and cardiovascular health in childhood. Pediatrics. 2008;122:198–208.
19. Dennison BA, Jenkins PL, Pearson TA. Challenges to implementing the current pediatric cholesterol screening guidelines into practice. Pediatrics. 1994;94:296–302.
20. Kelishadi R, Zadegan NS, Naderi GA, Asgary S, Bashardoust N. Atherosclerosis risk factors in children and adolescents with or without family history of premature coronary artery disease. Med Sci Monit. 2002;8: 425–9.
21. Romaldini CC, Issler H, Cardoso AL, Diament J, Forti N. Risk factors for atherosclerosis in children and adolescents with family history of premature coronary artery disease. J Pediatr (Rio J). 2004;80:135–40.
22. Surdacki A, Zawiślak B, Rakowski T, Wieczorek-Surdacka E, Fedak D, Dubiel JS. Parental history of premature coronary artery disease does not affect plasma levels of asymmetric dimethylarginine in young healthy adults. Pol Arch Med Wewn. 2012;122:487–93.
23. Marcovecchio ML, Tossavainen PH, Heywood JJ, Dalton RN, Dunger DB. An independent effect of parental lipids on the offspring lipid levels in a cohort of adolescents with type 1 diabetes. Pediatr Diabetes. 2012;13:463–9.
24. Mendes GA, Martinez TL, Izar MC, Amancio OM, Novo NF, Matheus SC, Bertolami MC, Fonseca FA. Lipid profile and nutrition counseling effects in adolescents with family history of premature coronary artery disease. Arq Bras Cardiol. 2006;86:361–5.
25. Kwiterovich PO. Recognition and management of dyslipidemia in children and adolescents. J Clin Endocrinol Metab. 2008;93:4200–9.
26. Guardamagna O, Abello F, Anfossi G, Pirro M. Lipoprotein(a) and family history of cardiovascular disease in children with familial dyslipidemias. J Pediatr. 2011;159:314–9.
27. Marquez A, Mendoza S, Carrasco H, Hamer T, Glueck CJ. High lipoprotein (a) in children from kindreds with parental premature myocardial infarction. Pediatr Res. 1993;34:670–4.
28. Wilcken DE, Wang XL, Greenwood J, Lynch J. Lipoprotein (a) and apolipoproteins B and A1 in children and coronary vascular events in their grandparents. J Pediatr. 1993;123:519–26.
29. Bailleul S, Couderc R, Rossignol C, Fermanian J, Boutouchent F, Farnier MA, Etienne J. Lipoprotein(a) in childhood: relation with other atherosclerosis risk factors and family history of atherosclerosis. Clin Chem. 1995;41:241–5.
30. Tonstad S, Refsum H, Sivertsen M, Christophers B, Ose L, Ueland PM. Relation of total homocysteine and lipid levels in children to premature cardiovascular death in male relatives. Pediatr Res. 1996;40:47–52.
31. Litwin M, Niemirska A. Intima-media thickness measurements in children with cardiovascular risk factors. Pediatr Nephrol. 2009;24:707–19.
32. Morrison KM, Conner DW, Helden E, Newkirk L, Yusuf S, Lonn E. Cardiovascular risk factors and non-invasive assessment of subclinical atherosclerosis in youth. Atherosclerosis. 2010;208:501–5.
33. Barra S, Gaeta G, Cuomo S, Guarini P, Foglia MC, Capozzi G, et al. Early increase of carotid intima-media thickness in children with parental history of premature myocardial infarction. Heart. 2009;95:642–5.

17

Health-related quality of life in paediatric arterial hypertension

Tadej Petek[1*], Tjaša Hertiš[1] and Nataša Marčun Varda[1,2]

Abstract

Background: The prevalence of paediatric hypertension is increasing worldwide, especially due to the childhood obesity epidemic, and is an important public-health concern. While the Health-Related Quality of Life (HRQoL) was already shown to be impaired in the adult hypertensive population, a scarcity of data still exists on HRQoL in paediatric hypertensive patients. Our purpose was thus to assess the HRQoL of children and adolescents with arterial hypertension, using self- and proxy-reports, and to determine the correlations between child and parent questionnaire scores.

Methods: The Paediatric Quality of Life Inventory™ 4.0 Generic Core Scales were administered via post to children and adolescents, aged 5-18 years, with primary or secondary arterial hypertension and parents as proxy-reports. Patients were recruited from a paediatric nephrology unit in a tertiary hospital, using an out-patient clinic visit registry. Healthy school children and adolescents from a local primary school, aged 6 to 15 years, and their parents formed the control group. HRQoL group comparisons were calculated with independent samples t-test and child-parent correlations with the Pearson's r correlation coefficient.

Results: In total we recruited 139 patient and 199 control group participants as self- and proxy-reports. Scores from self- as well as proxy-reports indicated a significantly lower overall HRQoL in the paediatric hypertensive population (95% CI for mean score difference: − 11.02, − 2.86 for self- and − 10.28, − 2.67 for proxy-reports; $p = .001$). In self-reports, lower physical (95% CI: -13.95, − 4.89; p = <.001), emotional (95% CI: -12.96, − 2.38; $p = .005$), school (95% CI: -11.30, − 0.42; $p = .035$), and psychosocial functioning scores were observed (95% CI: -10.34, − 1.89; $p = .005$). Parent proxy-reports were lower in physical (95% CI: -14.31, − 5.39; p = <.001), emotional (95% CI: -12.39, − 2.60; $p = .003$) and psychosocial scores (95% CI: -9.36, − 1.34; $p = .009$). Pearson's r values ranged between 0.62 to 0.79 in patient and 0.56 to 0.80 in control sample ($p < .001$). Interestingly, hypertensive children reported lower social functioning scores than hypertensive adolescents ($p < .001$).

Conclusions: This cross-sectional study gives insight into the detrimental impact of hypertension on children's and adolescents HRQoL, which may inform public health experts. Furthermore, it shows that clinicians should aim to improve patients' physical and psychosocial well-being throughout their development.

Keywords: Arterial hypertension, Paediatric, Health-related quality of life, PedsQL

* Correspondence: tadejpetek01@gmail.com
[1]Faculty of Medicine, University of Maribor, Taborska ulica 8, 2000 Maribor, Slovenia
Full list of author information is available at the end of the article

Background

Paediatric hypertension is becoming an increasing public-health concern, especially in light of the growing childhood obesity epidemic [1–3]. The prevalence rates of pre-hypertension and hypertension with repeated screenings are rising [4] and are estimated at 9-12% and 2.5–3%, respectively, which makes elevated blood pressure one of the most common paediatric health conditions [1].

It is well-established that children with elevated blood pressure are more likely to grow into hypertensive adults in the future [5]. In addition, it has been shown that target organ damage, including left ventricular hypertrophy and pathologic vascular changes, develops already early on in the disease process [2, 6]. Proper management of high blood pressure in children and adolescents is based on the recommendations of the European Society of Hypertension from 2009 [7], encompassing both lifestyle changes and in cases of symptomatic hypertension, secondary hypertension, hypertensive organ damage, or diabetes, pharmacological therapy.

As measures of Health-Related Quality of Life (HRQoL) have been increasingly developed in the recent years and have to some extent already come to use in paediatric clinical practice [8], several childhood chronic conditions have been shown to negatively influence HRQoL [9]. Whereas there is increasing knowledge regarding clinical aspects of childhood hypertension, a scarcity of data exists on the psychosocial aspects of the disease burden.

In the case of hypertension, paediatric and adult studies report conflicting results, with hypertensive children and adolescents in the "KiGGS" study in Germany [10] scoring higher with self- and parent-rated quality of life measures, as opposed to adults, who report a decrease in HRQoL [11]. Also, in children with mild-to-moderate chronic kidney disease, statistically (but not clinically) significant associations between elevated blood pressure and lower parent and child HRQoL scores were observed at baseline measurement, but did not persist over time [12].

Our aim was therefore to assess the HRQoL of hypertensive children and adolescents in comparison to a normotensive control sample. Based on comparison of several paediatric quality of life instruments [13–15], we have decided on the Slovene translation of the Paediatric Quality of Life Inventory™ (PedsQL) 4.0 [16–18], which is well-established in the paediatric quality of life research and provides good feasibility, reliability and validity of the results. In addition, we aimed to assess child-parent score correlations and finally, compare PedsQL™ scores of healthy children and adolescents to scores from neighbouring countries.

Methods

Study design and setting

The study was coordinated by the Nephrology Unit of the Department of Paediatrics, University Medical Centre Maribor, Slovenia. Using a cross-sectional design, we conducted a postal survey of children and adolescents with arterial hypertension and their parents as proxy-reports. The perception of patients' quality of life was compared to that of a control group, consisting of children and adolescents recruited from a local primary school and their parents. After gaining approval from the hospital Ethics Committee in October 2014 and obtaining permission to use the PedsQL™ 4.0 Questionnaires from Mapi Research Trust in November 2014, we have subsequently procured a list of paediatric hypertensive patient clinic visits from January 2010 to December 2014.

Patient sample

To be eligible to participate in the study, hypertensive children and adolescents had to be aged between 5 and 18 years at the time of the survey completion, have a diagnosis of primary or secondary arterial hypertension, defined as systolic or diastolic blood pressure above published age-, sex- and height adjusted 95th percentiles, based on measurements from at least 3 occasions [7], and be physically and mentally capable of answering the age-appropriate questionnaires, based on the child's health condition and parents' judgement. We did not include the stage of arterial hypertension, neither have we collected data on duration of the disease. Upon meeting eligibility criteria and obtaining oral consent from parents, we sent the families the self- and proxy-versions of the questionnaire, together with the information letter described below, in May 2015. We reached an adequate sample size by the end of the data collection period in December 2015.

We sent all study participants an information letter on the background of the study and the questionnaire administration guidelines, adopted from the PedsQL™ website [19]. The parents were especially advised to let their child fill in the questionnaire separately, without comparing their results. In each case, one parent and their child filled in the questionnaire. Parents of young children were given detailed instructions on administering the questionnaire to their child, in addition to a sheet with a 3-point smiley rating to clarify the meaning of the answers to their child.

Control sample

The control group consisted of healthy children and adolescents, aged 6 to 15 years, attending a local primary school. Based on reports of health, performed during routine preventive health programmes, we excluded children and adolescents with either a history of arterial hypertension, other chronic diseases or illnesses, and significant acute diseases which could affect one or more questionnaire scores. After gaining consent in November 2015, we have given the children the PedsQL™ questionnaires, together with a sheet with questions about the child's health in the past month and the before mentioned information letter. After completing the questionnaires, children returned them to the school social worker, who forwarded them to us by the end of December 2015.

Measures

For the purpose of the study, we used the Slovene translation of the PedsQL™ 4.0 Generic Core scales [19]. It assesses respondents' physical (8 items), emotional (5 items), social (5 items) and school functioning (5 items) and consists of parallel child self-report and parent proxy-report questionnaires with developmentally-appropriate child categories; ages 5-7 for young children, 8-12 years for children and 13-18 years for adolescents. The PedsQL™ 4.0 Child-Self Report and Parent-Proxy Report Questionnaires are available free of charge for not funded academic research via the ePROVIDE™ Mapi Research Trust website [20].

Asked about the frequency of a specific problem during the past 1 month, respondents could choose the appropriate answer on a 5-point response scale, except with the young child questionnaire, where a 3-point scale was used. Returned surveys were then anonymized and the survey items reverse-scored. Answers were combined into four Scale Scores (Physical Functioning, Emotional Functioning, Social Functioning and School Functioning Scale Score) ranging from 0 to 100, where higher scores indicate a better HRQoL. Two additional Summary Scores were calculated, the Total Scale Score and the Psychosocial Health Summary Score, the latter comprised of the Emotional, Social and School Functioning Scale Scores.

Outcomes

The primary interest of the study was performance on the Total Scale Score and the Psychosocial Health Summary Score. Secondary outcomes were performance on the Physical Functioning, Emotional Functioning, Social Functioning and School Functioning Scale Scores. Additionally, we calculated child-parent questionnaire score correlations and compared control sample PedsQL™ Scores to those of Slovenia's bordering countries.

Bias

We used an internationally accepted questionnaire with good psychometric properties in order to minimize information bias. Response bias was minimized by recalling the non-responders and resending them the questionnaires. Also, the control group had to fulfil specific criteria regarding their health status, thereby avoiding the assumption of "general well-being" in the school population.

Study size and statistical methods

To estimate the required number of participants, we have first decided on the "minimally clinically important difference" (MCID) of 5 PedsQL score points, taking into account the previously reported MCID's [16, 21]. Expecting a total score of approx. 8o points for the control group with an control group/patient group enrolment ratio of 1.5, a significance of $p = 0.05$ and a power of 80% ($\beta = 0.2$), the web-based ClinCalc Sample Size Calculator [22] suggested a total sample of 130 participants, with 52 participants in the patient and 78 participants in the control group.

For the statistical analyses, we used the IBM SPSS Statistics software (version 20), running on a personal computer with Windows 10 operating system. According to the PedsQL™ Scoring Algorithm, we would have to discard any questionnaire with more than 50% of the items in the scale missing, but that was not the case in any of the returned questionnaires. We calculated descriptive statistics with means and standard deviations for questionnaire scores and percentages for categorical variables (age, gender, and group). In comparing the means between patient and control groups from self- as also proxy-reports, we used the independent samples t-tests (Student's t-test in equal and Welch's t-test in cases of unequal variance). Pearson's r was calculated to estimate child-parent concordances.

Results

Sample characteristics

We have sent a total of 554 questionnaires (see Fig. 1). The hypertensive sample of 112 children and adolescents and their parents was obtained from a list of 510 clinic visits during the 2010-2014 time period. While all of the phone-contacted eligible parents were willing to participate, two children were not eligible due to a recent diagnosis of a brain tumour in one and an intellectual disability in the other case. In the hypertensive sample, a total of 70 children and adolescents (response rate 62. 5%) and 69 parents (response rate 61.6%) have answered the questionnaire. From the hypertensive participants, 17 (24.3%) were young children, 18 children (25.7%), and 35 adolescents (50.0%). Most ($n = 43$, 61.4%) were boys, with 10 (58.8%), 10 (58.8%) and 23 (65.7%) boys belonging to young child, child, and adolescent age groups, respectively.

From a total of 330 questionnaires given to children from a local primary school as control samples, we have received 99 self-reports (60.0% response rate) and 100 parent-proxy reports (60.6% response rate). Twelve children were not eligible as controls due to illnesses in the previous month. In control sample self-reports, 27 (27. 3%) were young children, 26 (26.3%) children and 46 (46.5%) adolescents. Among them, there were a total of

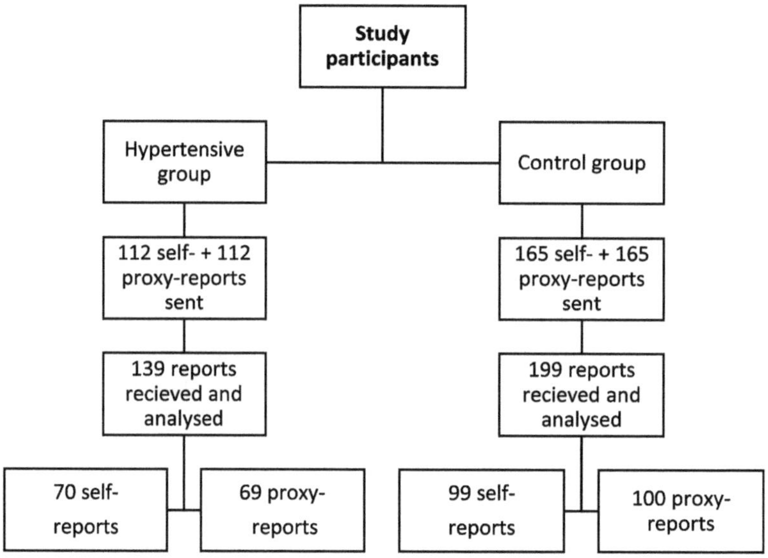

Fig. 1 Recruitment of study participants

46 (46.5%) boys, with 14 (51.9%), 10 (38.5%) and 22 (47.8%) boys belonging to young child, child, and adolescent age groups, respectively.

We did not exclude any questionnaires due to missing responses, as all participants had answered more than half of the items in a scale. In calculating Pearson's r correlations, we used 69 child-parent pairs in the hypertensive and 98 pairs in the control sample.

Outcomes

In comparing PedsQL™ scores of hypertensive children and adolescents to healthy control group using Student's and Welch's t-tests, several clinically and statistically important differences were found (see Table 1). Most importantly, self-reports in the patient group were 6.94 (SD = 2.06) points lower in the Total Score (95% CI: -11.02 to − 2.86; $p = .001$) and 6.11 (SD = 2.14) points lower in the Psychosocial Health Summary Score (95% CI: -10.32 to − 1.89; $p = .005$). Most affected health domains were the Physical Functioning Scores with a 9.41 score decrease (SD = 2.28; 95% CI: -13.95 to − 4.89; $p < .001$) and the Emotional Functioning scores with a 7.67 score decrease (SD = 2.67; 95% CI: -12.96 to − 2.38; p = .005). School Functioning Scores were lower by 5.86 score points (SD = 2.75; 95% CI: -11.30 to − 0.42; $p = .035$).

In parent proxy-reports, similar results were observed, with a 6.48 (SD = 1.93) score decrease in the Total Score (95% CI: -10.28 to − 2.67; $p = .001$) and a 9.85 (SD = 2.03) score decrease in the Psychosocial Health Summary Score in the patient sample (95% CI: -9.36 to − 1.34; $p = .009$). Physical Functioning domain was lower by 9.85 scores (SD = 2.25; 95% CI: -14.31 to − 5.39; $p = <.001$) and the Emotional Functioning domain by 7.49 scale scores (SD = 2.48; 95% CI: -12.39 to − 2.60; $p = .001$).

On further analysis we found no score differences between genders in patient and control groups. Comparing different age categories, age alone did not have an impact on the perceived HRQoL in most scores. However, hypertensive children aged 5-12 scored on average 18.00 (SD = 3.93) points lower in the Social Functioning Score, compared to hypertensive adolescents (95% CI: -25.87 to − 10.13; Hedges' $g = -1.10$; $t(53) = -4.59$; $p < .001$). On the basis of this, we compared Social Functioning scores (using Welch's t-test) between healthy and hypertensive children 5-12 years of age, and found a 12.52 (SD = 4.00) score decrease in hypertensive cases (95% CI: -20.42 to − 4.52; Hedges' $g = -0.77$; $t(58) = -3.13$; $p = .003$). We can consequently say that although Social Functioning scores were not impaired in the hypertensive child and adolescent sample as a whole, hypertensive children experience a significant decrease in social performance.

Calculation of Pearson's r correlation index revealed moderate to high correlations in child-parent pairs (see Table 2). In the patient sample, Pearson's r values ranged from $r = 0.62$ to $r = 0.79$, and in the control sample from $r = 0.56$ to $r = 0.80$. Both Total Scores and Psychosocial Health Summary Scores had a high correlation in the patient ($r = 0.79$ and $r = 0.75$, respectively) and control samples ($r = 0.79$ and $r = 0.80$, respectively).

Discussion

In our study, we have compared the Health-Related Quality of Life of hypertensive children and adolescents from patients' and parents' perspectives to a control sample of primary school children and their parents,

Table 1 Results of the Student's and Welch's t-tests, comparing hypertensive and control group scores

		Patient sample		Control sample		Mean Difference[a]	Effect size	Independent samples *t*-test			
PedsQL 4.0 Generic Core Scales	No. of items	N	Mean (SD)	N	Mean (SD)	Score Points (SED[b])	Hedges' *g*	t	df	*p*	95% CI for Mean Difference
Child Self-report											
Total Score	23	70	77.72 (14.57)	99	84.66 (11.00)	−6.94 (2.06)	0.55	−3.37	122	.001*	− 11.02; − 2.86
Psychosocial Health	15	70	76.29 (14.90)	99	82.41 (12.81)	−6.11 (2.14)	0.45	−2.86	167	.005	−10.34; − 1.89
Physical Functioning	8	70	82.00 (17.83)	99	91.41 (8.03)	−9.41 (2.28)	0.72	−4.13	89	<.001*	− 13.95; − 4.89
Emotional Functioning	5	70	71.57 (18.19)	99	79.24 (16.39)	−7.67 (2.67)	0.45	−2.86	167	.005	−12.96; −2.38
Social Functioning	5	70	81.86 (18.65)	99	86.67 (14.05)	−4.81 (2.64)	0.30	−1.82	122	.071*	− 10.03; 0.42
School Functioning	5	70	75.45 (19.39)	99	81.31 (16.28)	−5.86 (2.75)	0.33	−2.13	167	.035	−11.30; − 0.42
Parent Proxy-report											
Total Score	23	69	77.66 (13.99)	100	84.14 (11.00)	−6.48 (1.93)	0.53	−3.36	167	.001	−10.28; −2.67
Psychosocial Health	15	69	76.79 (14.52)	100	82.15 (11.79)	−5.36 (2.03)	0.41	−2.64	167	.009	−9.36; −1.34
Physical Functioning	8	69	80.26 (15.66)	100	90.11 (12.37)	−9.85 (2.25)	0.71	−4.37	123	<.001*	− 14.31; − 5.39
Emotional Functioning	5	69	70.91 (17.07)	100	78.40 (14.94)	−7.49 (2.48)	0.47	−3.02	167	.003	−12.39; − 2.60
Social Functioning	5	69	82.30 (18.88)	100	86.09 (14.52)	−3.79 (2.57)	0.23	−1.40	121	.163*	− 9.13; 1.55
School Functioning	5	69	77.17 (16.66)	100	81.95 (15.79)	−4.78 (2.53)	0.30	−1.89	167	.061	−9.77; 0.21

N number of participants, *SD* standard deviation, *df* degrees of freedom, *CI* confidence interval.
*Welch's t used due to unequal variances, according to Levene's Test for Equality of Variances
[a]Difference between patient and control sample mean scores
[b]Standard Error Difference

using a well-validated and frequently used PedsQL™ 4.0 Generic Core Scale Questionnaire [13, 15–18, 23]. Based on our results, both hypertensive children and adolescents as well as their parents as proxy-reports report lower overall HRQoL and Psychosocial Health, together with lower Physical and Emotional Functioning scores. Additionally, the patient sample had a significantly lower School Functioning score.

Calculation of Pearson's *r* revealed moderate ($r > 0.5$) to high ($r > 0.7$) positive correlations between child self- and parent proxy-reports, ranges in accordance with [24]. This is higher than the publication on school children by Varni [23], with Pearson's *r* values between 0.19 and 0.35, whereas some other studies have reported the correlation to be mostly in the moderate range; 0.69 in total scale scores in paediatric cancer patients [25] and from 0.36 to 0.64 in children with heart disease [26]. In contrast to experience in the literature [27], we did not find greater child-parent agreement in observable functioning (Physical HRQoL) in comparison to non-observable functioning (Psychosocial Health). Although the observed child-parent correlations in this study were higher than expected from literature, obtaining reports from both children and parents whenever possible is still advocated because of differences in correlations between studies.

Comparing the PedsQL™ 4.0 reports of our healthy control school-based sample to reports of Slovenia's neighbouring countries [21, 28–30], displayed in Table 3, our self-report sample had the highest scores in all but the Social Functioning scale. The parent proxy-reports were second-highest in all scales, with Austrian parents reporting the highest scores in five out of six scales. Although the selected primary school enrols children from different socioeconomic and ethnical backgrounds, with such high overall scores we cannot rule out a potential selection bias as well as the effect arising from a low sample size. Alternatively, the high score results may be a reflection of overall good self-reported health of Slovenian children, as reported by OECD [31].

On analysis of the size of mean differences between the patient and control groups, all the statistically significant differences also achieved the 5 points "cut-off" value for "minimally clinically significant difference". Therefore, we can assume our results to be important in the clinical setting. In scores where no significant difference was observed, the mean score differences were below 5 score points.

Considering previously published literature, a meta-analysis of cross-sectional studies on HRQoL in the adult hypertensive population reported a slightly worse quality of life compared to normotensive individuals [11], results concordant with our own. However, in adolescents, findings from the German "KiGGS" study suggested higher self- and parent-rated quality of life, as also lower parent-rated emotional, conduct and overall problems with elevated blood pressure [10]. The authors explained this by absence of confounding physical

Table 2 Concordance of child self- and parent proxy-reports

	Child self-report Mean (SD)	Parent proxy-report Mean (SD)	Pearson's r
Patient sample ($N = 69$)			
Total Score	77.85 (14.63)	77.66 (13.99)	0.79*
Psychosocial Health	76.51 (14.90)	76.79 (14.52)	0.75*
Physical Functioning	81.87 (17.93)	80.26 (15.66)	0.78*
Emotional Functioning	71.74 (18.27)	70.91 (17.07)	0.62
Social Functioning	81.88 (18.79)	82.30 (18.88)	0.78*
School Functioning	75.89 (19.18)	77.17 (16.66)	0.65
Control sample ($N = 98$)			
Total Score	84.90 (10.79)	84.44 (10.63)	0.79*
Psychosocial Health	82.69 (12.57)	82.38 (11.66)	0.80*
Physical Functioning	91.55 (7.95)	90.61 (11.11)	0.56
Emotional Functioning	79.69 (15.84)	78.62 (14.90)	0.75*
Social Functioning	86.79 (14.07)	86.21 (14.62)	0.71*
School Functioning	81.58 (16.14)	82.30 (15.50)	0.69

*Pearson's *r* showing a strong correlation (> 0.7) between the patient and control sample, $p < .001$ for all values of Pearson's *r*
SD standard deviation

comorbidity and the adolescents' unawareness of being hypertensive. The latter partially explains the discrepancy with our findings, as we only recruited patients from the clinic, who were thus mostly aware of their disease. In comparison to the study by Wong et al. [12] on paediatric chronic kidney disease patients, which found no significant associations between elevated blood pressure and HRQoL, a lack of hypertensive disease symptoms or more dominant chronic kidney disease symptoms might have masked the HRQoL impairments of hypertension [12]. In our study, hypertension was the primary disease under consideration, thereby avoiding the risk of symptom misattribution. As a majority of hypertensive children report some symptoms of hypertension, including headache, insomnia, fatigue and chest or abdominal pain [32], impaired HRQoL seems a likely consequence.

When comparing the patient and control sample self-reports regarding to gender, no differences were found. However, in comparing age categories, we have found greatly reduced social functioning in hypertensive children compared to adolescents. While chronically ill children have been shown before to have impaired social functioning, although not diagnosis specific, age alone was not related with measures of social functioning [33]. Even though the frequent hospital visits might play a role in this difference, further research might be needed to confirm this finding.

Limitations

Certain limitations regarding our study should be addressed. First, the standardized PedsQL Questionnaire did not contain questions regarding the duration or stage of the disease, treatment modality, nor gather information on socio-economic status or other social interactions at home or in school. However, in effort to preserve cross-study comparativeness of our results, no questions were added to the questionnaire that was standardized. The enrolled hypertensive participants were, however, from the same geographical region with similar socioeconomic backgrounds, in majority diagnosed with essential hypertension. In addition, they were mostly treated with lifestyle interventions, with a negligible number of cases necessitating drug therapy. Thus, we believe our participants have been similar in major characteristics. However, future studies on these topics influencing the quality of life with a high probability are needed.

Secondly, as it was a postal survey, we could not ensure that the parents followed the written instructions posted with the questionnaires. Especially important in this aspect is the high observed child-parent concordance, which might be the result of parents influencing their child's responses. Second, the patient and control sample differed in gender, most patients being male and controls female. Furthermore, even though obesity has been previously shown to negatively influence HRQoL [34, 35], we did not consider it a confounding factor, as it plays a major role in the development of hypertensive disease.

Finally, findings in the control population showed exceptional HRQoL in both self- and proxy-reports in relation to neighbouring countries. While we believe this to be connected to well-organized and publicly available

Table 3 Comparison of healthy population PedsQL™ scores with neighboring countries

Publication	Our Study	Felder-Puig et al. [20]	Berkes et al. [27]	Trapanotto et al. [28]	Jović et al. [29]
Region	Maribor, Slovenia	Vienna, Austria	Debrecen, Hungary	Padua, Italy	Zadar, Zagreb, Osijek and Split in Croatia
Sample Characteristics	99 Self- and 100 parent proxy-reports; ages 6 to 15 yr.; 46.5% boys, 53.5% girls	1412 children aged 8-12 yr.; 51.0% boys, 49.0% girls	366 Self- and 519 parent proxy-reports, ages 2-18 yr.; 55.5% boys, 44.5% girls	51 self- and 66 parent proxy-reports, aged 2-18 yr.; 21.2% boys, 78.8% girls	152 primary school children; 39.5% boys, 60.5% girls
	Mean (SD)	Mean (SD)	Mean (SD)	Mean (SD)	Mean (SD)
Patient sample					
Total Score	84.66 (11.00)	81.9 (12.6)	79.33 (12.35)	79.31 (10.00)	NA
Psychosocial Health	82.41 (12.81)	79.9 (14.1)	77.29 (13.39)	77.68 (10.56)	NA
Physical Functioning	91.41 (8.03)	87.8 (11.9)	83.12 (14.23)	82.54 (12.17)	77.85 (NA)
Emotional Functioning	79.24 (16.39)	76.9 (18.1)	72.10 (17.80)	72.16 (15.40)	68.08 (NA)
Social Functioning	86.67 (14.05)	82.6 (17.3)	83.81 (61.10)	80.98 (14.35)	90.47 (NA)
School Functioning	81.31 (16.28)	80.0 (16.7)	75.84 (16.65)	79.70 (12.58)	76.51 (NA)
Control sample					
Total Score	84.14 (11.00)	84.9 (10.5)	78.85 (13.18)	81.74 (11.21)	NA
Psychosocial Health	82.15 (11.79)	83.1 (11.6)	77.33 (13.69)	81.08 (11.63)	NA
Physical Functioning	90.11 (12.37)	90.6 (10.6)	81.03 (15.88)	82.99 (13.41)	NA
Emotional Functioning	78.4 (19.94)	79.4 (15.5)	71.79 (16.76)	75.53 (14.00)	NA
Social Functioning	86.09 (14.52)	88.1 (14.0)	84.45 (16.31)	83.79 (17.84)	NA
School Functioning	81.95 (15.79)	81.7 (14.2)	77.01 (16.93)	84.32 (13.67)	NA

NA Data not available, *yr.* years, *SD* standard deviation

healthcare, educational and other government systems, our findings suggest additional studies are needed to explain these unique observations. It should also be stressed that children in our country have regular preventive clinical examinations performed every 3 years including blood pressure measurements, meaning that children of control group should have been truly healthy.

Implications

The implications of our research are relevant in two aspects. First, we believe that the demonstrated study results give reason to assess the physical as well as psychosocial functioning of hypertensive children and adolescents, preferentially both from children's as also parent's perspectives. While the use of structured questionnaires measuring HRQoL in everyday paediatric clinical practice is under debate, according to Uzark et al. [36], utilizing such measures can facilitate patient-physician communication, improve patient/parent satisfaction, identify hidden morbidities, and assist in clinical decision-making. Moreover, it is advocated that specific interventions for deficits in HRQoL, including appropriate referrals, follow questionnaire findings, otherwise patient HRQoL outcomes might not be improved [8]. An example of such HRQoL-based interventions at a cardiology outpatient practice was presented by Uzark et al. [36]. Secondly, our findings indicate that hypertensive children differ from healthy controls in physical and psychosocial aspects. Therefore, special attention together with health-care fund allocation should be considered for this at-risk group of children, as early detection and intervention might prevent detrimental effects on psychosocial health and well-being later in life.

Conclusion

This study demonstrates a significant and clinically relevant association of hypertension with lower physical and psychosocial functioning in a paediatric child and adolescent hypertensive sample. We observed a moderate to high correlation between child and parent proxy-reports. From reasons not yet fully understood, hypertensive children reported lower social functioning scores than hypertensive adolescents. Scores of healthy primary school children were slightly higher than scores of healthy children from neighbouring countries. Based on our findings, we suggest an evaluation of HRQoL in paediatric hypertensive patients and appropriate interventions based on the findings. Also, further research is needed to evaluate the influence of disease severity, duration, antihypertensive therapy and patient-related factors (e. g. illness-awareness) on the HRQoL outcome. Furthermore, insight into the resilience of hypertensive adolescents in the social functioning domain might give us further information on potential "protective" factors for psychosocial well-being of hypertensive children.

Abbreviations

HRQoL: Health-related quality of life; PedsQL™ 4.0: Paediatric quality of life inventory version 4.0

Acknowledgments

We would like to specially thank University Medical Centre Maribor for providing access to their postal services and Ms. Karmen Obrul for providing administrative support and help regarding patient data retrieval.

Funding

This research has received no specific grant or funding from any funding source in the public, commercial, or not-for-profit sectors, and has therefore as non-funded academic research received the permission to use the PedsQL™ Questionnaires from copyright holder James W. Varni, Mapi Research Trust, Lyon, France, on a free-of-charge basis.

Authors' contributions

TP participated in the study design, performed the data collection, statistical analysis and wrote the first manuscript. TH participated in the study design, data collection and analysis, and helped draft the manuscript. NMV conceived of the study and its design, supervised data collection and the statistical analysis, and helped draft the manuscript. All authors have read and approved the final manuscript.

Competing interests

The authors declare that they have no competing interests.

Author details

[1]Faculty of Medicine, University of Maribor, Taborska ulica 8, 2000 Maribor, Slovenia. [2]Department of Paediatrics, University Medical Centre Maribor, Ljubljanska ulica 5, 2000 Maribor, Slovenia.

References

1. Flynn J. The changing face of pediatric hypertension in the era of the childhood obesity epidemic. Pediatr Nephrol. 2013;28:1059–66. https://doi.org/10.1007/s00467-012-2344-0.
2. Riley M, Bluhm B. High blood pressure in children and adolescents. Am Fam Physician. 2012;85:693–700. https://doi.org/10.1007/s00103-012-1638-5.
3. Bassareo PP, Mercuro G. Pediatric hypertension: an update on a burning problem. World J Cardiol. 2014;6:253–9. https://doi.org/10.4330/wjc.v6.i5.253.
4. Din-Dzietham R, Liu Y, Bielo MV, Shamsa F. High blood pressure trends in children and adolescents in national surveys, 1963 to 2002. Circulation. 2007;116:1488–96. https://doi.org/10.1161/CIRCULATIONAHA.106.683243.
5. Chen X, Wang Y. Tracking of blood pressure from childhood to adulthood: a systematic review and meta-regression analysis. Circulation. 2008;117: 3171–80. https://doi.org/10.1161/CIRCULATIONAHA.107.730366.
6. Karpettas N, Nasothimiou E, Kollias A, Vazeuo A, Stergiou GS. Ambulatory and home blood pressure monitoring in children and adolescents: diagnosis of hypertension and assessment of target-organ damage. Hypertens Res. 2013;36:285–92. https://doi.org/10.1038/hr.2012.220.
7. Lurbe E, Cifkova R, Cruickshank JK, Dillon MJ, Ferreira I, Invitti C, et al. Management of high blood pressure in children and adolescents: recommendations of the European Society of Hypertension. J Hypertens. 2009;27:1719–42. https://doi.org/10.1097/HJH.0b013e32832f4f6b.
8. Varni JW, Burwinkle TM, Lane MM. Health-related quality of life measurement in pediatric clinical practice: an appraisal and precept for future research and application. Health Qual Life Outcomes. 2005;3:34–43. https://doi.org/10.1186/1477-7525-3-34.
9. Ingerski LM, Modi AC, Hood KK, Pai AL, Zeller M, Piazza-Waggoner C, et al. Health-related quality of life across pediatric chronic conditions. J Pediatr. 2010;156:639–44. https://doi.org/10.1016/j.jpeds.2009.11.008.
10. Berendes A, Meyer T, Hulpke-Wette M, Herrmann-Lingen C. Association of elevated blood pressure with low distress and good quality of life: results from the nationwide representative German health interview and examination survey for children and adolescents. Psychosom Med. 2013;75: 422–8. https://doi.org/10.1097/PSY.0b013e31828ef0c2.
11. Trevisol DJ, Moreira LB, Kerkhoff A, Fuchs SC, Fuchs FD. Health-related quality of life and hypertension: a systematic review and meta-analysis of observational studies. J Hypertens. 2011;29:179–88. https://doi.org/10.1097/HJH.0b013e328340d76f.
12. Wong C, Gerson A, Hooper S, Matheson M, Lande M, Kupferman J, et al. Effect of elevated blood pressure on quality of life in children with chronic kidney disease. Pediatr Nephrol. 2016;31(7):1129–36. https://doi.org/10.1007/s00467-015-3262-8.
13. Hullmann SE, Ryan JL, Ramsey RR, Chaney JM, Mullins LL. Measures of general pediatric quality of life: child health questionnaire (CHQ), DISABKIDS chronic generic measure (DCGM), KINDL-R, pediatric quality of life inventory (PedsQL) 4.0 generic Core scales, and quality of my life questionnaire (QoML). Arthritis Care Res. 2011;63(Suppl 1):S420–30. https://doi.org/10.1002/acr.20637.
14. Davis E, Waters E, Mackinnon A, Reddihough D, Graham HK, Mehmet-Radji O, et al. Paediatric quality of life instruments: a review of the impact of the conceptual framework on outcomes. Dev Med Child Neurol. 2006;48:311–8. https://doi.org/10.1017/S0012162206000673.
15. Eiser C, Morse R. A review of measures of quality of life for children with chronic illness. Arch Dis Child. 2001;84:205–11. https://doi.org/10.1136/adc.84.6.487.
16. Varni JW, Limbers CA. The pediatric quality of life inventory: measuring pediatric health-related quality of life from the perspective of children and their parents. Pediatr Clin N Am. 2009;56:843–63. https://doi.org/10.1016/j.pcl.2009.05.016.
17. Varni JW, Seid M, Kurtin PS. PedsQL 4.0: reliability and validity of the pediatric quality of life inventory version 4.0 generic core scales in healthy and patient populations. Med. Care. 2001;39:800–12. https://doi.org/10.1097/00005650-200108000-00006.
18. Varni JW, Seid M, Rode CA. The PedsQL: measurement model for the pediatric quality of life inventory. Med Care. 1999;37:126–39. https://doi.org/10.1097/00005650-199902000-00003.
19. Varni JW. The PedsQL measurement model for the pediatric quality of life inventory. 2016. Available at: http://www.pedsql.org/about_pedsql.html. Accessed 13 Apr 2016.
20. ePROVIDE™. Pediatric Quality of Life Inventory™. 2018. Available at: https://eprovide.mapi-trust.org/instruments/pediatric-quality-of-life-inventory. Accessed 28 Mar 2018.
21. Felder-Puig R, Baumgartner M, Topf R, Gadner H, Formann AK. Health-related quality of life in Austrian elementary school children. Med Care. 2008;46:432–9. https://doi.org/10.1097/mlr.0b013e3181648e95.
22. Kane SP. Sample Size Calculator. Clin Calc. 2016. Available at: http://clincalc.com/Stats/SampleSize.aspx . Accessed 11 Feb 2016.
23. Varni JW, Burwinkle TM, Seid M. The PedsQL 4.0 as a school population health measure: feasibility, reliability, and validity. Qual. Life Res. 2006;15: 203–15. https://doi.org/10.1007/s11136-005-1388-z.
24. Mukaka MM. Statistics corner: a guide to appropriate use of correlation coefficient in medical research. Malawi Med J. 2012;24:69–71.
25. Chaudhry Z, Siddiqui S. Health related quality of life assessment in Pakistani paediatric cancer patients using PedsQL™ 4.0 generic core scale and PedsQL™ cancer module. Health Qual Life Outcomes. 2012;10:52.

26. Uzark K, Jones K, Burwinkle TM, Varni JW. The pediatric quality of life inventory™ in children with heart disease. Prog Pediatr Cardiol. 2003;18:141–9. https://doi.org/10.1016/S1058-9813(03)00087-0.
27. Eiser C, Morse R. Can parents rate their child's health-related quality of life? Results of a systematic review. Qual Life Res. 2001;10:347–57.
28. Uzark K, Jones K, Burwinkle TM, Varni JW, et al. Measuring health-related quality of life in Hungarian children with heart disease: psychometric properties of the Hungarian version of the pediatric quality of life inventory 4.0 generic Core scales and the cardiac module. Health Qual Life Outcomes. 2010;8 https://doi.org/10.1186/1477-7525-8-14.
29. Trapanotto M, Giorgino D, Zulian F, Benini F, Varni JW. The Italian version of the PedsQL in children with rheumatic diseases. Clin Exp Rheumatol. 2009;27:373–80.
30. Jović M, Vulić-Prtorić A, Baraban D, Grubić M, Brnović I, Padelin P. Coping strategies and health-related quality of life in children and adolescents with type 1 diabetes. Rev Psychol. 2009;16:29–36.
31. OECD. How's life in Slovenia? OECD Better Life Initiative; 2016. Available at http://www.oecd.org/slovenia/publicationsdocuments/reports/ . Accessed 13 Mar 2016.
32. Croix B, Feig DI. Childhood hypertension is not a silent disease. Pediatr Nephrol. 2006;21:527–32. https://doi.org/10.1007/s00467-006-0013-x.
33. Meijer SA, Sinnema G, Bijstra JO, Mellenbergh GJ, Wolters WHG. Social functioning in children with a chronic illness. J Child Psychol Psychiatry. 2000;41:309–17. https://doi.org/10.1017/S0021963099005211.
34. Pinhas-Hamiel O, Singer S, Pilpel N, Fradkin A, Modan D, Reichman B. Health-related quality of life among children and adolescents: associations with obesity. Int J Obes. 2006;30:267–72. https://doi.org/10.1038/sj.ijo.0803107.
35. Sikić-Pogačar M, Turk E, Dolinšek J, Marčun-Varda N, Mičetić-Turk D. Impact of obesity on health-related quality of life among children and adolescents in Slovenia. Health Med. 2013;7:2774–6.
36. Uzark K, King E, Spicer R, Beekman R, Kimball T, Varni JW. The clinical utility of health-related quality of life assessment in pediatric cardiology outpatient practice. Congenit Heart Dis. 2013;8:211–8.

18

Newborn weight change and childhood cardio-metabolic traits

Maria João Fonseca[1*], Milton Severo[1,2], Debbie A. Lawlor[3,4], Henrique Barros[1,2] and Ana Cristina Santos[1,2]

Abstract

Background: Newborn weight change (NWC) in the first 4 days represents short-term adaptations to external environment. It may be a key developmental period for future cardio-metabolic health, but this has not been explored. We aimed to determine the associations of NWC with childhood cardio-metabolic traits.

Methods: As part of Generation XXI birth cohort, children were recruited in 2005/2006 at all public units providing obstetrical and neonatal care in Porto. Birthweight was abstracted from clinical records and postnatal anthropometry was obtained by trained examiners during hospital stay. NWC was calculated as ((minimum weight - birthweight)/ birthweight) × 100. At age 4 and 7, children were measured and had a fasting blood sample collected. Fasting glucose, LDL-cholesterol, triglycerides, waist circumference, systolic and diastolic blood pressure were evaluated. This study included 312 children with detailed information on growth in very early life and subsequent cardio-metabolic measures. Path analysis was used to compute adjusted regression coefficients and 95% confidence intervals.

Results: NWC was not associated with any cardio-metabolic traits at ages 4 or 7. Strong associations were observed between each cardio-metabolic trait at 4 with the same trait at 7 years. The strongest associations were found for waist circumference [0.725 (0.657; 0.793)] and LDL-cholesterol [0.655 (0.575; 0.735)].

Conclusions: No evidence that NWC is related to childhood cardio-metabolic traits was found, suggesting that NWC should be faced in clinical practice as a short-term phenomenon, with no medium/long term consequences, at least in cardio-metabolic health. Our results show strong tracking correlations in cardio-metabolic traits during childhood.

Keywords: Cardio-metabolic risk, Metabolic syndrome, Newborn weight loss

Background

Hypertension, central adiposity, high glucose levels and adverse lipid profile are damaging cardio-metabolic traits that co-occur in adults and children and are associated with future type 2 diabetes and coronary heart disease [1, 2]. There is evidence that exposures during early development play an important role in the future risk of this adverse cardio-metabolic health. Barker's [3] initial description of an association between low birthweight and higher cardio-metabolic risk has been confirmed by other authors [4–7]. More recently, an association between higher birthweight and adverse cardio-metabolic health has also been reported, including in children [5, 8, 9]. Different patterns of postnatal weight change have also been found to associate with future cardio-metabolic health, and recent evidence suggests that body mass index (BMI) in childhood is more strongly related to adverse cardio-metabolic health than birthweight [10, 11].

These studies have not examined the association of weight change in the immediate postnatal period with later health outcomes, largely because few studies have such data. In the immediate postnatal period, newborns lose around 6% of their birthweight [12, 13]. Although this is considered a normal physiological process, there is considerable variation between newborns in the amount of weight lost during this period [12, 13]. Extreme values of newborn weight change (NWC) in the immediate postnatal period, which is mainly related to inadequate or

* Correspondence: mjoao.fonseca@ispup.up.pt; mjfonseca@med.up.pt
[1]EPIUnit - Instituto de Saúde Pública, Universidade do Porto, Rua das Taipas n° 135, 4050-600 Porto, Portugal
Full list of author information is available at the end of the article

excess hydration, are associated with adverse neonatal health [14, 15], but its association with subsequent cardio-metabolic health is unknown.

We hypothesized that NWC during the first 96 h is associated with cardio-metabolic traits in later childhood, through developmental adaptations occurring during this period, when newborns have to rapidly adapt their energy intake and expenditure to external conditions [6]. Accordingly, our primary aim was to evaluate the association of NWC with cardio-metabolic traits assessed at age 4 and 7 years. We also explored whether the associations of NWC with these traits at age 7 were direct or mediated by the same traits at age 4 as represented in Fig. 1, and estimated all the paths represented in the figure. To our knowledge this is the first study to examine the associations of NWC with later cardio-metabolic traits.

Methods

Participants

The participants of this study are part of the Generation XXI birth cohort [16], assembled between April 2005 and August 2006, after delivery, during the hospital stay, at the five public units providing obstetrical and neonatal care in the metropolitan area of Porto, Portugal. Follow-up assessments of the cohort have been undertaken when the children were aged 4 years (April 2009 – July 2011), and 7 (April 2012 – January 2014).

All newborns were routinely weighed at birth and, since November 2005, whenever possible, newborns additionally had a second weight measurement performed by a trained examiner during their hospital stay. Since November 2005, 5034 newborns were recruited to Generation XXI, of which 4449 were full-term singletons without known congenital anomalies. Of those 4449 children, a random sub-sample of 1806 newborns had the second neonatal weight measurement. This group of 1806 children were eligible for this study and of that 1806, 471 had missing information on exact time of measurement during hospital stay, 28 were measured after 96 h of life (the period of interest was the first 96 h of life) and 19 were considered outliers [1st/3rd quartile ±3 times the interquartile range corresponding to those with weight loss higher than 0.50% of birthweight per hour ($n = 15$) and those with weigh gain higher than 0.19% of birthweight per hour ($n = 4$)]. Of the remaining 1288, 312 children had complete data on all key variables and are the participants included in this study. Figure 2 shows the study flow chart of participants. Similar characteristics were found between participants and eligible non-participants (Additional file 1).

Baseline evaluation

The second weight measurement of the newborn was performed by trained examiners, during the hospital stay, but independently of routine procedures. Newborns were weighted after the questionnaire to the mother, without clothes or diaper. The same digital scales were used (seca®) to weight all newborns to the nearest 1 g, after waiting for the scale to stabilize. The date and time of measurement were registered. The measurement time varied from 6.3 to 96.0 h of life, mean of 45.3 (SD 19.4) hours. We calculated NWC using the formula:

NWC(%) = ((estimated minimum weight – birthweight) / birthweight) × 100.

where estimated minimum weight was the predicted weight at 52.3 h of life - the mean *nadir* time of lowest weight in the first 96 h in European infants [13]. This was estimated for each child using a cubic regression model as described in the statistical analysis section.

Information on family and personal history of disease, socio-demographic characteristics, maternal pre-pregnancy anthropometric parameters, and intra-uterine exposures were collected during a face-to-face interview conducted during the hospital stay by trained interviewers. These interviews took place 24 to 72 h after delivery. Data on delivery and newborn characteristics, including birthweight and gestational age, were abstracted from clinical records by the same interviewers.

Follow-up evaluations

At 4 and 7 years of age, trained researchers performed anthropometric and blood pressure measurements and obtained a fasting blood sample, according to standard procedures. Waist circumference measurements were taken with an inextensible tape measure to the nearest 0.1 cm, at the umbilicus level, with the child in a standing position, the abdomen relaxed, arms at the sides and feet positioned together [17]. Blood pressure was measured with an electronic sphygmomanometer (Omron®), with the child conformably sitting in a chair, with the cuff on the non-dominant arm, 2–3 cm above the elbow (without clothes compressing the arm). Two measurements of systolic (SBP) and diastolic (DPB) blood pressure, separated by at least 5 min, were taken after 10-min rest. If the

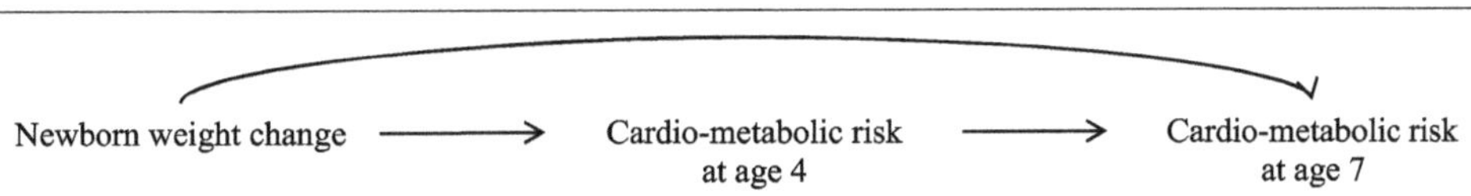

Fig. 1 Hypothesized mechanism linking newborn weight change with cardio-metabolic risk at ages 4 and 7 years: an overall effect with direct and indirect components

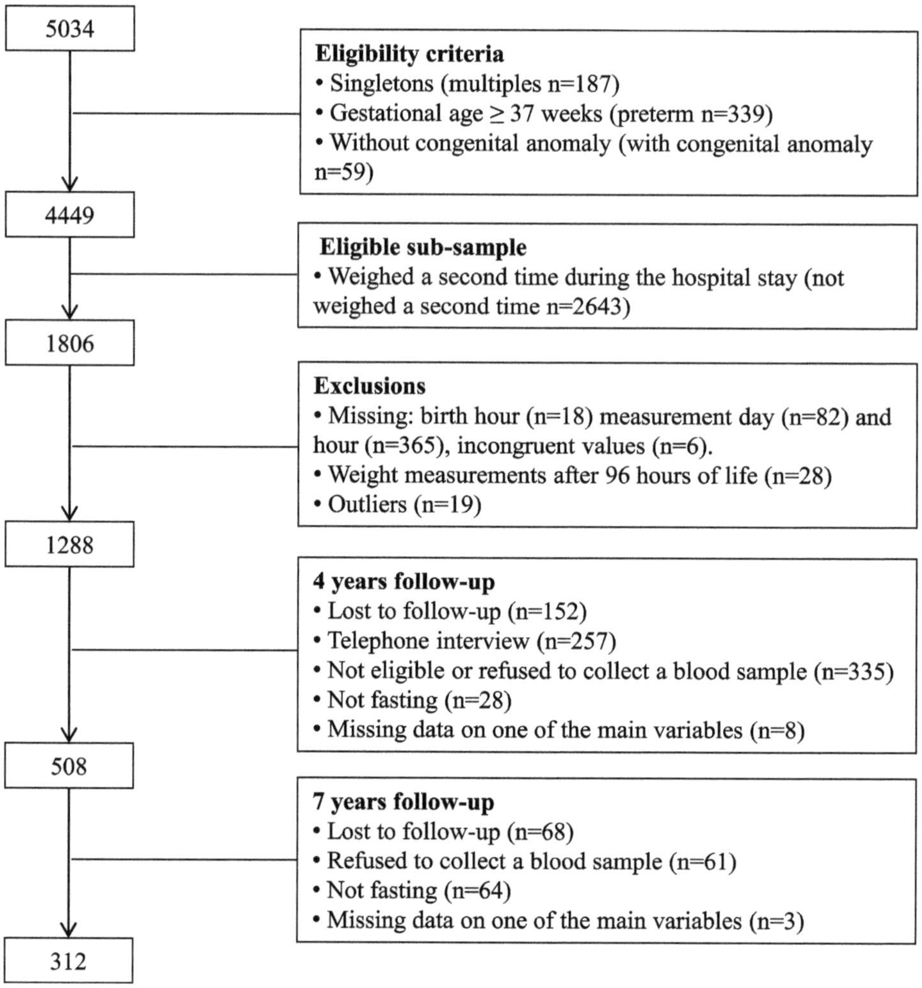

Fig. 2 Study flow chart of participants

difference between them was less than 5 mmHg for SBP or DBP, the mean was calculated. If the difference was larger than 5 mmHg a third measurement was taken and the mean of the 2 closest values was used [18]. After an overnight fast, a venous blood sample was collected before 11 a.m., according to standard procedures, after applying a topical analgesic cream (EMLA cream). This blood sample was centrifuged at 3500 rpm for 10 min and then the supernatant (serum) was stored at − 80 °C. Glucose was measured using UV enzymatic assay (hexokinase method), total and high density lipoprotein-cholesterol (for posterior calculation of LDL-C using Friedewald equation) [19], and triglycerides (TG) using an enzymatic colorimetric assay, in the Clinical Pathology Department of Centro Hospitalar São João, Porto, Portugal.

Our outcomes were: glucose, LDL-C, TG, waist circumference, SBP and DBP. In order to be able to compare magnitudes of association between different cardio-metabolic traits, we generated age- and sex-specific z-scores. For fasting glucose, LDL-C, TG and waist circumference this was done using the age- (in 6-months categories) and sex-specific means and standard deviations (SD) from the whole Generation XXI cohort. For SBP and DBP, we generated age-, sex- and height-specific z-scores using the means and standard deviations recommended by the American Academy of Pediatrics, in order to generate measures of BP that are independent of height (a major contribution to BP variation in children) [18]. High levels of the outcomes were considered when above the 90th percentile.

All the phases of the study complied with the Ethical Principles for Medical Research Involving Human Subjects expressed in the Declaration of Helsinki. The study was approved by the University of Porto Medical School/ Centro Hospitalar São João ethics committee and all parents or legal representative signed an informed consent according Helsinki.

STROBE checklist for the present manuscript can be found in Additional file 2.

Statistical analysis

The estimated *nadir* time was 52.3 h of life, thus, weights used to calculate NWC were birthweight and the weight estimated at 52.3 h of life. A cubic model with random intercept and slope by subject [$weight(t)$~3241.442 + (−9.378) × t + 0.119 × $t2$ + (−0.0004) × $t3$ + $b0$i + $b1$i × t] was used to estimate the weight according to the newborn's age represented as t in the formula (this analysis was performed using R version 2.14.1) [13].

Proportions were compared using the chi-square test, and means were compared using student's t-test or ANOVA (analysis performed using SPSS version 21.0). Pearson correlations were also computed. Crude and adjusted linear regression coefficients (β) and 95% confidence intervals (95% CI) were computed using path analysis. Full information maximum likelihood estimation was used to handle missing values, assuming missing at random [20]. We conducted path analysis based on the theoretical model depicted in Fig. 1 and tested the fit of the model with potential confounders. The final model included NWC, maternal education, maternal pre-pregnancy BMI, gestational age, and birthweight as explanatory variables. Path analysis was performed with Mplus software (version 7); 95% confidence intervals were calculated by bootstrapping. The fit of the models was assessed using different indexes: the Comparative Fit Index (CFI) [21], the Tucker–Lewis Index (TLI) [22], and the Root Mean Square Error of Approximation (RMSEA) [23]. A good model fit is indicated by a CFI and TLI values ≥0.90 and values of RMSEA close to 0.

Results

Table 1 shows the mean and standard deviation (or median and interquartile range for TG due to non-normal distribution) of NWC and all cardio-metabolic traits (glucose, LDL-C, TG, waist circumference, SBP and DBP) and also the number of children above the 90th percentile of the outcomes. Mean NWC was − 6.86% (ranging from − 15.03 and 5.30%). Mean values of all cardio-metabolic traits increased between 4 and 7 years, with the exception of LDL-C and TG which decreased.

Table 2 presents unadjusted correlations of NWC and cardio-metabolic trait z-scores in childhood. There was no strong evidence of association of NWC with any of the cardio-metabolic traits at age 4 or 7. There were correlations between some cardio-metabolic traits at each age and traits at age 4 were positively associated with the same trait at age 7.

Table 3 presents linear regression coefficients and 95% confidence intervals showing the adjusted total association of NWC with cardio-metabolic traits at ages 4 (model 1) and 7 (model 1) and the adjusted direct association of NWC with cardio-metabolic traits at age 7 (model 2), from the path analysis. These were consistent with the unadjusted association, with no strong evidence that NWC was associated with cardio-metabolic traits at age 4 or 7. Cardio-metabolic traits at age 4 were associated with the same trait at age 7, with the strongest associations observed for waist circumference [adjusted regression coefficient: 0.725 (0.657; 0.793)] and LDL-C [adjusted regression coefficient: 0.655 (0.575; 0.735)].

Discussion

We evaluated the association of NWC during the first 96 h of life with childhood cardio-metabolic outcomes. To our knowledge, no previous studies have longitudinally examined these associations. Similar to previous reports, we found that newborns lost on average 7% of their birthweight in the first 96 h of life. No robust evidence that NWC influenced childhood cardio-metabolic traits was

Table 1 Characteristics of the study sample at baseline, 4 and 7 years follow-up

	Baseline	4 years follow-up	7 years follow-up
Newborn weight change (%), mean (SD)	−6.86 (2.32)	–	–
Glucose (mg/dL), mean (SD)	–	77.9 (7.9)	83.0 (5.7)
High glucose, n (%)	–	22 (7.1)	27 (8.7)
LDL-C (mg/dL), mean (SD)	–	107.0 (23.5)	99.8 (22.2)
High LDL-C, n (%)	–	30 (9.6)	31 (9.9)
Triglycerides (mg/dL), median (IQR)	–	61.0 (25.0)	55.0 (28.0)
High triglycerides, n (%)	–	30 (9.6)	28 (9.0)
Waist circumference (cm), mean (SD)	–	52.0 (4.2)	58.3 (6.2)
High waist circumference, n (%)	–	20 (6.4)	25 (8.0)
Systolic blood pressure (mmHg), mean (SD)	–	97.3 (7.6)	105.0 (8.7)
High systolic blood pressure, n (%)	–	23 (7.4)	66 (21.2)
Diastolic blood pressure (mmHg), mean (SD)	–	56.1 (7.8)	69.2 (7.4)
High diastolic blood pressure, n (%)	–	21 (6.7)	102 (32.7)

Abbreviations: *LDL-C* low density lipoprotein cholesterol, *SD* standard deviation

Table 2 Correlations of newborn weight change (in first 96 h) and cardio-metabolic risk factors z-scores in childhood

		4 years						7 years					
		Glucose	LDL-C	TG	Waist circumf.	SBP	DBP	Glucose	LDL-C	TG	Waist circumf.	SBP	DBP
	NWC	0.015	0.041	0.014	−0.015	0.071	0.057	0.025	0.007	0.046	0.044	0.108	−0.020
4 years	Glucose	1	0.039	0.036	0.151**	0.039	0.019	**0.266*****	0.081	0.049	0.090	0.096	0.062
	LDL-C	–	1	0.053	0.031	0.041	−0.027	0.015	**0.667*****	0.042	−0.032	− 0.044	− 0.007
	TG	–	–	1	0.053	0.047	0.086	−0.119*	0.064	**0.295*****	0.047	−0.043	−0.002
	Waist circumf.	–	–	–	1	0.226***	0.344***	0.091	−0.007	0.133*	**0.776*****	0.160**	0.097
	SBP	–	–	–	–	1	0.369***	0.033	−0.007	0.000	0.207***	**0.367*****	0.307***
	DBP	–	–	–	–	–	1	0.033	−0.028	−0.013	0.242***	0.164**	**0.175****
7 years	Glucose	–	–	–	–	–	–	1	0.098	0.089	0.090	0.154**	0.116*
	LDL-C	–	–	–	–	–	–	–	1	0.120*	−0.020	0.047	0.078
	TG	–	–	–	–	–	–	–	–	1	0.135*	0.024	0.015
	Waist circumf.	–	–	–	–	–	–	–	–	–	1	0.262***	0.172**
	SBP	–	–	–	–	–	–	–	–	–	–	1	0.554***
	DBP	–	–	–	–	–	–	–	–	–	–	–	1

Abbreviations: *DBP* diastolic blood pressure, *LDL-C* low density lipoprotein cholesterol, *NWC* newborn weight change, *SBP* systolic blood pressure, *TG* triglycerides
*$p < 0.05$
**$p < 0.01$.
***$p < 0.001$.

found. Tracking correlation coefficients between ages 4 and 7 years were found for all cardio-metabolic traits, with the strongest being for waist circumference and LDL-C.

The prevalence of adverse levels of cardio-metabolic traits, such as central obesity, impaired glucose tolerance, dyslipidemia, and hypertension, has been increasing among children [1, 8]. Also, the co-occurrence of adverse levels of these cardio-metabolic traits, known as metabolic syndrome, has recently been identified in children, and its prevalence is around 3% but tending to increase [1, 24]. The tracking found in regards to all cardio-metabolic traits indicates that prevention should start as early as possible, because, according to our results, a 4-year-old child with adverse levels of cardio-metabolic traits will probably be a 7-year-old child also with adverse levels, and, according to previous studies, will probably have adverse levels across life [25]. Bearing in mind this remark, early screening of the levels of cardio-metabolic traits in children may indeed be justified from the point of view of cardio-metabolic chronic disease prevention. So, studies showing the normal cardio-metabolic traits distribution during childhood are of importance [26–28].

The biological mechanisms by which weight change during critical periods could lead to chronic diseases remain unclear. Theories of early programming hypothesize that under- or over- nutrition and other insults, when occurring during critical periods of development, may lead to permanent alterations in tissues' structure and functions, and in the neuroendocrine systems [6, 29]. Nevertheless, the exact timing of programming that contributes to the medium/long-term risk continues to be debated. There is some evidence that different early growth patterns may precede the development of adverse levels of cardio-metabolic traits later in life [5, 30–33], with a recent genetic study in 22,769 Europeans finding genetic evidence for a causal link between age and BMI at adiposity rebound and subsequent cardio-metabolic ill-health. However, the medium/long-term consequences of weight changes during the very first days of life had not been studied until now because very few studies have a second weight measure after birth within the first 96 h.

The nearest studies we could find to this very early period of rapid weight loss and major adaptation, were two recent studies, one of which examined weight change in the first week of life [34] and the second the first two weeks [35]; both found higher weight gain in these periods was associated with greater odds of overweight in adulthood and childhood, respectively. However, these studies considered a period when the NWC *nadir* had already occurred, so all newborns evaluated in those studies were already gaining weight. On the other hand, in our time frame, almost all newborns lost weight, because it focused in the first 96 h of life. Additionally, none of the studies examine NWC in relation to the cardio-metabolic traits analyzed in the present study.

Extreme values of NWC in the immediate postnatal period are associated with adverse health outcomes in the neonatal period, such as hypernatremic dehydration, which

Table 3 Adjusted associations between newborn weight change, cardio-metabolic indicators at age 4 and cardio-metabolic indicators at age 7 from path analysis

	NWC (%) β_1 (95%CI)	Cardio-metabolic indicators at age 4 (z-score) β_5 (95%CI)
Cardio-metabolic indicators at age 4		
Model 1		
Glucose z-score	0.004 (−0.043; 0.051)	–
LDL-cholesterol z-score	0.017 (−0.031; 0.065)	–
Triglycerides z-score	0.004 (−0.040; 0.049)	–
Waist circumference z-score	−0.003 (− 0.046; 0.039)	–
Systolic blood pressure z-score	0.017 (−0.016; 0.049)	–
Diastolic blood pressure z-score	0.015 (−0.018; 0.048)	–
Cardio-metabolic indicators at age 7		
Model 1		
Glucose z-score	0.008 (−0.035; 0.051)	–
LDL-cholesterol z-score	0.001 (−0.045; 0.047)	–
Triglycerides z-score	0.017 (−0.025; 0.060)	–
Waist circumference z-score	0.019 (−0.022; 0.060)	–
Systolic blood pressure z-score	0.031 (−0.006; 0.067)	–
Diastolic blood pressure z-score	−0.010 (− 0.040; 0.020)	–
Model 2		
Glucose z-score	0.007 (−0.035; 0.048)	0.235 (0.136; 0.334)*
LDL-cholesterol z-score	−0.012 (− 0.045; 0.022)	0.655 (0.575; 0.735)*
Triglycerides z-score	0.016 (−0.024; 0.057)	0.281 (0.180; 0.383)*
Waist circumference z-score	0.021 (−0.008; 0.025)	0.725 (0.657; 0.793)*
Systolic blood pressure z-score	0.025 (−0.009; 0.058)	0.369 (0.251; 0.488)*
Diastolic blood pressure z-score	−0.013 (− 0.042; 0.016)	0.153 (0.050; 0.256)*

Abbreviations: *NWC* newborn weight change, *LDL* low density lipoprotein, β regression coefficient, *CI* confidence interval
Cardio-metabolic indicator at age 4 (Model 1) ≈ $\beta_0 + \beta_1$ (NWC) + β_2 (maternal education) + β_3 (maternal pre-pregnancy BMI) + β_4 (gestational age) + β_5 (birth weight)
Cardio-metabolic indicator at age 7 (Model 1) ≈ $\beta_0 + \beta_1$ (NWC) + β_2 (maternal education) + β_3 (maternal pre-pregnancy BMI) + β_4 (birth weight)
Cardio-metabolic indicator at age 7 (Model 2) ≈ $\beta_0 + \beta_1$ (NWC) + β_2 (maternal education) + β_3 (maternal pre-pregnancy BMI) + β_4 (birth weight) + β5 (same cardio-metabolic indicator at 4)
*$p < 0.05$.

can cause serious medical complications, such as disseminated intravascular coagulation, cerebrovascular accidents and even death, or, on the other hand, over hydration and related morbidities such as bronchopulmonary dysplasia, intraventricular–periventricular hemorrhage, necrotizing enterocolitis and patent ductus arteriosus [14, 15]. Even though extreme values of NWC has adverse effects in the neonatal period, it does not appear to have long term adverse cardio-metabolic effects.

Limitations and strengths

A large proportion of the main cohort participants were not included in our analyses. However, distributions of maternal and neonatal characteristics between participants and eligible non-participants were similar. Our finding that NWC during the first 96 h was not associated with childhood cardio-metabolic traits might be due to lack of statistical power, but the point estimates were all close to the null and the 95%CI were narrow, suggesting that we had adequate power to obtain precise estimates and rule out an important association.

As weight measurements were not taken at regular periods for each newborn, it is possible that the precise *nadir* of NWC was not detected. Nevertheless, a systematic review [12] found a mean NWC ranged from – 5.7% to – 6.6% and a *nadir* around the 2nd and 3rd days following birth. These results support our methodology as we found a mean NWC of – 6.7% occurring at 52.3 h of life [13], suggesting that we correctly estimate the actual *nadir* in our sample.

We used path analysis to explore associations. This is an extension of regression analysis, which allows for simultaneous estimation of the interrelations between variables. We used it here because it is a useful method for comparing the magnitudes of effects between variables with complex interrelations or to test the plausibility of mediation effects [36].

Our exposure – NWC – measures the growth occurring within 96 h, which is a very narrow period. It is known that the measurement error on weight change is higher and the capacity to identify associations between growth periods and outcomes reduced, when the measurements are closer in time and the weight change is smaller [37]. Since measurement error in NWC is unlikely to be related to later child cardio-metabolic outcomes (the midwives and trained researchers who measured birth and later weight would have no way of knowing the future cardio-metabolic traits of the newborns they were assessing), the expectation would be for this random error to attenuate the observed associations, however the bias would also depend on relationships of the error to other explanatory variables in the model. We doubt it would fully explain the consistent null results we find across all traits.

Although cardio-metabolic traits in early childhood track throughout childhood (as we showed) and into adulthood, clinically abnormal values of cardio-metabolic risk factors, such as fasting glucose or SBP, are unusual in childhood [38], and it is possible that the medium/long--term effects of NWC on cardio-metabolic health are not yet fully evident at the ages we have assessed. Future research conducted as this population ages will enable this possibility to be explored.

Conclusions

We found no strong evidence that NWC is related to cardio-metabolic traits at age 4 or 7, suggesting that NWC does not influence the development of adverse cardio-metabolic outcomes at least up to age 7. Thus, NWC should be faced in clinical practice as a short-term phenomenon, with no medium/long term consequences, at least in cardio-metabolic health.

Additional files

Additional file 1: Comparison between participants and eligible non participants regarding maternal, pregnancy, delivery and newborn characteristics. Table with the comparison between participants and eligible non participants.

Additional file 2: STROBE Statement—Checklist of items that should be included in reports of cohort studies. A STROBE checklist for the present manuscript.

Abbreviations

BMI: Body mass index; DBP: Diastolic blood pressure; LDL-C: Low density lipoprotein cholesterol; NWC: Newborn weight change; SBP: Systolic blood pressure; TG: Triglycerides

Acknowledgements

The authors gratefully acknowledge the families enrolled in Generation XXI for their kindness, all members of the research team for their enthusiasm and perseverance and the participating hospitals and their staff for their help and support.

Funding

This work was supported by Programa Operacional de Saúde – Saúde XXI, Quadro Comunitário de Apoio III and Administração Regional de Saúde Norte (Regional Department of Ministry of Health); FEDER through the Operational Programme Competitiveness and Internationalization and national funding from the Foundation for Science and Technology – FCT (Portuguese Ministry of Science, Technology and Higher Education) [POCI-01- 0145-FEDER-016837], under the project "PathMOB.: Risco cardiometabólico na infância: desde o início da vida ao fim da infância" [Ref. FCT PTDC/DTP-EPI/3306/2014], and FCT Investigator contract [IF/01060/2015] - ACS; Unidade de Investigação em Epidemiologia - Instituto de Saúde Pública da Universidade do Porto (EPIUnit) [POCI-01-0145-FEDER-006862; Ref. UID/DTP/04750/2013]; Norte Portugal Regional Operational Programme (NORTE 2020), under the PORTUGAL 2020 Partnership Agreement, through the European Regional Development Fund (ERDF) - DOCnet (NORTE-01-0145-FEDER-000003); UK Medical Research Council [MC_UU_12013/5] and UK National
Institute of Health Research Senior Investigator [NF-SI-0611-10196] – DAL.

Authors' contributions

MJF conceptualized the study, carried out statistical analyses, drafted the initial manuscript, and approved the final manuscript as submitted. MS carried out statistical analyses, reviewed the manuscript, and approved the final manuscript as submitted. DAL critically reviewed and revised the manuscript, and approved the final manuscript as submitted. HB designed the data collection instruments, and coordinated and supervised data collection, critically reviewed the manuscript, and approved the final manuscript as submitted. ACS designed the data collection instruments, and coordinated and supervised data collection, conceptualized the study, reviewed and revised the manuscript, and approved the final manuscript as submitted.

Competing interests

The authors declare that they have no competing interests.

Author details

[1]EPIUnit - Instituto de Saúde Pública, Universidade do Porto, Rua das Taipas n° 135, 4050-600 Porto, Portugal. [2]Departamento de Ciências da Saúde Pública e Forenses e Educação Médica, Faculdade de Medicina, Universidade do Porto, Porto, Portugal. [3]Medical Research Council Integrative Epidemiology Unit at the University of Bristol, Bristol, UK. [4]School of Social and Community Medicine, University of Bristol, Bristol, UK.

References

1. Weiss R, Dziura J, Burgert TS, Tamborlane WV, Taksali SE, Yeckel CW, Allen K, Lopes M, Savoye M, Morrison J, et al. Obesity and the metabolic syndrome in children and adolescents. N Engl J Med. 2004;350(23):2362–74.
2. Lassale C, Tzoulaki I, Moons KGM, Sweeting M, Boer J, Johnson L, Huerta JM, Agnoli C, Freisling H, Weiderpass E, et al. Separate and combined associations of obesity and metabolic health with coronary heart disease: a pan-European case-cohort analysis. Eur Heart J. 2018;39(5):397–406.
3. Barker DJ, Hales CN, Fall CH, Osmond C, Phipps K, Clark PM. Type 2 (non-insulin-dependent) diabetes mellitus, hypertension and hyperlipidaemia (syndrome X): relation to reduced fetal growth. Diabetologia. 1993;36(1):62–7.

4. Lakshmy R. Metabolic syndrome: role of maternal undernutrition and fetal programming. Rev Endocr Metab Disord. 2013;14(3):229–40.
5. Chiavaroli V, Marcovecchio ML, de Giorgis T, Diesse L, Chiarelli F, Mohn A. Progression of cardio-metabolic risk factors in subjects born small and large for gestational age. PLoS One. 2014;9(8):e104278.
6. Hales CN, Barker DJ. The thrifty phenotype hypothesis. Br Med Bull. 2001;60:5–20.
7. Wells JC. The programming effects of early growth. Early Hum Dev. 2007;83(12):743–8.
8. Beilin L, Huang RC. Childhood obesity, hypertension, the metabolic syndrome and adult cardiovascular disease. Clin Exp Pharmacol Physiol. 2008;35(4):409–11.
9. Boney CM, Verma A, Tucker R, Vohr BR. Metabolic syndrome in childhood: association with birth weight, maternal obesity, and gestational diabetes mellitus. Pediatrics. 2005;115(3):e290–6.
10. Hardy R, Lawlor DA, Kuh D. A life course approach to cardiovascular aging. Futur Cardiol. 2014;11(1):101–13.
11. Howe LD, Tilling K, Benfield L, Logue J, Sattar N, Ness AR, Smith GD, Lawlor DA. Changes in ponderal index and body mass index across childhood and their associations with fat mass and cardiovascular risk factors at age 15. PLoS One. 2011;5(12):e15186.
12. Noel-Weiss J, Courant G, Woodend AK. Physiological weight loss in the breastfed neonate: a systematic review. Open Med. 2008;2(4):e99–e110.
13. Fonseca MJ, Severo M, Santos AC. A new approach to estimating weight change and its reference intervals during the first 96 hours of life. Acta Paediatr. 2015;104(10):1028–34.
14. Bell EF, Warburton D, Stonestreet BS, Oh W. Effect of fluid administration on the development of symptomatic patent ductus arteriosus and congestive heart failure in premature infants. N Engl J Med. 1980;302(11):598–604.
15. van Dommelen P, van Wouwe JP, Breuning-Boers JM, van Buuren S, Verkerk PH. Reference chart for relative weight change to detect hypernatraemic dehydration. Arch Dis Child. 2007;92(6):490–4.
16. Larsen PS, Kamper-Jorgensen M, Adamson A, Barros H, Bonde JP, Brescianini S, Brophy S, Casas M, Charles MA, Devereux G, et al. Pregnancy and birth cohort resources in europe: a large opportunity for aetiological child health research. Paediatr Perinat Epidemiol. 2013;27(4):393–414.
17. Gibson RS. Principles of nutritional assessment, 2nd edn. New York, NY, USA: Oxford University Press; 2005.
18. National High Blood Pressure Education Program Working Group on High Blood Pressure in C, Adolescents. The fourth report on the diagnosis, evaluation, and treatment of high blood pressure in children and adolescents. Pediatrics. 2004;114(2 Suppl 4th Report):555–76.
19. Friedewald WT, Levy RI, Fredrickson DS. Estimation of the concentration of low-density lipoprotein cholesterol in plasma, without use of the preparative ultracentrifuge. Clin Chem. 1972;18(6):499–502.
20. Yuan KH, Bentler PM. Three likelihood-based methods for mean and covariance structure analysis with nonnormal missing data. In: Sobel, Becker, editors. *Sociological Methodology*; 2000. p. 165–200.
21. Bentler PM. Comparative fit indexes in structural models. Psychol Bull. 1990;107(2):238–46.
22. Tucker L, Lewis C. A reliability coefficient for maximum likelihood factor analysis. Psychometrika. 1973;38:1–10.
23. Steiger JH. Structural model evaluation and modification. An interval estimation approach. Multivar Behav Res. 1990;25:173–80.
24. Friend A, Craig L, Turner S. The prevalence of metabolic syndrome in children: a systematic review of the literature. Metab Syndr Relat Disord. 2013;11(2):71–80.
25. Camhi SM, Katzmarzyk PT. Tracking of cardiometabolic risk factor clustering from childhood to adulthood. Int J Pediatr Obes : IJPO : an official journal of the International Association for the Study of Obesity. 2010;5(2):122–9.
26. De Henauw S, Michels N, Vyncke K, Hebestreit A, Russo P, Intemann T, Peplies J, Fraterman A, Eiben G, de Lorgeril M, et al. Blood lipids among young children in Europe: results from the European IDEFICS study. Int J Obes. 2014;38(Suppl 2):S67–75.
27. Jolliffe CJ, Janssen I. Distribution of lipoproteins by age and gender in adolescents. Circulation. 2006;114(10):1056–62.
28. Mascarenhas LP, Leite N, Titski AC, Brito LM, Boguszewski MC. Variability of lipid and lipoprotein concentrations during puberty in Brazilian boys. J Pediatr Endocrino Metab : JPEM. 2015;28(1–2):125–31.
29. Lawlor DA. The Society for Social Medicine John Pemberton Lecture 2011. Developmental overnutrition–an old hypothesis with new importance? Int J Epidemiol. 2013;42(1):7–29.
30. Ekelund U, Ong KK, Linne Y, Neovius M, Brage S, Dunger DB, Wareham NJ, Rossner S. Association of weight gain in infancy and early childhood with metabolic risk in young adults. J Clin Endocrinol Metab. 2007;92(1):98–103.
31. Eriksson JG, Forsen T, Tuomilehto J, Osmond C, Barker DJ. Early growth and coronary heart disease in later life: longitudinal study. BMJ. 2001; 322(7292):949–53.
32. Eriksson JG, Forsen T, Tuomilehto J, Osmond C, Barker DJ. Early adiposity rebound in childhood and risk of type 2 diabetes in adult life. Diabetol. 2003;46(2):190–4.
33. Ong KK, Ahmed ML, Emmett PM, Preece MA, Dunger DB. Association between postnatal catch-up growth and obesity in childhood: prospective cohort study. BMJ. 2000;320(7240):967–71.
34. Stettler N, Stallings VA, Troxel AB, Zhao J, Schinnar R, Nelson SE, Ziegler EE, Strom BL. Weight gain in the first week of life and overweight in adulthood: a cohort study of European American subjects fed infant formula. Circulation. 2005;111(15):1897–903.
35. Andersen LG, Holst C, Michaelsen KF, Baker JL, Sorensen TI. Weight and weight gain during early infancy predict childhood obesity: a case-cohort study. Int J Obes. 2012;36(10):1306–11.
36. Gamborg M, Andersen PK, Baker JL, Budtz-Jorgensen E, Jorgensen T, Jensen G, Sorensen TI. Life course path analysis of birth weight, childhood growth, and adult systolic blood pressure. Am J Epidemiol. 2009;169(10):1167–78.
37. Wells JC, Hallal PC, Wright A, Singhal A, Victora CG. Fetal, infant and childhood growth: relationships with body composition in Brazilian boys aged 9 years. Int J Obes. 2005;29(10):1192–8.
38. Expert panel on integrated guidelines for cardiovascular health and risk reduction in children and adolescents: summary report. Pediatrics. 2012; 128(Suppl 5):S213–56.

19

Genetic variation in folate metabolism is associated with the risk of conotruncal heart defects in a Chinese population

Xike Wang[1†], Haitao Wei[1†], Ying Tian[1], Yue Wu[1] and Lei Luo[2*]

Abstract

Background: Conotruncal heart defects (CTDs) are a subgroup of congenital heart defects that are considered to be the most common type of birth defect worldwide. Genetic disturbances in folate metabolism may increase the risk of CTDs.

Methods: We evaluated five single-nucleotide polymorphisms (SNPs) in genes related to folic acid metabolism: methylenetetrahydrofolate reductase (MTHFR C677T and A1298C), solute carrier family 19, member 1 (SLC19A1 G80A), methionine synthase (MTR A2576G), and methionine synthase reductase (MTRR A66G), as risk factors for CTDs including various types of malformation, in a total of 193 mothers with CTD-affected offspring and 234 healthy controls in a Chinese population.

Results: Logistic regression analyses revealed that subjects carrying the TT genotype of MTHFR C677T, the C allele of MTHFR A1298C, and the AA genotype of SLC19A1 G80A had significant 2.47-fold (TT vs. CC, OR [95% CI] = 2.47 [1.42–4.32], $p = 0.009$), 2.05–2.20-fold (AC vs. AA, 2.05 [1.28–3.21], $p = 0.0023$; CC vs AA, 2.20 [1.38–3.58], $p = 0.0011$), and 1.68-fold (AA vs. GG, 1.68 [1.02–2.70], $p = 0.0371$) increased risk of CTDs, respectively. Subjects carrying both variant genotypes of MTHFR A1298C and SLC19A1 G80A had a higher (3.23 [1.71–6.02], $p = 0.0002$) increased risk for CTDs. Moreover, the MTHFR C677T, MTHFR A1298C, and MTRR A66G polymorphisms were found to be significantly associated with the risk of certain subtypes of CTD.

Conclusions: Our data suggest that maternal folate-related SNPs might be associated with the risk of CTDs in offspring.

Keywords: Conotruncal heart defect, Single-nucleotide polymorphism, Methionine synthase, Methylenetetrahydrofolate reductase, Solute carrier family 19

Background

Congenital heart defects (CHDs) are the most common type of birth defect and are associated with significant morbidity and mortality. CHDs occur in approximately 0.4–1% of children born alive [1, 2]. CHDs include a broad range of different forms of structural malformations that are developmentally and clinically heterogeneous [3, 4]. Among the identified subgroups of CHDs, conotruncal heart defects (CTDs) account for 25–33% of all patients [4]. This CHD subgroup involves cardiac structures that are partially derived from cell lineages [5], and includes malformations such as tetralogy of Fallot (TOF), pulmonary atresia with ventricular septal defect (PA/VSD), double outlet of right ventricle (DORV), transposition of the great arteries (TGA), persistent truncus arteriosus (PTA), and interrupted aortic arch (IAA). CTD was considered to be a folate-sensitive birth defect because women who take multivitamins containing folic acid early in pregnancy are at approximately a 30–40% reduced risk of delivering offspring with these heart defects [6, 7]. Although the protective mechanism of folic acid is unclear, evidence has been reported that genetic variations that alter the activity of key enzymes in the folate pathway could influence the risk of such heart defects [8–10].

Although the folic acid cycle is highly complex in mammals, various genes controlling folate metabolism, such as

* Correspondence: linzhongyueliang@163.com
†Xike Wang and Haitao Wei contributed equally to this work.
[2]Department of science and education, Guizhou Provincial People's Hospital, Guiyang 550002, China
Full list of author information is available at the end of the article

methylenetetrahydrofolate reductase (MTHFR), solute carrier family 19, member 1 (SLC19A1), methionine synthase (MTR), and methionine synthase reductase (MTRR), have been proven to play crucial roles in this metabolic pathway. For example, the MTHFR gene, located on chromosome 1p36.3, encodes an enzyme that catalyzes the reduction of 5,10-methylenetetrahydrofolate to 5-methyltetrahydrofolate [11], which is essential for folate-mediated one-carbon metabolism. SLC19A1 has also been referred to as reduced folate carrier-1 (RFC1), which is involved in the active transport of 5-methyltetrahydrofolate from the plasma to the cytosol and the regulation of intracellular concentrations of folate [12]. MTR catalyzes the remethylation of homocysteine to methionine [13], while MTRR catalyzes the regeneration of the cobalamin cofactor of MTR, thus maintaining MTR in an active state [14]. A single-nucleotide polymorphism (SNP) is a variation in a single nucleotide that is present to some appreciable degree within a population. Many studies have investigated associations between SNPs in the above-mentioned genes and the risk of CHD/CTD. Among them, the MTHFR C677T variant (TT), MTHFR A1298C variant (CC), SLC19A1 G80A variant (AG or AA), MTR A2576G variant (GG), and MTRR A66G variant (GG) have been extensively investigated. Although these gene variants would theoretically influence the risk of CHD/CTD, studies have yielded conflicting results on this issue in different populations [10, 12, 15–19].

Based on the results of previously published studies, we concluded that polymorphisms in genes that encode these key enzymes in the folate pathway would alter its activity, but there is debate on whether these genetic variants affect the risk of heart defects. In the present study, we thus aimed to determine whether the maternal polymorphisms of MTHFR C677T, MTHFR A1298C, SLC19A1 G80A, MTR A2576G, and MTRR A66G in a Chinese population are associated with various types of CTD.

Methods

Patients and controls

The present study was approved by the ethics committee of Guizhou Provincial People's Hospital. All participants provided written informed consent to approve the use of their blood samples for research purposes. A total of 193 mothers of echocardiographically proven CTD-affected children (CTD group, mean age: 29.4 ± 5.1) and 234 mothers of healthy children (control group, mean age: 29.1 ± 5.1) were recruited in the study between January 2017 and January 2018. All participants were genetically unrelated ethnic Han Chinese. For 193 mothers in the CTD group, each had only one child with CTD, as summarized in Table 1; different types of CTD in the children included TOF (90 cases), PA/VSD (31 cases), DORV (35 cases), TGA (10 cases), PTA (14 cases), and IAA (13 cases). For each mother, 5 ml of peripheral blood was collected in EDTA tubes, and within 5 h, genomic DNA was isolated from whole blood using the QIAamp DNA Blood Mini Kit (QIAGEN, Germany), in accordance with the manufacturer's protocol. Then, the genomic DNA was either stored at − 80 °C or SNP genotyping was conducted on it immediately.

Table 1 Conotruncal heart defects affecting the children

Type of conotruncal heart defect	No. (%)
Tetralogy of Fallot	90 (46.6)
Pulmonary atresia with ventricular septal defect	31 (16.1)
Double outlet of right ventricle	35 (18.1)
Transposition of the great arteries	10 (5.2)
Persistent truncus arteriosus	14 (7.3)
Interrupted aortic arch	13 (6.7)
Total	193

Polymorphism detection

The polymorphisms of five selected genetic variants were determined by the Taqman SNP Genotyping Assay (Thermo Fisher, USA), Briefly, 50 ng of DNA was amplified using Taqman Genotyping Master Mix (Thermo Fisher, USA) and commercial probes (Thermo Fisher, USA) for MTHFR C677T (rs1801133), MTHFR A1298C (rs1801131), SLC19A1 G80A (rs1051266), MTR A2576G (rs1805087), and MTRR A66G (rs1801394) in a final volume of 25 μL. PCR thermal cycling conditions were as follows: 10 min at 95 °C for AmpliTaq Gold, UP Enzyme activation, and then 40 cycles of denaturation at 95 °C for 15 s and annealing/extension at 65 °C for 1 min.

Statistical analysis

The statistical analyses were performed using SPSS version 19.0 software. The differences in allele frequencies between patients and controls were evaluated using chi-squared test. The associations between genotypes and the risk of CTD were estimated by calculating the odds ratio (OR) and the 95% confidence interval (CI) from logistic regression analyses.

Results

Allele frequencies

The distribution of allele frequencies did not differ for MTR A2576G and MTRR A66G between the CTD and control groups (Table 2). However, statistically significant differences were observed in the distribution of the mutated allele for MTHFR C677T, MTHFR A1298C, and SLC19A1 G80A, in which the frequencies of the T allele (48.7% vs. 38.9%, $p = 0.004$), C allele (52.1% vs. 38.7%, $p < 0.001$), and A allele (46.9% vs. 40.2%, $p = 0.0485$) were higher in the CTD group. These deviations could have been due to genetic associations with CTDs.

Table 2 Allele frequencies of the CTD and control groups

Genotyped SNPs	Controls (*n* = 234) % (No.)	CTD (*N* = 193) % (No.)	*p*-Value for HWE test
MTHFR C677T (rs1801133)			
C	61.1(286)	51.3(198)	0.004*
T	38.9(182)	48.7(188)	
MTHFR A1298C (rs1801131)			
A	61.3(287)	47.9(185)	< 0.001*
C	38.7(181)	52.1(201)	
SLC19A1 G80A (rs1051266)			
G	59.8(280)	53.1(205)	0.0485*
A	40.2(188)	46.9(181)	
MTR A2576G (rs1805087)			
A	41.5(194)	61.9(239)	0.7862
G	58.5(174)	38.1(147)	
MTRR A66G (rs1801394)			
A	56.8(266)	60.6(234)	0.2639
G	43.2(202)	39.4(152)	

HWE Hardy-Weinberg equilibrium
*means *p*-value< 0.05

Association of folate-related SNPs with risk of CTDs

The associations between the risk of CTDs and the homozygous variant genotype, heterozygous variant genotype, and variant allele were evaluated for each of the five folate-related SNPs (Table 3). In the single-locus analyses, the genotype frequencies of MTHFR C677T were 33.68% (CC), 35.23% (CT), and 31.09% (TT) in the CTD group and 35.47% (CC), 51.28% (CT), and 13.25% (TT) in the control group, and the difference was significant for the TT genotype ($p = 0.0009$), when using the CC genotype as a reference point. Logistic regression analyses revealed that subjects carrying the TT genotype had a significant 2.47-fold (OR: 2.47, 95% CI: 1.42–4.32) increased risk of CTDs, compared with the subjects carrying the CC genotype. Moreover, subjects carrying the C allele of MTHFR A1298C had a significant 2.05–2.20-fold increased risk of CTDs (AC vs. AA, OR: 2.05, 95% CI: 1.28–3.21, $p = 0.0023$; CC vs. AA, OR: 2.20, 95% CI: 1.38–3.58, $p = 0.0011$). There was also a significantly higher frequency of the AA genotype for SLC19A1 G80A in the CTD group than in the controls (OR: 1.68, 95% CI: 1.02–2.70, $p = 0.0371$), when using the GG genotype as a reference. However, none of MTR A2576G and MTRR A66G exhibited a statistically significant difference in the genotype distributions between the two groups.

Table 3 Genotype frequencies among controls and CTD cases

Genotype	Controls (n = 234) No. (%)	CTD (N = 193) No. (%)	OR (95% CI)	*p*-Value
MTHFR C677T				
CC	83(35.47)	65(33.68)	1.00	
CT	120(51.28)	68(35.23)	0.72(0.47–1.11)	0.1493
TT	31(13.25)	60(31.09)	2.47(1.42–4.32)	0.0009*
CT + TT	151(64.53)	128(66.32)	1.08(0.73–1.62)	0.6987
MTHFR A1298C				
AA	110(47.01)	57(29.53)	1.00	
AC	67(28.63)	71(36.79)	2.05(1.28–3.21)	0.0023*
CC	57(24.36)	65(33.68)	2.20(1.38–3.58)	0.0011*
AC + CC	124(52.99)	136(70.47)	2.12(1.40–3.19)	0.0002*
SLC19A1 G80A				
GG	102(43.59)	68(35.23)	1.00	
AG	82(35.04)	69(35.75)	1.26(0.82–1.96)	0.3031
AA	50(21.37)	56(29.02)	1.68(1.02–2.70)	0.0371*
AG + AA	132(56.41)	125(64.77)	1.42(0.96–2.09)	0.0791
MTR A2756G				
AA	87(37.18)	66(34.20)	1.00	
AG	120(51.28)	107(55.44)	1.18(0.77–1.76)	0.4426
GG	27(11.54)	20(10.36)	0.98(0.51–1.92)	0.9436
AG + GG	147(62.82)	127(65.80)	1.14(0.77–1.70)	0.5224
MTRR A66G				
AA	75(32.05)	71(36.79)	1.00	
AG	116(49.57)	92(47.67)	0.84(0.55–1.28)	0.4136
GG	43(18.38)	30(15.54)	0.74(0.42–1.32)	0.2917
AG + GG	159(67.95)	122(63.21)	0.81(0.54–1.21)	0.3045

OR odds ratio, *CI* confidence interval
*means *p*-value< 0.05

Association of folate-related SNPs with risk of TOF, PA/VSD, DORV, TGA, PTA, and IAA

We also performed stratification analyses to evaluate the effects of five folate-related SNPs on certain types of CTD (Table 4). Our results suggest that subjects carrying the TT genotype of MTHFR C677T had significantly increased risks of TOF (OR: 2.33, 95% CI: 1.18–4.39, $p = 0.0111$), DORV (OR: 3.87, 95% CI: 1.55–9.32, $p = 0.0034$), and IAA (OR: 4.02, 95% CI: 1.09–13.12, $p = 0.0297$). The C allele of MTHFR A1298C was also associated with an increased risk of TOF (AC vs. AA, OR: 2.01, 95% CI: 1.11–3.70, $p = 0.0201$; CC vs. AA, OR: 2.14, 95% CI: 1.14–3.88, $p = 0.0133$), while it was only statistically significant in homozygote comparisons for DORV (OR: 2.51, 95% CI: 1.00–6.13, $p = 0.0369$) and IAA (OR: 6.75, 95% CI: 1.41–32.67, $p = 0.008$). Moreover, the GG genotype of MTRR A66G was associated with significantly decreased risks of TOF (OR: 0.39, 95% CI: 0.17–0.88, $p = 0.026$) and PA/VSD (OR: 0.12, 95% CI:

Table 4 Genotype frequencies among controls, TOF, PA/VSD, DORV, TGA, PTA and IAA cases

Genotype	Controls (n = 234)	TOF ($n = 90$)		*p*-Value	PA/VSD ($n = 31$)		*p*-Value	DORV ($n = 35$)		*p*-Value	TGA ($n = 10$)		*p*-Value	PTA ($n = 14$)		*p*-Value	IAA ($n = 13$)		*p*-Value
	No. (%)	No. (%)	OR (95% CI)		No. (%)	OR (95% CI)		No. (%)	OR (95% CI)		No. (%)	CR (95% CI)		No. (%)	OR (95% CI)		No. (%)	OR (95% CI)	
MTHFR C677T																			
CC	83(35.47)	31(34.44)	1.00		13(41.94)	1.00		9(25.71)	1.00		2(20.00)	1.00		6(42.86)	1.00		4(30.77)	1.00	
CT	120(51.28)	32(35.56)	0.71 (0.41–1.24)	0.2347	11(35.48)	0.59 (0.26–1.39)	0.2130	13(37.14)	0.99 (0.40–2.39)	0.9984	5(50.00)	1.73 (0.36–8.84)	0.5140	4(28.57)	0.46 (0.14–1.80)	0.2315	3(23.08)	0.52 (0.13–1.98)	0.3906
TT	31(13.25)	27(30.00)	2.33 (1.18–4.39)	0.0111*	7(22.58)	1.44 (0.56–3.90)	0.4749	13(37.14)	3.87 (1.55–9.32)	0.0034*	3(30.00)	4.02 (0.78–23.14)	0.1120	4(28.57)	1.79 (0.54–6.38)	0.3883	6(46.15)	4.02 (1.09–13.12)	0.0297*
CT + TT	151(64.53)	59(65.56)	1.05 (0.64–1.72)	0.8625	18(58.06)	0.76 (0.36–1.59)	0.4816	26(74.29)	1.59 (0.70–3.60)	0.2565	8(80.00)	2.20 (0.52–10.46)	0.3147	8(57.14)	0.73 (0.24–2.21)	0.5757	9(69.23)	1.24 (0.38–3.72)	0.7298
MTHFR A1298C																			
AA	110(47.01)	27(30.00)	1.00		11(35.48)	1.00		10(28.57)	1.00		4(40.00)	1.00		3(21.43)	1.00		2(15.38)	1.00	
AC	67(28.63)	33(36.67)	2.01 (1.11–3.70)	0.0201*	13(41.94)	1.94 (0.80–4.39)	0.1255	12(34.29)	1.97 (0.85–4.87)	0.1313	2(20.00)	0.82 (0.15–3.61)	0.8222	7(50.00)	3.83 (1.00–13.90)	0.0431*	4(30.77)	3.28 (0.74–17.52)	0.1543
CC	57(24.36)	30(33.33)	2.14 (1.14–3.88)	0.0133*	7(22.58)	1.23 (0.47–3.39)	0.6869	13(37.14)	2.51 (1.00–6.13)	0.0369*	4(40.00)	1.93 (0.54–6.80)	0.3575	4(28.57)	2.57 (0.67–10.43)	0.2113	7(53.85)	6.75 (1.41–32.67)	0.008*
AC + CC	124(52.99)	63(70.00)	2.07 (1.22–3.50)	0.0055*	20(64.52)	1.61 (0.76–3.63)	0.2261	25(71.43)	2.22 (1.02–4.61)	0.0407*	6(60.00)	1.33 (0.35–4.26)	0.6635	11(78.57)	3.25 (0.97–11.09)	0.0619	11(84.62)	4.88 (1.15–22.36)	0.0258*
SLC19A1 G80A																			
GG	102(43.59)	29(32.22)	1.00		13(41.94)	1.00		15(42.86)	1.00		3(30.00)	1.00		3(21.43)	1.00		5(38.46)	1.00	
AG	82(35.04)	35(38.89)	1.62 (0.93–2.87)	0.0987	12(38.71)	1.24 (0.51–2.90)	0.6163	10(28.57)	0.89(0.38–2.06)	0.7983	1(10.00)	0.45 (0.03–3.06)	0.4786	5(35.71)	2.24 (0.57–8.62)	0.2691	6(46.15)	1.61 (0.45–4.84)	0.4416
AA	50(21.37)	26(28.89)	1.63 (0.88–2.99)	0.1205	6(19.35)	0.84 (0.31–2.26)	0.7387	10(28.57)	1.21 (0.51–2.85)	0.6593	6(60.00)	3.64 (0.96–13.59)	0.0593	6(42.86)	3.64 (0.96–13.59)	0.0593	2(15.38)	0.73 (0.14–3.58)	0.7094
AG + AA	132(56.41)	61(67.78)	1.63 (0.96–2.70)	0.0618	18(58.06)	1.07 (0.51–2.22)	0.8614	20(57.14)	1.03 (0.50–2.12)	0.9350	7(70.00)	1.80 (0.49–6.53)	0.3953	11(78.57)	2.83 (0.84–9.67)	0.1031	8(61.54)	1.24 (0.38–3.44)	0.7165
MTR A2756G																			
AA	87(37.18)	33(36.67)	1.00		13(41.94)	1.00		10(28.57)	1.00		2(20.00)	1.00		3(21.43)	1.00		5(38.46)	1.00	
AG	120(51.28)	46(51.11)	1.01 (0.59–1.70)	0.9686	15(48.39)	0.84 (0.39–1.83)	0.6585	21(60.00)	1.52 (0.70–3.29)	0.3018	6(60.00)	2.18 (0.52–10.77)	0.3373	11(78.57)	2.66 (0.78–9.10)	0.1289	8(61.54)	1.16 (0.35–3.24)	0.8003
GG	27(11.54)	11(12.22)	1.07 (0.50–2.37)	0.8623	3(9.68)	0.74 (0.21–2.60)	0.6609	4(11.43)	1.29 (0.42–4.40)	0.6871	2(20.00)	3.22 (0.43–21.06)	0.2295	0(0.00)	NA	NA	0(0.00)	NA	NA
AG + GG	147(62.82)	57(63.33)	1.02 (0.61–1.72)	0.9318	18(58.06)	0.82 (0.39–1.71)	0.6077	25(71.43)	1.48 (0.67–3.10)	0.3226	8(80.00)	2.37 (0.56–11.26)	0.2691	11(78.57)	2.17 (0.64–7.42)	0.2338	8(61.54)	0.95 (0.29–2.64)	0.9259
MTRR A66G																			
AA	75(32.05)	36(40.00)	1.00		14(45.16)	1.00		12(34.29)	1.00		3(30.00)	1.00		2(14.29)	1.00		4(30.77)	1.00	
AG	116(49.57)	46(51.11)	0.83 (0.48–1.38)	0.4747	16(51.61)	0.74 (0.33–1.54)	0.4423	11(31.43)	0.59 (0.26–1.36)	0.2338	3(30.00)	0.65 (0.15–2.83)	0.5966	9(64.29)	0.29 (0.73–13.68)	0.1615	7(53.85)	1.13 (0.34–3.55)	0.8478
GG	43(18.38)	8(8.89)	0.39 (0.17–0.88)	0.026*	1(3.23)	0.12 (0.01–0.71)	0.021*	12(34.29)	1.74 (0.75–4.03)	0.2139	4(40.00)	2.33 (0.60–9.50)	0.2719	3(21.43)	2.62 (0.51–15.07)	0.2862	2(15.38)	0.87 (0.16–3.88)	0.8773
AG + GG	159(67.95)	54(60.00)	0.71 (0.43–1.18)	0.1769	17(54.84)	0.57 (0.27–1.19)	0.1464	23(65.71)	0.90 (0.42–1.91)	0.7921	7(70.00)	1.10 (0.29–4.00)	0.8917	12(85.71)	2.83 (0.69–12.93)	0.1629	11(84.62)	1.06 (0.44–3.81)	0.9232

OR odds ratio, *CI* confidence interval
*means *p*-value< 0.05

0.01–0.71, $p = 0.021$). In addition, subjects carrying the AC genotype of MTHFR A1298C had a significant 3.83-fold increased risk of PTA (OR: 3.83, 95% CI: 1.00–13.9, $p = 0.0431$). However, none of the folate-related SNPs was found to be associated with the risk of TGA.

MTHFR C677T, A1298C, and SLC19A1 G80A combined genotype frequencies and risk of CTDs

We investigated the association between three combined genotypes (MTHFR C677T and A1298C, and SLC19A1 G80A) and the risk of CTDs (Table 5). Significant differences were only observed in the combined genotype distributions of MTHFR A1298C and SLC19A1 G80A. Subjects carrying either one variant genotype (OR: 1.9, 95% CI: 1.05–3.4, $p = 0.0382$) or both variant genotypes (OR: 3.23, 95% CI: 1.71–6.02, $p = 0.0002$) of these two folate-related SNPs had a significant 1.9–3.23-fold increased risk of CTDs. Moreover, none of the other comparisons produced significant results.

Discussion

Folate is known to play a crucial role in preventing birth defects during pregnancy, including CHD [20]. Thus, genetic variations in components of the folate pathway could influence the risk of CHD. However, the results of studies on the association between folate-related gene polymorphisms and CHD risk are inconclusive and contradictory [9, 12, 17–19]. It was hypothesized that these gene variants may be only associated with specific subsets of CHD, leading to conflicting results when study samples included heterogeneous disease phenotypes [10]. CTDs are the most prevalent congenital anomalies, accounting for approximately one-third of all CHDs, and they play a significant role in fetal morbidity and mortality. To the best of our knowledge, the present study is the first to provide reliable evidence about the association between folate-related gene polymorphisms and the risk of CTDs, specifically including various subtypes of CTD in a Chinese population. This study particularly focused on the maternal genotype. Maternal genetic effects behave as environmental risk factors for offspring [21]. However, it is easier to identify the maternal genotype during pregnancy, so it would be more convenient to translate this approach into a clinical context. For women carrying high-risk genotypes, clinicians could suggest targeted risk reduction strategies aimed at increasing folic acid supplementation.

In this hospital-based case–control study, we analyzed the involvement of five gene variants (MTHFR C677T, MTHFR A1298C, SLC19A1 G80A, MTR A2576G, and MTRR A66G) related to the metabolism of folic acid as risk factors for CTDs. Our results demonstrated that genotypes for MTHFR C677T, MTHFR A1298C, and SLC19A1 G80A might be associated with the risk of CTDs. For certain types of CTD, the genotypes of MTHFR C677T and MTHFR A1298C were also found to be associated with the risks of TOF, DORV, PTA, and IAA, and the GG genotype of MTRR A66G was associated with decreased risks of TOF and PA/VSD.

Because the MTHFR gene plays a key role in folate metabolism through affecting global DNA methylation, which is essential for embryonic development and the formation of the cardiovascular system [22], it has attracted the most attention as an etiological factor for CHDs. Although many studies have indicated that MTHFR C677T and MTHFR A1298C are not strongly related to the risk of CHDs [18, 23, 24], in two recent meta-analyses, Li et al. evaluated 19 eligible studies concerning the MTHFR C677T polymorphism and CHD, comprising 4219 cases and 20,123 controls. They found a significant association between the MTHFR C677T polymorphism and CHD risk in the maternal analysis (OR: 1.52, 95% CI: 1.09–2.11, $p = 0.01$) [25]. In another study by Yu et al., 16 eligible studies concerning MTHFR A1298C polymorphism and CHD, involving 2207 cases and 2364 controls, were included in the meta-analysis; the results suggested that the CC genotype of MTHFR A1298C is a risk factor for CHDs [26]. As well as these previous studies, our results demonstrated that the MTHFR C677T and MTHFR A1298C polymorphisms are also strongly related to the risks of CTDs and of certain types of CTD, including TOF, DORV, PTA, and IAA.

Regarding the MTR and MTRR genes, which play key roles in the second step of folate metabolism and may confer protective effects against CHDs, a recent meta-analysis has also evaluated the associations of MTR A2576G and MTRR A66G polymorphisms with the risk of CHDs. Cai et al. evaluated nine eligible studies comprising 914 cases and 964 controls [27]. The results showed that the MTRR 66G allele significantly increased the risk of CHDs compared with the MTRR 66A allele (OR: 1.35, 95% CI: 1.14–1.59, $p < 0.001$), but no significant differences were found in the MTR A2576G polymorphism between the groups. However, the present results indicate that the allele frequencies of MTR A2576G and MTRR A66G did not differ between the CTD and control groups, except for the MTRR A66G polymorphism, for which the frequency of the GG genotype was significantly lower in the TOF and PA/VSD groups. Moreover, the number of studies focusing on the association of the SLC19A1 G80A polymorphism with the risk of CHDs is small, and the reported results are disputable. For example, Koshy et al. demonstrated that the SLC19A1 G80A polymorphism is not significantly associated with the risk of CTDs in an Indian population [17]. However, Christensen et al. reported that the AG and GG genotypes were associated with decreased odds ratios for heart defects in a Canadian population [28]. By contrast, Gong et al. found that the AG genotype was associated with

Table 5 Combined genotype frequencies of MTHFR C677T, A1298C and SLC19A1 G80A among controls and CTD cases

Genotype	Controls (n = 234)	CTD (N = 193)		*p*-Value
	No. (%)	No. (%)	OR (95% CI)	
MTHFR C677T and A1298C combinations				
677CC, 1298AA	32(13.68)	23(11.92)	1.00	
677CC, 1298 AC + CC	51(21.79)	42(21.76)	1.15(0.60–2.23)	0.6921
1298AA, 677CT + TT	78(33.33)	34(17.62)	0.61(0.32–1.17)	0.1421
Either one variant genotype	129(55.13)	76(39.38)	0.82(0.44–1.49)	0.5199
Both variant genotypes	73(31.20)	94(48.70)	1.79(0.95–3.33)	0.0623
MTHFR C677T and SLC19A1 G80A combinations				
677CC, 80GG	35(14.96)	21(10.88)	1.00	
677CC, 80AG + AA	48(20.51)	44(22.80)	1.53(0.76–3.03)	0.2196
80GG, 677CT + TT	67(28.63)	47(24.35)	1.17(0.60–2.23)	0.6410
Either one variant genotype	115(49.15)	91(47.15)	1.32(0.72–2.44)	0.3706
Both variant genotypes	84(35.90)	81(41.97)	1.61(0.85–3.05)	0.1327
MTHFR A1298C and SLC19A1 G80A combinations				
1298AA, 80GG	46(19.66)	18(9.33)	1.00	
1298AA, 80AG + AA	64(27.35)	39(20.21)	1.56(0.79–3.14)	0.1969
80GG, 1298 AC + CC	56(23.93)	50(25.91)	2.28(1.18–4.53)	0.0141*
Either one variant genotype	120(51.28)	89(46.11)	1.90(1.05–3.40)	0.0382*
Both variant genotypes	68(29.06)	86(44.56)	3.23(1.71–6.02)	0.0002*
MTHFR C677T, A1298C and SLC19A1 G80A combinations				
677CC, 1298AA, 80GG	12(5.13)	10(5.18)	1.00	
677CC, 1298AA, 80AG + AA	20(8.55)	11(5.70)	0.66(0.20–2.09)	0.4646
677CC, 80GG, 1298 AC + CC	23(9.83)	11(5.70)	0.57(0.18–1.77)	0.3226
1298AA, 80GG, 677CT + TT	34(14.53)	10(5.18)	0.35(0.11–1.06)	0.0582
Either one variant genotype	77(32.91)	32(16.58)	0.50(0.20–1.34)	0.1400
677CC, 1298 AC + CC, 80AG + AA	28(11.97)	31(16.06)	1.33(0.48–3.32)	0.5704
677CT + TT, 1298AA, 80AG + AA	44(18.80)	26(13.47)	0.71(0.26–1.78)	0.4859
677CT + TT, 1298 AC + CC, 80GG	33(14.10)	39(20.21)	1.42(0.54–3.52)	0.4740
Either two variant genotypes	105(44.87)	96(49.74)	1.10(0.48–2.67)	0.8370
All variant genotypes	40(17.09)	55(28.50)	1.65(0.66–4.40)	0.2900

OR odds ratio, *CI* confidence interval
*means *p*-value< 0.05

a significantly increased risk of CHD in a Han Chinese population [10]. As well as the present results on MTR A2576G and MTRR A66G polymorphisms being the opposite of those of several studies concerning CHDs, our results show that the AA genotype of SLC19A1 G80A is associated with a significantly increased risk of CTDs, which also differs from the finding of the previous study by Gong et al. These discrepancies might have arisen because the study samples included different disease phenotypes. Otherwise, the subjects exhibited differences in the regular intake of folic acid because the gene polymorphisms might influence the risk of CTDs only in situations in which the intake of folic acid is insufficient. However, further studies on these issues are required. In addition, we also found a significant genotype interaction between MTHFR A1298C and SLC19A1 G80A. Mothers carrying both variant genotypes of these two SNPs had a higher increased risk for CTDs compared with mothers carrying single variant genotypes. The mechanism linking these factors remains unclear, so further studies of this issue are also required.

The present study had several limitations. First, it was a hospital-based case–control study, so the recruited subjects may not be representative of the general population. Second, there was a lack of information on maternal folate status, so we could not determine whether the gene polymorphisms could influence the risk of CTDs if sufficient folic acid were consumed, and whether this variable was a cause of the heterogeneity of the results among different studies. Third, the sample size was moderate in this study, and in the subgroup analyses including PA/VSD, DORV, TGA, PTA, and IAA there were relatively small numbers of cases in each group. Therefore, further studies with larger sample sizes are required to confirm the present findings.

Conclusions

Our results demonstrated that maternal genotypes of MTHFR C677T, MTHFR A1298C, and SLC19A1 G80A might be associated with the risk of CTDs. In addition, the maternal genotypes for MTHFR C677T, MTHFR A1298C, and MTRR A66G might be associated with the risk of certain types of CTD, including TOF, PA/VSD, DORV, PTA, and IAA.

Abbreviations

CHD: Congenital heart defect; CTD: Conotruncal heart defect; DORV: Double outlet of right ventricle; IAA: Interrupted aortic arch.;
MTHFR: Methylenetetrahydrofolate reductase; MTR: Methionine synthase;
MTRR: Methionine synthase reductase; PA/VSD: Pulmonary atresia with ventricular septal defect; PTA: Persistent truncus arteriosus; SLC19A1: Solute carrier family 19, member 1; SNP: Single nucleotide polymorphism;
TGA: Transposition of the great arteries; TOF: Tetralogy of fallot

Acknowledgements

The authors thank the patients and their parents who participated in this study.

Funding

This study was supported by Science and Technology Project of Guizhou Province in China (no.[2016]7141 and [2017]1106), Science and Technology Innovation Talent Team Project of Guizhou Province (no.[2015]4019) and high-level innovative talents training project of Guizhou Province (no.GZSYQCC[2016]004).

Authors' contributions

XW and HW contributed to the conception, design, sample processing, statistical analysis, and interpretation of data. YT and YW contributed to the collection of human samples and clinical and demographic data, sample processing, data analysis, and interpretation of data. LL contributed to the conception, interpretation of data, the draft and critical revision of the manuscript. All authors read and approved the final manuscript.

Competing interests

The authors declare that they have no competing interests.

Author details

[1]Department of paediatrics, Guizhou Provincial People's Hospital, Guiyang 550002, China. [2]Department of science and education, Guizhou Provincial People's Hospital, Guiyang 550002, China.

References

1. Botto LD, Correa A, Erickson JD. Racial and temporal variations in the prevalence of heart defects. Pediatrics. 2001;107(3):E32.
2. Marelli AJ, Mackie AS, Ionescu-Ittu R, Rahme E, Pilote L. Congenital heart disease in the general population: changing prevalence and age distribution. Circulation. 2007;115(2):163–72.
3. Botto LD, Lin AE, Riehle-Colarusso T, Malik S, Correa A. National Birth Defects Prevention Study. Seeking causes: classifying and evaluating congenital heart defects in etiologic studies. Birth Defects Res A Clin Mol Teratol. 2007;79(10):714–27.
4. Debrus S, Berger G, de Meeus A, Sauer U, Guillaumont S, Voisin M, et al. Familial non-syndromic conotruncal defects are not associated with a 22q11 microdeletion. Hum Genet. 1996;97(2):138–44.
5. Hutson MR, Kirby ML. Model systems for the study of heart development and disease. Cardiac neural crest and conotruncal malformations. Semin Cell Dev Biol. 2007;18(1):101–10.
6. Shaw GM, O'Malley CD, Wasserman CR, Tolarova MM, Lammer EJ. Maternal periconceptional use of multivitamins and reduced risk for conotruncal heart defects and limb deficiencies among offspring. Am J Med Genet. 1995;59(4):536–45.
7. Botto LD, Khoury MJ, Mulinare J, Erickson JD. Periconceptional multivitamin use and the occurrence of conotruncal heart defects: results from a population-based, case-control study. Pediatrics. 1996;98(5):911–7.
8. Hobbs CA, James SJ, Parsian A, Krakowiak PA, Jernigan S, Greenhaw JJ, et al. Congenital heart defects and genetic variants in the methylenetetrahydroflate reductase gene. J Med Genet. 2006;43(2):162–6.
9. Goldmuntz E, Woyciechowski S, Renstrom D, Lupo PJ, Mitchell LE. Variants of folate metabolism genes and the risk of conotruncal cardiac defects. Circ Cardiovasc Genet. 2008;1(2):126–32.
10. Gong D, Gu H, Zhang Y, Gong J, Nie Y, Wang J, et al. Methylenetetrahydrofolate reductase C677T and reduced folate carrier 80 G> a polymorphisms are associated with an increased risk of conotruncal heart defects. Clin Chem Lab Med. 2012;50(8):1455–61.
11. Goyette P, Sumner JS, Milos R, Duncan AM, Rosenblatt DS, Matthews RG, et al. Human methylenetetrahydrofolate reductase: isolation of cDNA mapping and mutation identification. Nat Genet. 1994;7(4):551.
12. Chango A, Emery-Fillon N, de Courcy GP, Lambert D, Pfister M, Rosenblatt DS, et al. A polymorphism (80G-> a) in the reduced folate carrier gene and its associations with folate status and homocysteinemia. Mol Genet Metab. 2000;70(4):310–5.
13. Brandalize AP, Bandinelli E, Borba JB, Félix TM, Roisenberg I, Schüler-Faccini L. Polymorphisms in genes MTHFR, MTR and MTRR are not risk factors for cleft lip/palate in South Brazil. Braz J Med Biol Res. 2007;40(6):787–91.
14. Yamada K, Gravel RA, Toraya T, Matthews RG. Human methionine synthase reductase is a molecular chaperone for human methionine synthase. Proc Natl Acad Sci U S A. 2006;103(25):9476–81.
15. Chango A, Boisson F, Barbé F, Quilliot D, Droesch S, Pfister M, et al. The effect of 677C--> T and 1298A--> C mutations on plasma homocysteine and 5,10-methylenetetrahydrofolate reductase activity in healthy subjects. Br J Nutr. 2000;83(6):593–6.
16. van Beynum IM, den Heijer M, Blom HJ, Kapusta L. The MTHFR 677C-> T polymorphism and the risk of congenital heart defects: a literature review and meta-analysis. QJM. 2007;100(12):743–53.
17. Koshy T, Venkatesan V, Perumal V, Hegde S, Paul SF. The A1298C methylenetetrahydrofolate reductase gene variant as a susceptibility gene for non-syndromic Conotruncal heart defects in an Indian population. Pediatr Cardiol. 2015;36(7):1470–5.
18. Sahiner UM, Alanay Y, Alehan D, Tuncbilek E, Alikasifoglu M. Methylene tetrahydrofolate reductase polymorphisms and homocysteine level in heart defects. Pediatr Int. 2014;56(2):167–72.
19. Tetik Vardarlı A, Zengi A, Bozok Çetintaş V, Karadeniz M, Tamsel S, Küçükaslan AŞ, et al. An association study between gene polymorphisms of folic acid metabolism enzymes and biochemical and hormonal parameters in acromegaly. Genet Test Mol Biomarkers. 2015;19(8):431–8.
20. Bailey LB, Berry RJ. Folic acid supplementation and the occurrence of congenital heart defects, orofacial clefts, multiple births, and miscarriage. Am J Clin Nutr. 2005;81(5):1213S–7S.
21. Doolin MT, Barbaux S, McDonnell M, Hoess K, Whitehead AS, Mitchell LE. Maternal genetic effects, exerted by genes involved in homocysteine remethylation, influence the risk of spina bifida. Am J Hum Genet. 2002; 71(5):1222–6.

22. Henderson GI, Perez T, Schenker S, Mackins J, Antony AC. Maternal-to-fetal transfer of 5-methyltetrahydrofolate by the perfused human placental cotyledon: evidence for a concentrative role by placental folate receptors in fetal folate delivery. J Lab Clin Med. 1995;126(2):184–203.
23. Pereira AC, Xavier-Neto J, Mesquita SM, Mota GF, Lopes AA, Krieger JE. Lack of evidence of association between MTHFR C677T polymorphism and congenital heart disease in a TDT study design. Int J Cardiol. 2005;105(1):15–8.
24. Shaw GM, Lu W, Zhu H, Yang W, Briggs FB, Carmichael SL, et al. 118 SNPs of folate-related genes and risks of spina bifida and conotruncal heart defects. BMC Med Genet. 2009;10:49.
25. Li Z, Jun Y, Zhong-Bao R, Jie L, Jian-Ming L. Association between MTHFR C677T polymorphism and congenital heart disease. A family-based meta-analysis. Herz. 2015;40(Suppl 2):160–7.
26. Yu D, Zhuang Z, Wen Z, Zang X, Mo X. MTHFR A1298C polymorphisms reduce the risk of congenital heart defects: a meta-analysis from 16 case-control studies. Ital J Pediatr. 2017;43(1):108.
27. Cai B, Zhang T, Zhong R, Zou L, Zhu B, Chen W, et al. Genetic variant in MTRR, but not MTR, is associated with risk of congenital heart disease: an integrated meta-analysis. PLoS One. 2014;9(3):e89609.
28. Christensen KE, Zada YF, Rohlicek CV, Andelfinger GU, Michaud JL, Bigras JL, et al. Risk of congenital heart defects is influenced by genetic variation in folate metabolism. Cardiol Young. 2013;23(1):89–98.

20

Percentile curves for cardiometabolic disease markers in Canadian children and youth

Nicole Ata[1], Bryan Maguire[2], David C Hamilton[1] and Stefan Kuhle[1*]

Abstract

Background: The objective of this study to develop percentile curves for cardiometabolic disease markers in a population-based sample of Canadian children and youth.

Methods: The analysis used data from 6116 children and adolescents between 6 and 19 years of age who participated in the Canadian Health Measures Survey cycles 1 (2007/2009), 2 (2009/2011), and 3 (2012/2013). Total cholesterol, HDL cholesterol, and hemoglobin A1c levels as well as fasting levels of triglycerides, insulin, and homeostasis model assessment insulin resistance were measured using standardized procedures. Age- and sex-specific centiles for all markers were calculated using Cole and Green's LMS method.

Results: With the exception of hemoglobin A1c, all markers showed age- and sex-related differences during childhood and adolescence.

Conclusions: We have developed centile curves for cardiometabolic disease markers in Canadian children and adolescents and demonstrated age and sex differences that should be considered when evaluating these markers in this age group.

Keywords: Child, Adolescent, Metabolism, Obesity, Development, Diabetes

Background

Cardiovascular disease (CVD) is currently the leading cause of death worldwide [1]. With the exception of congenital heart disease, CVD manifests in adulthood, but its risk factors are already detectable in childhood. Abnormal blood lipids and diabetes are among the risk factors for the development of CVD [2, 3]. An abnormal lipid profile can include elevated total cholesterol, elevated triglycerides, and low high-density lipoprotein (HDL) cholesterol. Insulin resistance plays an important role in the development of youth-onset type 2 diabetes, an emerging disease in children and youth [4]. Homeostasis model assessment estimates insulin resistance (HOMA-IR) from fasting levels of insulin and glucose [5]; other measures that have been used to identify insulin resistance or diabetes include fasting insulin and glycosylated hemoglobin (HbA1c), respectively [6–8].

Levels of these markers vary by sex and across age in childhood and adolescence, and percentile curves have been developed to describe their physiologic development. Percentile curves have been published for lipids and markers of insulin resistance in various populations [9–14]. Since these curves are specific to populations and there are no percentile curves for the levels of these markers in Canadian children, the objective of this study was to develop percentile curves for cardiometabolic markers in a population-based sample of Canadian children and youth.

Methods

Study design

This study used data of children and youth aged 6 to 19 years from the Canadian Health Measures Survey (CHMS) cycles 1 to 3, a representative, cross-sectional survey assessing health and wellness in Canadians [15–17]. The survey includes a household interview to

* Correspondence: stefan.kuhle@dal.ca
[1]Departments of Pediatrics and Obstetrics & Gynaecology, Dalhousie University, Halifax, NS, Canada
Full list of author information is available at the end of the article

obtain sociodemographic and health information and a visit to a mobile examination centre to perform physical measurements and tests. The sampling frame of the Canadian Labour Force Survey was used to identify the collection sites for the mobile examination centres. Within each collection site, households were selected using the 2006 Census as the sampling frame. Interviews and examinations for the CHMS Cycle 1 were performed between 2007 and 2009, for Cycle 2 between 2009 and 2011, and for Cycle 3 between 2012 and 2013. Household response rates were 69.6, 75.9, and 74.1%, respectively; final response rates in the 3 cycles were 51.7, 55.7 and 51.7%, respectively [15–17]. We combined data from the 3 cycles as per Statistics Canada guidelines [18]. A total of 11,999 persons participated in physical examination part of the three survey cycles. The present analysis uses data from 6116 children and adolescents between 6 and 19 years of age.

The Health Canada Research Ethics Board gave approval for the CHMS. All participants gave written informed consent; parents or guardians consented on behalf of children aged 6 to 13 years, and the child provided their assent to participate; youth 14 to 17 years consented on their own, but their parents or guardians had to give verbal permission for the household interview [15]. The current project was approved by the IWK Health Centre Research Ethics Board, Halifax, NS, Canada (File # 1014413).

Laboratory measurements

Blood for measurement of cardiometabolic markers was collected by standard venipuncture. Fasted blood samples for measurement of insulin, glucose, and triglycerides were taken in a randomly selected sample of participants. The sample was obtained by randomly offering each respondent a clinic appointment either in the morning (after an overnight fast) or in the afternoon (non-fasted) [15]. Blood samples were centrifuged within 2 h and aliquoted within 4 h of collection. The samples were stored either in the refrigerator or in the freezer until shipping. Samples were shipped once a week to the Health Canada reference laboratory in Ottawa. Participants with diabetes were excluded from the analysis of insulin, HOMA-IR, and HbA1c; participants taking lipid-lowering medication were excluded from the analysis of lipids. Levels of total cholesterol, HDL cholesterol, triglycerides, and glucose were measured using a colorimetric test and HbA1c was measured using a immunoturbidimetric test on the Vitros 5,1FS (Ortho Clinical Diagnostics, Markham, ON, Canada). Fasting insulin levels were determined using a solid-phase, two-site chemiluminescent immunometric assay on the Advia Centaur XP (Siemens, Erlangen, Germany). Since insulin measurements in cycle 1 were performed using a different method and had a considerable proportion of levels below the test's limit of detection, we only used insulin measurements from cycles 2 and 3 in the present analysis. Fasting insulin and glucose levels were used to calculate HOMA-IR as (fasting insulin [μU/L] x glucose [mmol/L]) / 22.5 [19].

Statistical analysis

Percentile curves for total cholesterol, HDL cholesterol, triglycerides, insulin, HOMA-IR, and HbA1c were modeled using the LMS method by Cole and Green [20]. We have described the LMS method in

Table 1 Characteristics of 6116 Canadian children and youth aged 6 to 19 years in the Canadian Health Measures Survey Cycles 1 to 3

	Prevalence [%]
Sex	
Male	51.6
Female	48.4
Region of Canada	
Atlantic Canada	6.7
Québec	22.5
Ontario	40.5
Prairies	18.2
British Columbia	12.2
Racial origin	
White	80.9
Black	5.9[a]
Asian	10.7[a]
Other	2.4[a]
Weight status (IOTF)	
Underweight	7.5
Normal weight	65.6
Overweight	17.4
Obese	9.5
Household education	
Secondary school or less	15.7
College	46.6
University	37.6
Household income	
\$30,000 or less	15.1
\$30,001 - \$60,000	22.8
\$60,001 - \$80,000	18.3
\$80,001 - \$100,000	16.3
> \$100,000	27.5

Abbreviations: *IOTF* International Obesity Task Force
[a]Coefficient of variation between 16.6 and 33.3%; interpret with caution as per Statistics Canada sampling variability reporting guidelines

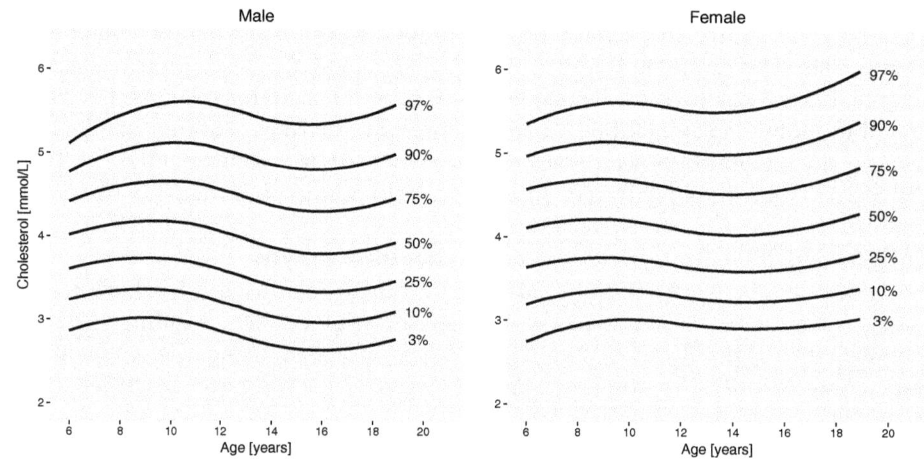

Fig. 1 Percentile curves for total cholesterol levels for male and female Canadian children and youth aged 6 to 19 years

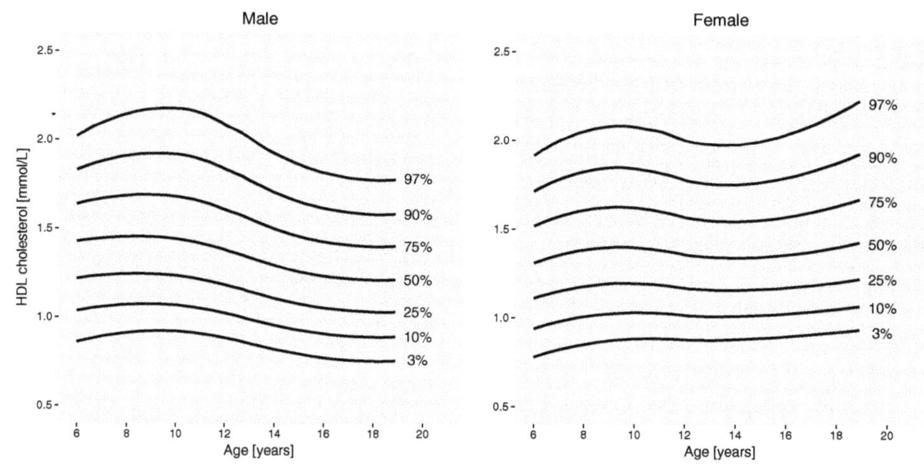

Fig. 2 Percentile curves for high-density lipoprotein (HDL) cholesterol levels for male and female Canadian children and youth aged 6 to 19 years

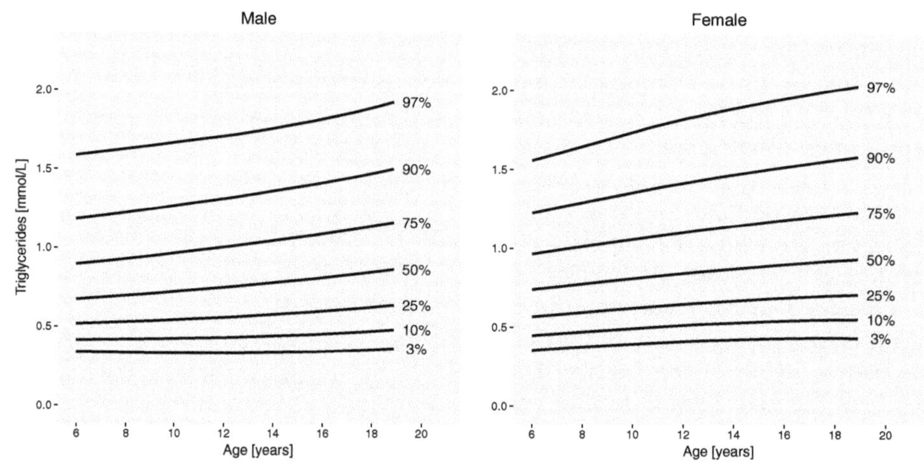

Fig. 3 Percentile curves for triglyceride levels for male and female Canadian children and youth aged 6 to 19 years

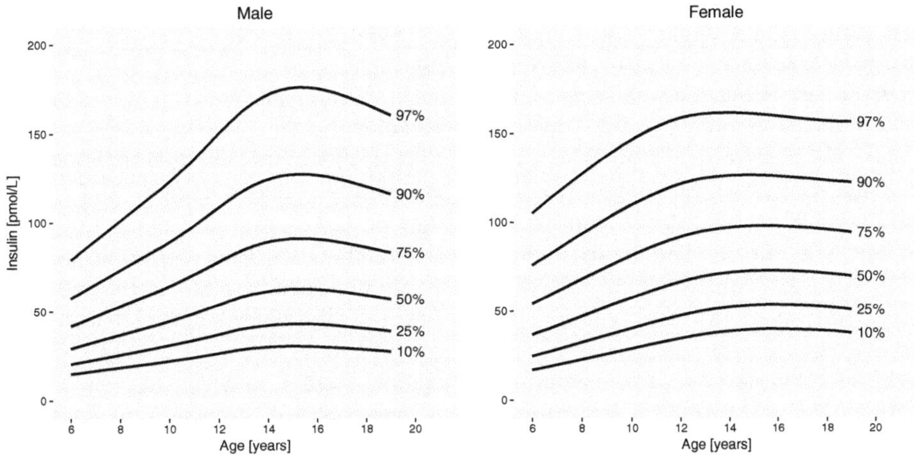

Fig. 4 Percentile curves for insulin levels for male and female Canadian children and youth aged 6 to 19 years

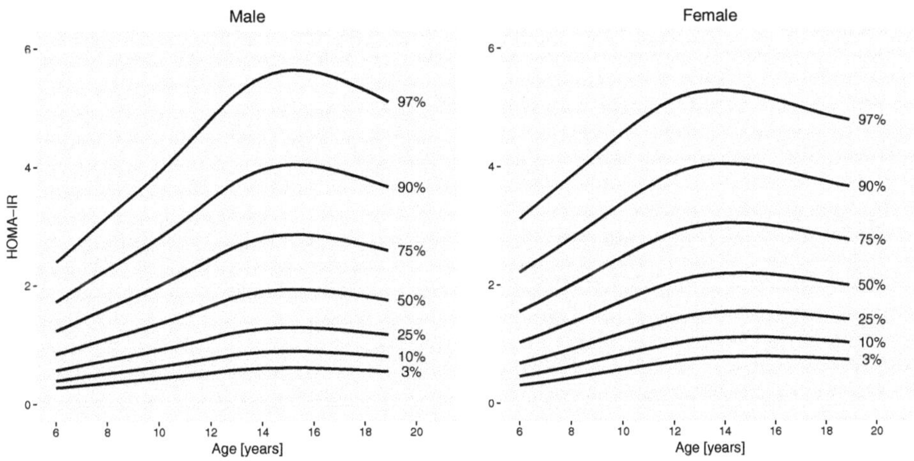

Fig. 5 Percentile curves for homeostasis model assessment insulin resistance (HOMA-IR) levels for male and female Canadian children and youth aged 6 to 19 years

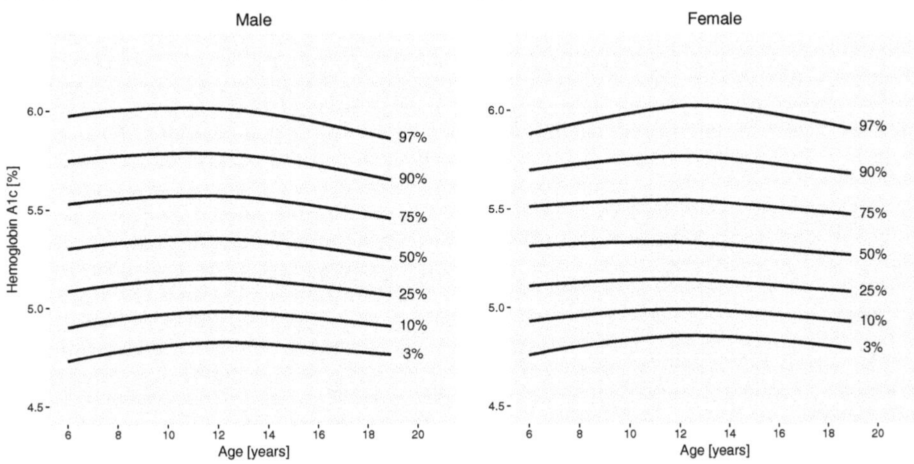

Fig. 6 Percentile curves for hemoglobin A1c levels for male and female Canadian children and youth aged 6 to 19 years

detail elsewhere [21]. Briefly, the method uses a Box-Cox transformation to normalize the data and models the mean (M), variance (S), and skewness (L) as parameters over age using cubic splines. Centiles and z-scores for the truncated standard normal distribution can then be determined from the three parameters at each age [20]. We calculated the 3rd, 10th, 25th, 50th, 75th, 90th, and 97th centile for each marker. Models were fit to data from respondents up to age 30 years to avoid unusual behaviour of the spline functions near the end of the age range. The goodness of fit for each model was assessed using residual quantile plots ("worm plots") [22]. All calculations were performed using sample weights provided by Statistics Canada to account for the design effect and reduce non-response bias. The statistical software package R [23] with the *gamlss* package [24] was used to perform the statistical analyses.

Results

Sociodemographic characteristics of the sample are summarized in Table 1. Figures 1, 2, 3, 4, 5 and 6 and Tables 2, 3, 4, 5, 6 and 7 show the percentile curves and their values for total cholesterol, HDL cholesterol, triglycerides, insulin, HOMA-IR, and HbA1c.

Total cholesterol curves had a bimodal distribution for both boys and girls. Overall, cholesterol levels were slightly higher in girls than in boys. Median levels at 6 years were 4.1 mmol/L in girls and 4.0 mmol/L in boys. In boys, the 50th centile peaked at age 10 years (4.2 mmol/L). The lowest median cholesterol level in

Table 2 L, M, and S values, and percentiles of total cholesterol [mmol/L] by age and sex for Canadian children and youth aged 6 to 19 years

Sex	Age	n	L	M	S	3rd	10th	25th	50th	75th	90th	97th
Female	6	203	1.2662	4.0824	0.1676	2.73	3.18	3.61	4.08	4.54	4.94	5.32
	7	184	1.0339	4.1657	0.1666	2.85	3.27	3.70	4.17	4.63	5.05	5.46
	8	215	0.7986	4.2255	0.1654	2.96	3.35	3.76	4.23	4.70	5.14	5.58
	9	233	0.5790	4.2369	0.1645	3.01	3.38	3.78	4.24	4.72	5.17	5.63
	10	256	0.3985	4.2026	0.1642	3.02	3.37	3.75	4.20	4.68	5.14	5.62
	11	283	0.2725	4.1427	0.1646	3.00	3.33	3.70	4.14	4.62	5.09	5.58
	12	187	0.2000	4.0742	0.1658	2.95	3.28	3.64	4.07	4.55	5.02	5.51
	13	178	0.1564	4.0321	0.1673	2.92	3.24	3.60	4.03	4.51	4.98	5.48
	14	170	0.1308	4.0222	0.1691	2.91	3.23	3.59	4.02	4.50	4.98	5.49
	15	175	0.1173	4.0342	0.1717	2.90	3.23	3.59	4.03	4.53	5.01	5.54
	16	178	0.1121	4.0701	0.1746	2.91	3.24	3.61	4.07	4.58	5.08	5.62
	17	186	0.1066	4.1326	0.1769	2.94	3.28	3.66	4.13	4.65	5.17	5.73
	18	168	0.1017	4.2050	0.1788	2.99	3.33	3.72	4.21	4.74	5.27	5.85
	19	152	0.0901	4.2612	0.1809	3.02	3.37	3.77	4.26	4.81	5.36	5.96
Male	6	203	1.1968	4.0369	0.1508	2.86	3.24	3.62	4.04	4.44	4.80	5.15
	7	211	0.8365	4.0884	0.1523	2.95	3.30	3.67	4.09	4.51	4.90	5.29
	8	232	0.5410	4.1350	0.1551	3.01	3.35	3.71	4.13	4.58	4.99	5.42
	9	239	0.3792	4.1691	0.1597	3.03	3.37	3.73	4.17	4.63	5.08	5.54
	10	263	0.3624	4.1766	0.1651	3.00	3.35	3.73	4.18	4.66	5.12	5.61
	11	277	0.3556	4.1469	0.1703	2.95	3.30	3.69	4.15	4.64	5.12	5.62
	12	207	0.3332	4.0711	0.1757	2.87	3.22	3.61	4.07	4.57	5.06	5.57
	13	207	0.3217	3.9598	0.1801	2.77	3.12	3.50	3.96	4.46	4.95	5.46
	14	205	0.2648	3.8546	0.1833	2.69	3.02	3.40	3.85	4.35	4.84	5.36
	15	184	0.1878	3.7910	0.1863	2.64	2.97	3.34	3.79	4.29	4.79	5.32
	16	208	0.1426	3.7735	0.1886	2.62	2.95	3.32	3.77	4.28	4.79	5.33
	17	183	0.1015	3.7992	0.1883	2.65	2.98	3.34	3.80	4.31	4.82	5.38
	18	144	0.0557	3.8565	0.1873	2.70	3.03	3.40	3.86	4.37	4.90	5.47
	19	139	0.0083	3.9299	0.1869	2.76	3.09	3.46	3.93	4.46	4.99	5.58

Abbreviations: *L* lambda (skewness); *M* mu (mean); *S* sigma (variance)

Table 3 L, M, and S values, and percentiles of HDL cholesterol [mmol/L] by age and sex for Canadian children and youth aged 6 to 19 years

Sex	Age	n	L	M	S	3rd	10th	25th	50th	75th	90th	97th
Female	6	203	0.6653	1.2995	0.2301	0.78	0.94	1.10	1.30	1.51	1.70	1.90
	7	184	0.5810	1.3513	0.2315	0.82	0.98	1.15	1.35	1.57	1.78	1.99
	8	215	0.4894	1.3925	0.2317	0.85	1.01	1.18	1.39	1.62	1.84	2.07
	9	233	0.4025	1.4128	0.2304	0.88	1.03	1.20	1.41	1.64	1.87	2.11
	10	256	0.3317	1.4069	0.2269	0.89	1.04	1.20	1.41	1.63	1.86	2.10
	11	283	0.2946	1.3835	0.2222	0.89	1.03	1.19	1.38	1.60	1.82	2.05
	12	187	0.2932	1.3527	0.2180	0.87	1.01	1.16	1.35	1.56	1.77	1.99
	13	178	0.2666	1.3372	0.2152	0.87	1.00	1.15	1.34	1.54	1.74	1.96
	14	170	0.1991	1.3404	0.2145	0.88	1.01	1.16	1.34	1.55	1.75	1.98
	15	175	0.1202	1.3502	0.2156	0.89	1.02	1.17	1.35	1.56	1.77	2.01
	16	178	0.0477	1.3590	0.2180	0.90	1.03	1.17	1.36	1.57	1.79	2.04
	17	186	−0.0261	1.3764	0.2213	0.91	1.04	1.19	1.38	1.60	1.83	2.09
	18	168	−0.0758	1.4019	0.2258	0.92	1.05	1.20	1.40	1.63	1.88	2.16
	19	152	−0.0551	1.4209	0.2316	0.92	1.06	1.22	1.42	1.66	1.92	2.21
Male	6	203	0.8228	1.4346	0.2226	0.86	1.04	1.22	1.43	1.65	1.85	2.06
	7	211	0.6385	1.4440	0.2207	0.89	1.06	1.23	1.44	1.66	1.87	2.09
	8	232	0.4626	1.4509	0.2215	0.91	1.07	1.24	1.45	1.68	1.89	2.12
	9	239	0.3069	1.4533	0.2256	0.92	1.07	1.24	1.45	1.69	1.92	2.17
	10	263	0.1937	1.4465	0.2296	0.92	1.07	1.24	1.45	1.68	1.93	2.19
	11	277	0.1465	1.4230	0.2297	0.91	1.05	1.22	1.42	1.66	1.90	2.16
	12	207	0.1687	1.3827	0.2281	0.89	1.02	1.18	1.38	1.61	1.84	2.09
	13	207	0.2352	1.3335	0.2266	0.85	0.99	1.14	1.33	1.55	1.77	2.00
	14	205	0.3157	1.2882	0.2251	0.82	0.95	1.10	1.29	1.49	1.70	1.92
	15	184	0.3915	1.2523	0.2244	0.79	0.92	1.07	1.25	1.45	1.64	1.85
	16	208	0.4549	1.2270	0.2256	0.77	0.90	1.05	1.23	1.42	1.61	1.81
	17	183	0.4843	1.2122	0.2260	0.75	0.89	1.03	1.21	1.40	1.59	1.78
	18	144	0.4698	1.2062	0.2245	0.75	0.89	1.03	1.21	1.40	1.58	1.77
	19	139	0.4299	1.2084	0.2234	0.76	0.89	1.03	1.21	1.40	1.58	1.78

Abbreviations: *L* lambda (skewness); *M* mu (mean); *S* sigma (variance)

boys was seen at 16 years of age (3.8 mmol/L), after which it increased to 3.9 mmol/L at 19 years. In girls, the 50th centile for cholesterol had a peak at 9 years (4.2 mmol/L), decreased to a trough at 15 years (4.0 mmol/L) and increased again to 4.3 mmol/L at 19 years of age. **HDL cholesterol** showed a bimodal distribution in girls, but only one peak in boys. In boys, the median levels were highest before 11 years (1.5 mmol/L) and then steadily declined until 19 years (1.2 mmol/L). Median HDL cholesterol in girls peaked at age 10 years (1.4 mmol/L) and after a trough (1.3 mmol/L) increased again to 1.4 mmol/L at 19 years. Median levels of **triglycerides** exhibited a steady linear increase from 6 years (0.7 mmol/L) to 19 years (0.9 mmol/L) for both sexes. **Insulin** levels were overall higher in girls than in boys. For both sexes, median levels increased until about 14 years of age (62 and 72 pmol/L in boys and girls, respectively), after which they slightly decreased to 57 pmol/L in boys and 70 pmol/L in girls at 19 years of age. Centile curves for **HOMA-IR** largely mirrored those for insulin with the 50th percentile peaking at 15 years for both sexes (1.9 for boys and 2.2 for girls). Median **HbA1c** levels held nearly constant around 5.3% from 6 to 19 years for both sexes.

Discussion

The objective of this study was to develop percentile curves for total cholesterol, HDL cholesterol, triglycerides, insulin, HOMA-IR, and HbA1c in a population-based

Table 4 L, M, and S values, and percentiles of triglycerides [mmol/L] by age and sex for Canadian children and youth aged 6 to 19 years

Sex	Age	n	L	M	S	3rd	10th	25th	50th	75th	90th	97th
Female	6	78	−0.0198	0.7390	0.3934	0.35	0.45	0.57	0.74	0.96	1.23	1.56
	7	85	− 0.0360	0.7567	0.3932	0.36	0.46	0.58	0.76	0.99	1.26	1.60
	8	98	−0.0522	0.7744	0.3931	0.37	0.47	0.60	0.77	1.01	1.29	1.65
	9	127	−0.0680	0.7922	0.3931	0.39	0.48	0.61	0.79	1.04	1.32	1.69
	10	114	−0.0821	0.8100	0.3931	0.40	0.49	0.62	0.81	1.06	1.35	1.74
	11	139	−0.0928	0.8273	0.3932	0.40	0.51	0.64	0.83	1.08	1.39	1.78
	12	93	−0.0987	0.8438	0.3935	0.41	0.52	0.65	0.84	1.10	1.42	1.82
	13	88	− 0.0996	0.8593	0.3942	0.42	0.52	0.66	0.86	1.13	1.44	1.86
	14	88	−0.0958	0.8738	0.3954	0.43	0.53	0.67	0.87	1.14	1.47	1.89
	15	91	−0.0874	0.8874	0.3972	0.43	0.54	0.68	0.89	1.16	1.49	1.92
	16	91	−0.0746	0.9003	0.3996	0.43	0.54	0.69	0.90	1.18	1.52	1.95
	17	89	−0.0581	0.9125	0.4026	0.43	0.55	0.70	0.91	1.20	1.54	1.98
	18	74	−0.0389	0.9240	0.4061	0.44	0.55	0.70	0.92	1.22	1.56	2.01
	19	72	−0.0180	0.9346	0.4102	0.43	0.55	0.71	0.93	1.23	1.58	2.03
Male	6	102	−0.2816	0.6737	0.4053	0.34	0.41	0.52	0.67	0.90	1.18	1.59
	7	98	−0.2348	0.6849	0.4111	0.34	0.42	0.52	0.68	0.91	1.20	1.61
	8	116	−0.1881	0.6961	0.4169	0.33	0.42	0.53	0.70	0.93	1.22	1.63
	9	120	−0.1418	0.7075	0.4227	0.33	0.42	0.54	0.71	0.95	1.24	1.64
	10	133	−0.0967	0.7195	0.4281	0.33	0.42	0.54	0.72	0.96	1.26	1.66
	11	135	−0.0544	0.7322	0.4329	0.33	0.42	0.55	0.73	0.98	1.29	1.68
	12	96	−0.0165	0.7459	0.4368	0.33	0.43	0.56	0.75	1.00	1.31	1.71
	13	112	0.0157	0.7606	0.4395	0.33	0.43	0.57	0.76	1.02	1.33	1.73
	14	97	0.0421	0.7763	0.4412	0.33	0.44	0.58	0.78	1.04	1.36	1.75
	15	93	0.0630	0.7927	0.4422	0.34	0.45	0.59	0.79	1.07	1.38	1.78
	16	103	0.0788	0.8098	0.4428	0.34	0.45	0.60	0.81	1.09	1.41	1.81
	17	92	0.0899	0.8275	0.4431	0.35	0.46	0.61	0.83	1.11	1.44	1.85
	18	78	0.0968	0.8457	0.4435	0.35	0.47	0.62	0.85	1.14	1.47	1.89
	19	74	0.0999	0.8642	0.4441	0.36	0.48	0.64	0.86	1.16	1.50	1.93

Abbreviations: L lambda (skewness); *M* mu (mean); *S* sigma (variance)

sample of Canadian children and youth. We found age- and sex-related differences in blood levels for all markers except for HbA1c.

A bimodal shape of the centile curves for total cholesterol levels has been described in various Western populations [9, 11, 13, 25]. A pre-adolescent peak at around 8 to 10 years of age that is more pronounced in boys is followed by a decrease during adolescence and another peak in late adolescence and young adulthood. The same pattern, but without a post-pubertal rise in boys, can be seen for HDL cholesterol [9, 11, 13]. The pubertal trough of cholesterol levels may be the result of the well described insulin resistance during puberty [26]. Clinicians should be aware of these physiologic changes when interpreting cholesterol levels. However, it should also be acknowledged that median levels of cholesterol in our study as well as in other studies varied by 10% or less in either direction during childhood and adolescence [9, 11, 13, 25].

Median triglyceride levels in our sample showed a nearly linear increase by about 30% from around 0.7 to 0.9 mmol/L in both sexes during childhood and adolescence. Some investigators previously described a bimodal pattern in girls with peaks at around 12 and 19 years of age [9, 11], while others also reported the linear increase we found [13]. These differences may be explained by different degrees of smoothing applied during the modeling process.

Median fasting insulin levels were higher in girls than in boys, and levels in both sexes peaked at around 15 years of age followed by a slight decrease

Table 5 L, M, and S values, and percentiles of insulin [pmol/L] by age and sex for Canadian children and youth aged 6 to 19 years

Sex	Age	n	L	M	S	3rd	10th	25th	50th	75th	90th	97th
Female	6	74	0.0810	36.8032	0.5822	11.69	17.05	24.69	36.80	54.17	75.94	105.08
	7	85	0.0832	41.9738	0.5661	13.77	19.86	28.47	41.97	61.13	84.90	116.43
	8	95	0.0861	47.1805	0.5505	15.95	22.79	32.35	47.18	68.00	93.58	127.19
	9	124	0.0909	52.4480	0.5352	18.25	25.83	36.33	52.45	74.82	102.02	137.42
	10	110	0.0997	57.6269	0.5201	20.59	28.91	40.32	57.63	81.35	109.87	146.55
	11	136	0.1121	62.4301	0.5044	22.90	31.91	44.13	62.43	87.17	116.52	153.78
	12	92	0.1263	66.5218	0.4884	25.06	34.66	47.52	66.52	91.86	121.50	158.64
	13	88	0.1414	69.6293	0.4734	26.89	36.93	50.22	69.63	95.15	124.61	161.05
	14	86	0.1553	71.6632	0.4607	28.26	38.58	52.12	71.66	97.07	126.08	161.58
	15	86	0.1652	72.6769	0.4515	29.11	39.56	53.17	72.68	97.82	126.30	160.90
	16	90	0.1703	72.8110	0.4465	29.42	39.88	53.45	72.81	97.67	125.70	159.62
	17	86	0.1707	72.2282	0.4460	29.21	39.58	53.04	72.23	96.85	124.61	158.18
	18	74	0.1665	71.1378	0.4500	28.57	38.80	52.10	71.14	95.65	123.38	157.03
	19	71	0.1592	69.7465	0.4583	27.60	37.65	50.80	69.75	94.31	122.28	156.42
Male	6	98	−0.0050	29.2964	0.5269	10.90	14.93	20.54	29.30	41.81	57.62	79.12
	7	95	−0.0012	33.2034	0.5309	12.24	16.82	23.21	33.20	47.50	65.58	90.17
	8	116	0.0028	37.0587	0.5348	13.54	18.66	25.83	37.06	53.14	73.49	101.18
	9	118	0.0065	40.8164	0.5385	14.78	20.44	28.37	40.82	58.67	81.26	112.00
	10	130	0.0097	44.7223	0.5419	16.06	22.28	31.01	44.72	64.42	89.36	123.31
	11	129	0.0126	49.2160	0.5451	17.54	24.40	34.05	49.22	71.02	98.66	136.29
	12	95	0.0153	54.1827	0.5477	19.18	26.75	37.41	54.18	78.32	108.91	150.58
	13	110	0.0178	58.6671	0.5499	20.65	28.87	40.44	58.67	84.91	118.19	163.49
	14	95	0.0203	61.7110	0.5519	21.61	30.27	42.47	61.71	89.42	124.55	172.38
	15	91	0.0232	62.9131	0.5539	21.91	30.75	43.23	62.91	91.27	127.21	176.13
	16	102	0.0271	62.5506	0.5561	21.65	30.46	42.90	62.55	90.85	126.71	175.45
	17	91	0.0318	61.1922	0.5583	21.03	29.67	41.90	61.19	88.97	124.15	171.90
	18	76	0.0370	59.3041	0.5602	20.25	28.65	40.54	59.30	86.30	120.44	166.70
	19	74	0.0431	57.1325	0.5615	19.39	27.51	39.00	57.13	83.18	116.05	160.46

Abbreviations: *L* lambda (skewness); *M* mu (mean); *S* sigma (variance)

towards late adolescence. Similar age and sex differences have also been reported by others [13, 27]. The peak in puberty reflects the physiologically reduced insulin sensitivity and concomitant increase in insulin secretion during that period [28, 29]. The median insulin levels in our study and others [12, 13, 27] varied with pubertal levels ranging from 52 to 63 pmol/L in boys and from 65 to 73 pmol/L in girls. These differences may be explained by differences in the insulin assay used [30] or differences in the body composition, ethnicity, and puberty stage of the children in the sample. The shape of the HOMA-IR curves was similar to those for fasting insulin. Schwartz et al. found a significant correlation between fasting insulin and HOMA-IR but found both only modestly correlated with the insulin resistance measurement gold standard, the euglycemic-hyperinsulinemic glucose clamp [31]. HOMA-IR still is among the most commonly used surrogate measure of insulin resistance to date. Given the variation over sex and age, in particular the physiologic insulin resistance in puberty, the use of an age- and sex-specific percentile-based cutoff for HOMA-IR is warranted. Unfortunately, such a cutoff has not been established to date [32].

Glycosylated hemoglobin or HbA1c is an established marker for long-term glycemic control in patients with diabetes [33]. HbA1c has been proposed as a screening tool for undiagnosed diabetes in adults [6] and children with overweight or obesity [8], but the evidence is still very limited. We found very little change in HbA1c levels from childhood to late adolescence, and there was no difference between the sexes.

Table 6 L, M, and S values, and percentiles of HOMA-IR by age and sex for Canadian children and youth aged 6 to 19 years

Sex	Age	n	L	M	S	3rd	10th	25th	50th	75th	90th	97th
Female	6	74	0.0680	1.0304	0.6120	0.31	0.46	0.68	1.03	1.55	2.21	3.12
	7	85	0.0816	1.1930	0.5955	0.37	0.54	0.79	1.19	1.77	2.50	3.48
	8	95	0.0953	1.3607	0.5795	0.43	0.63	0.91	1.36	2.00	2.79	3.84
	9	124	0.1090	1.5413	0.5642	0.50	0.73	1.04	1.54	2.24	3.09	4.21
	10	110	0.1226	1.7284	0.5496	0.57	0.83	1.18	1.73	2.48	3.40	4.57
	11	136	0.1354	1.9044	0.5360	0.64	0.93	1.31	1.90	2.71	3.67	4.90
	12	92	0.1467	2.0481	0.5235	0.71	1.01	1.43	2.05	2.89	3.88	5.14
	13	88	0.1557	2.1435	0.5125	0.75	1.07	1.50	2.14	3.00	4.01	5.26
	14	86	0.1619	2.1886	0.5036	0.78	1.11	1.54	2.19	3.05	4.04	5.28
	15	86	0.1645	2.1908	0.4970	0.79	1.12	1.55	2.19	3.04	4.02	5.23
	16	90	0.1635	2.1612	0.4930	0.79	1.11	1.54	2.16	2.99	3.94	5.12
	17	86	0.1591	2.1092	0.4916	0.78	1.09	1.50	2.11	2.91	3.84	5.00
	18	74	0.1514	2.0465	0.4928	0.75	1.05	1.46	2.05	2.83	3.74	4.87
	19	71	0.1411	1.9837	0.4965	0.73	1.02	1.41	1.98	2.75	3.65	4.77
Male	6	98	0.0558	0.8427	0.5725	0.28	0.40	0.57	0.84	1.23	1.73	2.40
	7	95	0.0576	0.9718	0.5752	0.32	0.46	0.66	0.97	1.43	2.00	2.78
	8	116	0.0595	1.1004	0.5778	0.36	0.52	0.74	1.10	1.62	2.27	3.15
	9	118	0.0610	1.2255	0.5802	0.40	0.57	0.82	1.23	1.80	2.54	3.52
	10	130	0.0617	1.3545	0.5823	0.44	0.63	0.91	1.35	2.00	2.81	3.91
	11	129	0.0619	1.5014	0.5841	0.48	0.70	1.01	1.50	2.22	3.12	4.35
	12	95	0.0618	1.6614	0.5855	0.53	0.77	1.11	1.66	2.45	3.46	4.82
	13	110	0.0618	1.8031	0.5864	0.58	0.84	1.21	1.80	2.67	3.76	5.24
	14	95	0.0619	1.8974	0.5873	0.60	0.88	1.27	1.90	2.81	3.96	5.52
	15	91	0.0627	1.9332	0.5883	0.61	0.89	1.29	1.93	2.86	4.04	5.63
	16	102	0.0646	1.9204	0.5896	0.61	0.89	1.28	1.92	2.84	4.02	5.60
	17	91	0.0673	1.8754	0.5910	0.59	0.86	1.25	1.88	2.78	3.93	5.48
	18	76	0.0705	1.8126	0.5922	0.57	0.83	1.21	1.81	2.69	3.80	5.30
	19	74	0.0747	1.7406	0.5929	0.54	0.80	1.16	1.74	2.58	3.64	5.08

Abbreviations: *L* lambda (skewness); *M* mu (mean); *S* sigma (variance)

To the best of our knowledge, only three previous studies have examined HbA1c levels during childhood [12, 14, 34]. Only Peplies et al. in the European IDEFICS cohort developed percentile curves to describe the changes in levels across age and found a 15% increase in median HbA1c levels between 7 and 11 years for both sexes [12].

The strengths of our study include the use of a large population-based sample and the use of standardized protocols and procedures for the measurement of the cardiometabolic marker levels. A shortcoming of the use of cross-sectional data is that it is not clear if the trajectories of individual children follow this pattern; longitudinal data may be more accurate in describing age-related changes but are considerably more resource intensive to collect at the population level. Due to the relatively small proportion of visible minority children in the sample (< 20%), we were not able to investigate ethnic differences in marker levels and trajectories. Another limitation of our study is that we were unable to take puberty stage, which may influence insulin and lipid levels, into account as this information was not available in the CHMS. By contrast to some of the previous studies in this area, we did not restrict our analysis to children with a healthy weight [9, 12], as our goal was to describe population-based trajectories. Since the inclusion of overweight and obese children in our sample may have influenced lipid and insulin levels, our percentiles cannot be considered as reference values.

Table 7 L, M, and S values, and percentiles of hemoglobin A1c by age and sex for Canadian children and youth aged 6 to 19 years

Sex	Age	n	L	M	S	3rd	10th	25th	50th	75th	90th	97th
Female	6	192	0.6293	0.0531	0.0565	0.0476	0.0493	0.0511	0.0531	0.0552	0.0570	0.0589
	7	178	0.0341	0.0532	0.0563	0.0478	0.0495	0.0512	0.0532	0.0552	0.0571	0.0591
	8	204	−0.5398	0.0532	0.0561	0.0480	0.0496	0.0513	0.0532	0.0553	0.0573	0.0593
	9	224	−1.0745	0.0533	0.0560	0.0482	0.0497	0.0513	0.0533	0.0553	0.0574	0.0596
	10	248	−1.5959	0.0533	0.0560	0.0484	0.0498	0.0514	0.0533	0.0554	0.0575	0.0598
	11	275	−2.1144	0.0533	0.0559	0.0485	0.0499	0.0514	0.0533	0.0554	0.0576	0.0600
	12	184	−2.5527	0.0533	0.0558	0.0486	0.0499	0.0514	0.0533	0.0554	0.0577	0.0602
	13	172	−2.8025	0.0532	0.0557	0.0486	0.0499	0.0514	0.0532	0.0554	0.0576	0.0603
	14	166	−2.8388	0.0531	0.0555	0.0485	0.0498	0.0513	0.0531	0.0553	0.0575	0.0601
	15	167	−2.7545	0.0530	0.0553	0.0484	0.0497	0.0512	0.0530	0.0551	0.0574	0.0599
	16	172	−2.6052	0.0529	0.0551	0.0483	0.0496	0.0511	0.0529	0.0550	0.0572	0.0597
	17	177	−2.4044	0.0528	0.0550	0.0481	0.0495	0.0509	0.0528	0.0549	0.0570	0.0595
	18	165	−2.1906	0.0527	0.0550	0.0480	0.0494	0.0509	0.0527	0.0548	0.0569	0.0593
	19	149	−2.0342	0.0527	0.0552	0.0479	0.0493	0.0508	0.0527	0.0548	0.0569	0.0592
Male	6	195	−0.4642	0.0530	0.0619	0.0473	0.0490	0.0509	0.0530	0.0553	0.0575	0.0598
	7	205	−0.5917	0.0532	0.0612	0.0476	0.0492	0.0510	0.0532	0.0554	0.0576	0.0599
	8	227	−0.7384	0.0533	0.0605	0.0478	0.0494	0.0512	0.0533	0.0555	0.0577	0.0600
	9	229	−0.8769	0.0534	0.0598	0.0480	0.0496	0.0513	0.0534	0.0556	0.0578	0.0601
	10	256	−0.9903	0.0535	0.0591	0.0481	0.0497	0.0514	0.0535	0.0557	0.0578	0.0601
	11	267	−1.0740	0.0535	0.0584	0.0482	0.0498	0.0515	0.0535	0.0557	0.0579	0.0602
	12	204	−1.1009	0.0535	0.0580	0.0483	0.0498	0.0515	0.0535	0.0557	0.0578	0.0601
	13	201	−1.0887	0.0535	0.0577	0.0483	0.0498	0.0515	0.0535	0.0556	0.0578	0.0600
	14	203	−1.0467	0.0534	0.0574	0.0482	0.0497	0.0514	0.0534	0.0555	0.0576	0.0599
	15	180	−1.0081	0.0532	0.0571	0.0481	0.0496	0.0512	0.0532	0.0554	0.0574	0.0596
	16	205	−0.9894	0.0530	0.0567	0.0479	0.0494	0.0511	0.0530	0.0551	0.0572	0.0594
	17	180	−1.0085	0.0528	0.0561	0.0478	0.0493	0.0509	0.0528	0.0549	0.0569	0.0591
	18	138	−1.0586	0.0527	0.0555	0.0477	0.0492	0.0508	0.0527	0.0547	0.0567	0.0588
	19	135	−1.1174	0.0526	0.0549	0.0477	0.0491	0.0507	0.0526	0.0546	0.0566	0.0587

Abbreviations: *L* lambda (skewness); *M* mu (mean); *S* sigma (variance)

Conclusions

Our study has developed percentile curves for cardiometabolic disease markers in Canadian children and adolescents. We have demonstrated age- and sex-related differences in marker levels for lipids, insulin, and HOMA-IR that should be considered when evaluating these markers in children and adolescents.

Abbreviations

CHMS: Canadian Health Measures Survey; CVD: Cardiovascular disease; HbA1c: Hemoglobin A1c; HDL: High-density lipoprotein; HOMA-IR: Homeostasis model assessment insulin resistance; LMS: Lambda Mu Sigma

Acknowledgements

The analysis presented in this paper was conducted at the Atlantic Research Data Centre, which is part of the Canadian Research Data Centre Network (CRDCN). The services and activities provided by the Atlantic Research Data Centre are made possible by the financial or in-kind support of the SSHRC, the CIHR, the CFI, Statistics Canada, and Dalhousie University. The views expressed in this paper do not necessarily represent the views of the CRDCN or its partners.

Funding

This work was supported by an IWK Health Centre (http://www.iwk.nshealth.ca) Establishment Grant awarded to Dr. Stefan Kuhle (FRN 09020). The funder had no role in the design of the study and collection, analysis, and interpretation of data and in writing the manuscript.

Availability of data and materials

The data that support the findings of this study are available from Statistics Canada through the Statistics Canada Research Data Centres program to researchers who meet the criteria for access to confidential data. The application process is described at http://www.statcan.gc.ca/eng/rdc/process In brief, researchers submit an application form and project proposal to the Statistics Canada Research Data Centres Program. Upon approval they have to undergo a security check. Once completed, they get access to one of the Research Data Centres in Canada to analyze the data. Only aggregated data can be released, and all output produced at the centres must be vetted by a Statistics Canada analyst before release.

Authors' contributions

NA, BM, DCH, and SK conceived and designed the experiments. BM and SK analyzed the data. NA wrote the manuscript. BM, DCH, and SK critically revised the manuscript. All authors read and approved the final manuscript.

Competing interests
The authors declare that they have no competing interests.

Author details
[1]Departments of Pediatrics and Obstetrics & Gynaecology, Dalhousie University, Halifax, NS, Canada. [2]Department of Mathematics and Statistics, Dalhousie University, Halifax, NS, Canada.

References

1. World Health Organization. Cardiovascular diseases (CVDs). Fact sheet No. 317. Geneva: World Health Organization; 2017.
2. Linton MF, Yancey PG, Davies SS, Jerome WGJ, Linton EF, Vickers KC. The role of lipids and lipoproteins in atherosclerosis. In: De Groot LJ, Chrousos G, Dungan K, Feingold KR, Grossman A, Hershman JM, et al., editors. Endotext. South Dartmouth: MDText.com, Inc.; 2000.
3. Thomas JE, Foody JM. The pathophysiology of cardiovascular disease in diabetes mellitus and the future of therapy. J Cardiometab Syndr. 2007;2: 108–13.
4. Nadeau KJ, Anderson BJ, Berg EG, Chiang JL, Chou H, Copeland KC, et al. Youth-onset type 2 diabetes consensus report: current status, challenges, and priorities. Diab Care. 2016;39:1635–42.
5. Wallace TM, Levy JC, Matthews DR. Use and abuse of HOMA modeling. Diab Care. 2004;27:1487–95.
6. Rohlfing CL, Little RR, Wiedmeyer HM, England JD, Madsen R, Harris MI, et al. Use of GHb (HbA1c) in screening for undiagnosed diabetes in the U.S. population. Diab Care. 2000;23:187–91.
7. American Diabetes Association. Consensus Development Conference on Insulin Resistance. 5–6 November 1997. American Diabetes Association. Diab Care. 1998;21:310–4.
8. Ehehalt S, Wiegand S, Körner A, Schweizer R, Liesenkötter KP, Partsch CJ, et al. Diabetes screening in overweight and obese children and adolescents: choosing the right test. Eur J Pediatr. 2017;176:89–97.
9. Skinner AC, Steiner MJ, Chung AE, Perrin EM. Cholesterol curves to identify population norms by age and sex in healthy weight children. Clin Pediatr (Phila). 2012;51:233–7.
10. Dathan-Stumpf A, Vogel M, Hiemisch A, Thiery J, Burkhardt R, Kratzsch J, et al. Pediatric reference data of serum lipids and prevalence of dyslipidemia: results from a population-based cohort in Germany. Clin Biochem. 2016;49:740–9.
11. Cook S, Auinger P, Huang TT. Growth curves for cardio-metabolic risk factors in children and adolescents. J Pediatr. 2009;155:S6.e15–26.
12. Peplies J, Jiménez-Pavón D, Savva SC, Buck C, Günther K, Fraterman A, et al. Percentiles of fasting serum insulin, glucose, HbA1c and HOMA-IR in pre-pubertal normal weight European children from the IDEFICS cohort. Int J Obes. 2014;38(Suppl 2):S39–47.
13. Mellerio H, Alberti C, Druet C, Capelier F, Mercat I, Josserand E, et al. Novel modeling of reference values of cardiovascular risk factors in children aged 7 to 20 years. Pediatrics. 2012;129:e1020–9.
14. Rödöö P, Ridefelt P, Aldrimer M, Niklasson F, Gustafsson J, Hellberg D. Population-based pediatric reference intervals for HbA1c, bilirubin, albumin, CRP, myoglobin and serum enzymes. Scand J Clin Lab Invest. 2013;73:361–7.
15. Statistics Canada. Canadian health measures survey (CHMS) data user guide: cycle 1. Ottawa: Statistics Canada; 2011.
16. Statistics Canada. Canadian health measures survey (CHMS) data user guide: cycle 2. Ottawa: Statistics Canada; 2013.
17. Statistics Canada. Canadian health measures survey (CHMS) data user guide: cycle 3. Ottawa: Statistics Canada; 2015.
18. Statistics Canada. Canadian Health Measures Survey (CHMS): Instructions for combining cycle 1 and cycle 2 data. Otttawa; 2013.
19. Matthews DR, Hosker JP, Rudenski AS, Naylor BA, Treacher DF, Turner RC. Homeostasis model assessment: insulin resistance and beta-cell function from fasting plasma glucose and insulin concentrations in man. Diabetologia. 1985;28:412–9.
20. Cole TJ, Green PJ. Smoothing reference centile curves: the LMS method and penalized likelihood. Stat Med. 1992;11:1305–19.
21. Kuhle S, Maguire B, Ata N, Hamilton D. Percentile curves for anthropometric measures for Canadian children and youth. PLoS One. 2015;10:e0132891.
22. van Buuren S, Fredriks M. Worm plot: a simple diagnostic device for modelling growth reference curves. Stat Med. 2001;20:1259–77.
23. R Core Team. R: A language and environment for statistical computing. Vienna: R Foundation for Statistical Computing; 2016.
24. Rigby RA, Stasinopoulos DM. Using the box-cox t distribution in GAMLSS to model skewness and kurtosis. Stat Modelling. 2006;6:209–29.
25. Loh TP, Metz MP. Trends and physiology of common serum biochemistries in children aged 0-18 years. Pathology. 2015;47:452–61.
26. Goran MI, Gower BA. Longitudinal study on pubertal insulin resistance. Diabetes. 2001;50:2444–50.
27. Ford ES, Li C, Imperatore G, Cook S. Age, sex, and ethnic variations in serum insulin concentrations among U.S. youth: findings from the National Health and nutrition examination survey 1999-2002. Diab Care. 2006;29:2605–11.
28. Savage MO, Smith CP, Dunger DB, Gale EA, Holly JM, Preece MA. Insulin and growth factors adaptation to normal puberty. Horm Res. 1992;37(Suppl 3):70–3.
29. Ball GD, Huang TT, Gower BA, Cruz ML, Shaibi GQ, Weigensberg MJ, et al. Longitudinal changes in insulin sensitivity, insulin secretion, and beta-cell function during puberty. J Pediatr. 2006;148:16–22.
30. Robbins DC, Andersen L, Bowsher R, Chance R, Dinesen B, Frank B, et al. Report of the American Diabetes Association's task force on standardization of the insulin assay. Diabetes. 1996;45:242–56.
31. Schwartz B, Jacobs DR, Moran A, Steinberger J, Hong CP, Sinaiko AR. Measurement of insulin sensitivity in children: comparison between the euglycemic-hyperinsulinemic clamp and surrogate measures. Diab Care. 2008;31:783–8.
32. Fox C, Bernardino L, Cochran J, Essig M, Bridges KG. Inappropriate use of homeostasis model assessment cutoff values for diagnosing insulin resistance in pediatric studies. J Am Osteopath Assoc. 2017;117:689–96.
33. Diabetes Control and Complications Trial Research Group, Nathan DM, Genuth S, Lachin J, Cleary P, Crofford O, et al. The effect of intensive treatment of diabetes on the development and progression of long-term complications in insulin-dependent diabetes mellitus. N Engl J Med. 1993; 329:977–86.
34. Saaddine JB, Fagot-Campagna A, Rolka D, Narayan KM, Geiss L, Eberhardt M, et al. Distribution of HbA(1c) levels for children and young adults in the U. S.: third National Health and nutrition examination survey. Diab Care. 2002; 25:1326–30.

21

Kawasaki disease: two case reports from the Aga Khan Hospital, Dar es Salaam-Tanzania

Mariam Noorani* and Nuruddin Lakhani

Abstract

Background: Kawasaki disease is a common childhood vasculitis which may result in cardiovascular morbidity if not adequately treated. Its epidemiology in the African region is not well described. Its features may mimic other childhood infections and hemoglobinopathies and it is rarely diagnosed in the East African region. These are the first reports of this disease from Tanzania.

Case presentation: We present two cases of complete Kawasaki disease seen over a 2 year period and diagnosed as per the criteria defined by the American Heart Association. One child was and infant and the other a 3 year old. Both of them presented with a prolonged fever and mucocutaneous findings. None of the children developed coronary artery aneurysms. One was treated with aspirin alone and the other with both aspirin and intravenous immunoglobulin. Both children had complete recovery and did not have any cardiovascular sequelae.

Conclusion: Kawasaki disease may be more common in the East African region than previously thought. It should be considered as a differential diagnosis in children who present with a prolonged fever of greater than 5 days and mucocutaneous findings. More awareness about this condition, its epidemiology, diagnosis and management are required in order to prevent the cardiovascular morbidity associated with it.

Keywords: Kawasaki, Vasculitis, Coronary aneurysms, Tanzania, Intravenous immunoglobulin, Rash, Fever

Background

Kawasaki disease is one of the most common vasculitides in childhood. It occurs predominantly in infants and young children and has long term cardiovascular morbidity due to coronary artery lesions if not adequately treated [1]. It is the leading cause of acquired heart disease in children in developed countries. The highest incidence is in Asia with almost 1 in a 100 children in Japan having the disease by age 5 [2]. In Africa, two cases were reported in South Africa in Caucasian children in 1980 but the first case in an African child was reported in Ivory Coast in 1981. Despite of sporadic cases being reported across many countries in Africa, mainly North Africa and the West African region, the epidemiological data for KD is limited for African countries [3–5].

The etiology of the disease remains unknown and several hypothesis exist in trying to explain the cause. Epidemiologic data suggest that an infectious agent may be causing the disease in genetically susceptible individuals [6]. The classic presentation of the disease occurs in children below 5 years. This suggests that there is an environmental trigger to which children mount an immune response after which the disease no longer manifests [7]. Postulated infectious agents include variants of normal flora which are induced by environmental factors such as improved hygiene [8]. Pathogenetic mechanisms postulated to result in endothelial injury include that of a protein homeostasis system in which immune cells target pathogenic proteins bound to endothelial cells resulting in host cell injury [9].

The initial symptoms are of a febrile illness lasting longer than 5 days with other mucocutaneous features including a rash, conjuctivitis and adenopathy. Diagnostic criteria exist to make a diagnosis of both complete and incomplete forms of disease [10]. If left untreated, the symptoms resolve in about 10 days. However, the coronary artery lesions may lead to long term cardiovascular complications

* Correspondence: mariam.noorani@akhst.org
Aga Khan Hospital, Dar es Salaam, Tanzania

including myocardial infarction, heart failure and arrhythmias. Treatment in the acute phase reduces the incidence of coronary artery lesions from 25 to 30% to 3–5% [11]. Currently, the recommended treatment is intravenous immunoglobulin in addition to acetylsalicylic acid at high doses [10].

In sub-saharan Africa, children suffer from many tropical and infectious diseases that present with symptoms similar to those of kawasaki disease such as fever, irritability and a rash. Common conditions include malaria, typhoid fever, meningitis and viral exanthems such as measles and roseola infantum. Other conditions that may mimic this disease include sickle cell dactylitis and infection with group A beta hemolytic streptococcus. A high index of suspicion is hence required to identify cases of kawasaki disease and institute early treatment.

We report here 2 cases of kawasaki disease seen at our institution that met diagnostic criteria defined by the American Heart Association. These are the first reports in published literature from the East African region.

Case presentations

Case 1

A.M was a 3 year old female child of African ethnicity who presented in July 2012 with a 8 day history of high grade fever and a 1 day history of swelling of the hands and feet. (Table 1 – timeline of case 1). She had received oral antibiotics, anti malarials and antihistamines with no improvement in symptoms. Her past medical history had been uneventful and her vaccinations were uptodate.

On examination, she was alert, had dry, red lips and non pitting edema on her hands and feet. She had cervical nodes measuring about 0.5 cm. Her cardiovascular exam was normal. She was admitted for further work up for the cause of her fever.

Her results showed an elevated WBC count of 36,000/μl, Hb of 9.1 g/dl and platelets of 380,000/μl. Her CRP was 173 mg/l. Malaria antigen and slide were both negative. Her urinalysis was normal. She was started empirically on ceftriaxone for presumed bacteremia and blood and urine cultures were sent. A differential diagnosis of sickle cell anaemia with dactylitis was also made and a peripheral smear, reticulocyte count and sickling test were requested. The reticulocyte count was low with a percentage of 0.38. Sickling test was negative and the peripheral smear was normal.

She continued to have fever spikes despite the antibiotics and then developed a maculopapular hyperemic rash on her chest. A diagnosis of incomplete kawasaki disease was now made which met 3 out of the 5 required criteria. An echocardiogram was done which showed normal coronary arteries. High dose aspirin was started at 80 mg/kg/day. IVIG was not available at the institution at that time. A repeat complete blood count showed some improvement in white blood cells (28000/μl) but elevated platelets of 644000/μl. The blood and urine culture were both reported as negative after 48 h.

The child was then flown out to Nairobi, Kenya for IVIG treatment which she received uneventfully. She was discharged on low dose aspirin and subsequent echocardiograms remained normal.

Case 2

W.I was an 8 month old infant of African ethnicity who presented in August 2013 with a 6 day history of a high grade fever with temperatures upto 39 degrees celsius. (Table 2 – Timeline of case 2). This was associated with redness of the eyes, lips and mouth. He had been treated at various health facilities with antimalarials and 2 antibiotics: cefalexin and coamoxiclav. He had also received paracetamol, ibuprofen and diclofenac injections to control the fever. His past medical history was uneventful and his vaccines were uptodate. He had attained milestones appropriately.

On examination, the child was irritable and difficult to console. He was febrile with a temperature of 38.5 ^{0} C and was not pale. He had dry, cracked, hyperemic lips and conjuctival injection bilaterally. Cervical nodes were not palpable. He had a papular rash on the neck and at the site of the BCG scar. The rest of his physical exam was normal.

A presumptive diagnosis of incomplete kawasaki disease was made meeting 3 of the five criteria required in addition to the fever. A complete blood count showed mild anaemia with normal platelet count. (WBC: 9.07 $*10^3$/μl, Hb: 9.3 g/dl, platelets:190,000/μl). Malaria antigen and blood slide were both negative. He was started on high dose aspirin at 90 mg/kg/day as IV IG was not available in our institution at that time. An echocardiogram was done which showed normal coronary arteries and normal cardiac function.

His fever resolved after 72 h and he developed swelling of the hands and feet which now confirmed the diagnosis of complete kawasaki disease. The aspirin dose was reduced to 5 mg/kg/day after the fever subsided. The platelet count was repeated and it showed elevated platelets of 742,000/μl. The CRP was also high: 153 mg/l.

On follow up after a week, the limb swelling had reduced and he had skin exfoliation. His CRP had reduced to 60 mg/l and the platelets were 605,000/μl.

A follow up echo done after 1 month was normal and the aspirin was stopped after the hematological parameters had normalised. He has subsequently remained well with no cardiovascular sequelae.

Discussion and conclusions

Both cases described above presented to us after a prolonged duration of fever and failure to respond to

Table 1 Timeline of Case 1

Dates	Relevant past medical history and interventions		
	Previously well child with no chronic disease, growth and development appropriate for age, vaccinations complete as per schedule		
Date	Summary from initial and follow up visits	Diagnostic testing	Interventions
July 2012 – Day 1	8 days of fever 1 day of swollen hands and feet Received antibiotics, antimalarials, antihistamines On examination: dry lips, non-pitting edema, cervical nodes Diagnosis – probable sickle cell anaemia	WBC – 36,000/μl, platelets – 380,000/μl, hemoglobin-9.1 g/dl Blood cultures – negative (results on day 5) Sickling test – negative Peripheral smear – normal Reticulocyte count - normal	IV ceftriaxone
Day 3	Persistent fever. Maculopapular rash on chest. Diagnosis – probable Kawasaki meeting 3 of 5 criteria	Echocardiogram – normal coronary arteries Repeat blood count: elevated platelets – 644,000/μl	High dose aspirin –80 mg/kg/day
Day 5	Persistent fever		Flew to Nairobi for IVIG treatment
Day 7	Fever resolved	Repeat Echo normal	Discharged on low dose aspirin – 5 mg/kg/day
September 2012	Follow up visit – no signs and symptoms	Echo – normal WBC and platelets – normal	Aspirin stopped

antimalarials and antibiotics. This is a common presentation also described in case reports from Ghana [3].

The first case was 3 year old child while the second was an infant. This is in keeping with epidemiologic studies from Algeria and Japan which have shown that more than 90% of children are less than 5 years of age [2, 5].

The children had the classical mucocutaneous features that are key to making the diagnosis. The first child had limb swelling, a skin rash and oral mucosal changes. The limb swelling was initialy thought to be sickling dactylitis which is a common condition seen in our environment and is one of the presenting signs of sickle cell disease [12].

The second child had non purulent conjuctivitis, swelling of limbs and the skin rash with involvement of the BCG scar which has been described previously [13]. Hematologic parameters are not diagnostic of kawasaki disease, however they can assist to confirm or support the diagnosis. Both our children were admitted with normal platelet counts which subsequently became elevated. This is a common finding in the second week of illness and is used as an adjunct in making diagnosis of incomplete kawasaki disease [10]. The first child had an elevated WBC count leading to a diagnosis of bacteremia and initiation of parenteral antibiotics. However, the blood culture eventually ruled out a bacteremia. The CRP was raised for both the cases as expected and eventually reduced after initiation of aspirin.

The first case was treated with both aspirin and IVIG while the second received only aspirin. The role of aspirin remains uncertain in the current era of use of IVIG, however it still remains as part of the standard

Table 2 Timeline of Case 2

Dates	Relevant past medical history and interventions		
	Previously well child with no chronic disease, growth and development appropriate for age, vaccinations complete as per schedule		
Date	Summary from initial and follow up visits	Diagnostic testing (including dates)	Interventions
August 2013 – day 1	Fever for 6 days and redness of eyes, lips and mouth. Treated with antimalarials, antibiotics with no relief On examination: dry cracked lips, conjuctival injection, rash at BCG scar site and on the neck Diagnosis: incomplete kawasaki	Platelets: normal – 190,000/μl Malaria negative Echo: normal coronary arteries	High dose aspirin – 90 mg/kg/day
Day 3	Fever resolved Swelling of hands and feet Diagnosis: complete kawasaki	Platelets elevated – 743,000/μl CRP elevated: 153 mg/l	Aspirin reduced to 5 mg/kg/day
Day 7	Swelling subsided Skin exfoliation	Repeat platelet count: 605,000/μl CRP: reduced to 60 mg/l	Aspirin continued
Day 30	Follow up visit – no signs and symptoms	Repeat echo: normal CRP - < 5 mg/l Platelets: normal range	Aspiring stopped

treatment protocols. The current treatment: IVIG is an expensive drug that is not readily available or affordable to most families in our population. A single vial of 5 g costs as much as 1 million tanzanian shillings which is about 450 US dollars. This hampers effective treatment which is essential to reduce the cardiovascular sequelae.

Other treatment options that could be considered are use of corticosteroids. A cochrane review of 7 trials showed benefits of reducing cardiac complications by using steroids as adjunct therapy to IVIG early in the course of illness [14]. Use of steroids alone without IVIG has not been studied. However, in low resource settings where IVIG is not available, steroids could be used to reduce the cardiovascular morbidity [15]. Other agents such as infliximab have shown promise as adjuncts to IVIG but are also not widely available in sub – saharan Africa [16].

The echocardiograms for both children were normal at baseline and on subsequent follow ups. This was reassuring since the incidence of coronary abnormalities is as high as 25–30% in patients who are not treated with IVIG [11]. Echo is a vital modality to follow up the cardiac sequelae in chidlren with kawasaki disease. However, it is not widely available in most resource limited settings and requires specialised training to operate. In Tanzania, it is only available at a few referral hospitals in the cities. This is yet another challenge in providing long-term care to children with kawasaki disease.

Kawasaki disease has not commonly been described in sub-saharan Africa. However, these 2 cases were seen over a 2 year period at a single tertiary institution. This raises concern about how many missed cases there may be which are not diagnosed or managed effectively since the fever and mucocutaneous changes eventually resolve within 3 weeks even without specific treatment. The subsequent devastating cardiovascular morbidity of this condition in children with missed diagnosis remains unknown.

The pattern of disease in the setting of tropical infections like malaria also remains unknown. Kawasaki like syndromes have been described in adults with HIV infection especially with severe immunosupression [17]. Similar illness in children infected with HIV has not been described but may also occur.

We recommend that a diagnosis of kawasaki disease be entertained for any febrile illness lasting longer than 5 days and presenting with mucocutaneous findings. Any child presenting with a prolonged fever should promptly be referred to and evaluated at a tertiary centre. Doctors and other care providers should be made familiar with this condition in order to diagnose, treat and prevent the cardiovascular morbidity and mortality.

Cases that are seen at other institutions should be published in literature so that the spectrum of the disease, its epidemiologic characteristics and its outcomes in sub-saharan Africa can be described. Equally important is that IVIG be made available at a subsidised and more affordable cost in order to benefit patients with kawasaki disease and other autoimmune conditions where it is indicated.

Abbreviations

CBC: Complete blood count; IVIG: Intravenous immunoglobulin; WBC: White blood cells

Authors' contributions

MN reviewed the case records and wrote the manuscript, NL reviewed and contributed to the final version. Both authors read and approved the final manuscript.

Competing interests

The authors declare that they have no competing interests.

References

1. Burns JC, Glodé MP. Kawasaki syndrome. Lancet. 2004;364:533.
2. Nakamura Y, Yashiro M, Uehara R, et al. Epidemiologic features of Kawasaki disease in Japan: results of the 2007-2008 nationwide survey. J Epidemiol. 2010;20:302.
3. Badoe EV, Neequaye J, Oliver-Commey JO, et al. Kawasaki disease in Ghana: case reports from Korle Bu teaching hospital. Ghana Med J. 2011;45:38.
4. Chemli J, Kchaou H, Amri F, Belkadhi A, Essoussi AS, Gueddiche N, Harbi A. Clinical features and course of Kawasaki disease in central Tunisia: a study about 14 cases collected over a period of three years (2000-2002). Tunis Med. 2005;83(8):477–83.
5. Boudiaf H, Achir M. The clinical profile of Kawasaki disease in Algerian children: a single institution experience. J Trop Pediatr. 2016;62(2):139–43.
6. Kim KY, Kim DS. Recent advances in Kawasaki disease. Yonsei Med J. 2016; 57(1):15–21.
7. Burgner D, Harnden A. Kawasaki disease: what is the epidemiology telling us about the etiology? Int J Infect Dis. 2005;9:185–94.
8. Lee KY, Han JW, Lee JS. Kawasaki disease may be a hyperimmune reaction of genetically susceptible children to variants of normal environmental flora. Med Hypotheses. 2007;69(3):642–51.
9. Lee KY, Rhim JW, Kang JH. Kawasaki disease: laboratory findings and an immunopathogenesis on the premise of a "protein homeostasis system". Yonsei Med J. 2012;53(2):262–75.
10. Newburger JW, Takahashi M, Gerber MA, et al. Diagnosis, treatment, and long-term management of Kawasaki disease: a statement for health professionals from the committee on rheumatic fever, endocarditis and Kawasaki disease, council on cardiovascular disease in the young, American Heart Association. Circulation. 2004;110(17):2747–71.
11. Terai M, Shulman ST. Prevalence of coronary artery abnormalities in Kawasaki disease is highly dependent on gamma globulin dose but independent of salicylate dose. J Pediatr. 1997;131(6):888.
12. Bainbridge R, Higgs DR, Maude GH, Serjeant GR. Clinical presentation of homozygous sickle cell disease. J Pediatr. 1985;106(6):881.
13. Uehara R, Igarashi H, Yashiro M, Nakamura Y, Yanagawa H. Kawasaki disease patients with redness or crust formation at the Bacille Calmette-Guérin inoculation site. Pediatr Infect Dis J. 2010;29(5):430.
14. Wardle AJ, Connolly GM, Seager MJ, Tulloh RM. Corticosteroids for the treatment of Kawasaki disease in children. Cochrane Database Syst Rev. 2017;1:CD011188.
15. Singh S, Newburger JW, Kuijpers T, Burgner D. Management of Kawasaki disease in resource-limited settings. Pediatr Infect Dis J. 2015;34(1):94–6.
16. Jone PN, Anderson MS, Mulvahill MJ, Heizer H, Glodé MP, Dominguez SR. Infliximab plus intravenous immunoglobulin (IVIG) versus IVIG alone as initial therapy in children with Kawasaki disease presenting with coronary artery lesions: is dual therapy more effective? Pediatr Infect Dis J. 2018; 37(10):976–80.

Rare presentation of an atrial myxoma in an adolescent patient

Eduardo Macias[1*], Elizabeth Nieman[2], Kentaro Yomogida[3], Orlando Petrucci[4], Cylen Javidan[5], Kevin Baszis[3] and Shafkat Anwar[1]

Abstract

Background: Cardiac tumors are uncommon in the pediatric population. When present, cardiac manifestations stem from the tumor causing inflow or outflow obstruction. While common in adults, cardiac myxomas presenting with generalized systemic illness or peripheral emboli especially with no cardiac or neurological symptoms are rare in children.

Case presentation: We report a case of a previously healthy adolescent girl who presented with a 6-month history of constitutional symptoms and a purpuric rash with no cardiac or neurologic symptoms, found to have a cardiac myxoma.

Conclusions: A vasculopathic rash in the setting of atrial myxomas has been shown be a precursor to significant morbidity and mortality. Due to the rarity of this entity, the time elapsed from onset of non-cardiac symptoms until diagnosis of a myxoma is usually prolonged with interval development of irreversible neurological sequelae and death reported in the literature. Therefore, we highlight the importance of including cardiac myxomas and paraneoplastic vasculitis early in the differential diagnosis for patients presenting with a purpuric rash and systemic symptoms.

Keywords: Myxoma, Purpuric rash, Systemic symptoms, Neurological sequelae, Paraneoplastic vasculitis, Embolic phenomena

Background

Cardiac tumors are rare in the pediatric population, found in less than 0.5% of children evaluated for cardiac disease [1]. Atrial myxomas are the most common cardiac tumor in adults, most commonly presenting with cardiac symptoms. Embolic phenomena, and constitutional or systemic signs [2, 3] follow cardiac symptoms in frequency. In pediatrics, myxomas comprise less than 15% of cardiac tumors [1, 4–6] and presentation with non-cardiac, constitutional symptoms is rare. Thus, we report a case of an adolescent girl who presented with a rash, fever, purpura, and elevated inflammatory markers found to have to a cardiac myxoma. Our case establishes a unique precedent of a diagnosis of cardiac myxoma manifesting with systemic symptoms and a vasculopathic rash, but no neurological embolic phenomena.

* Correspondence: e.macias@wustl.edu
[1]Division of Cardiology, Department of Pediatrics, Washington University School of Medicine in St. Louis, One Children's Place, Campus Box 8116-NWT, St. Louis, MO 63110, USA
Full list of author information is available at the end of the article

Case presentation

A 13-year-old previously healthy girl presented to the emergency department (ED) for evaluation of fever, bilateral foot pain, and rash. Her symptoms began 6 months prior to presentation, occurring 1–2 times per month, lasting for 2–3 days, and improving with ibuprofen. A few weeks prior to ED presentation, she noted onset of fatigue, pain in her hip and calf, which she attributed to her competitive soccer playing, and acute abdominal pain with diarrhea and emesis.

Patient denied fever, headaches, visual changes, oral ulcers, muscle pain, or changes in bowel and bladder

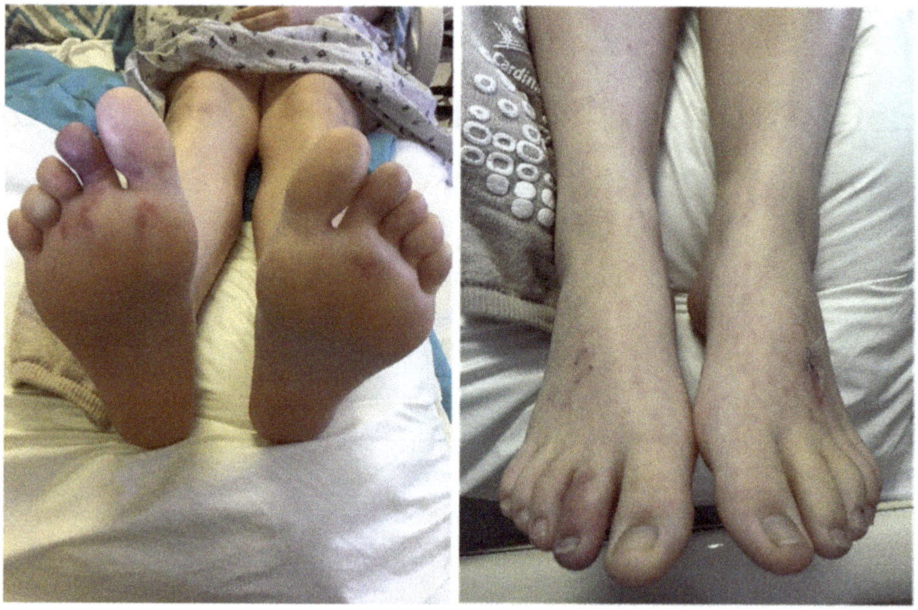

Fig. 1 Skin findings at presentation, including retiform patches, purpura and duskiness of right 2nd toe. Left foot dorsum with biopsy sutures in place

functions. She had no other medication use or recent travel. Her family history was negative for autoimmune diseases.

Her vital signs upon presentation showed a temperature of 39.2 degrees Celsius, heart rate of 90 beats per minute, respiratory rate of 20 breaths per minute, blood pressure of 114/62 mmHg, and 97% oxygen saturation on room air. She had a blanchable, retiform, violaceous patches with few areas of true purpura on her bilateral lower extremities and duskiness of her right second toe (Fig. 1). The remainder of her physical exam was unremarkable: a regular heart rate and rhythm with normal S1, S2 and no murmurs, rubs, or gallops; 2+ symmetric peripheral pulses; and joints with full range of motion without effusion or warmth. Her neurological exam was normal with no focal deficits. Her inflammatory markers were elevated (Table 1) and she was admitted for further evaluation.

Initial diagnostic considerations were vasculitis, including cutaneous polyarteritis nodosa, leukocytoclastic vasculitis (associated with lupus erythematosus, infection or idiopathic), versus a vasculopathy due to antiphospholipid antibody syndrome, cryoglobulinemia, coagulopathy or septic emboli (Table 2).

Skin biopsy of a non-palpable purpuric area on the dorsum of her left foot demonstrated subtle ischemia, vascular congestion, purpura, and focal eccrine gland necrosis without evidence of vasculitis, which was concerning for a vasculopathic process. Direct immunofluorescence of the skin biopsy was negative. Extensive systemic work-up was unremarkable and included: hepatitis panel, cryoglobulins, lupus anticoagulant panel, cardiolipins, beta-2-microglobulin, beta-2-glycopreotin, complements 3 and 4, antistreptolysin O (ASO) titers, anti-DNAse B, and aldolase. Abdominal and renal Doppler ultrasounds were also unremarkable.

During her hospital course, she developed recurrent fevers that were treated with acetaminophen at typical doses. In addition, she received a 1-time dose IV methylprednisolone 1 mg/kg after her battery of laboratory tests and skin biopsy.

An echocardiogram was performed to screen for intra-cardiac thrombus and assess for coronary abnormalities due to concerns for vasculitis. The echocardiogram revealed a 2.5 by 3-cm (cm) mass in the left

Table 1 Inflammatory markers at initial presentation

Laboratory	Value	Reference Range
Creatinine Kinase	1076	< 300 U/L
LDH	1216	100-250 U/L
CRP	48.8	< 10.0 mg/L
ESR	16	< 20.0 mm/hr
AST/ALT	164/89	10-50 U/L; 10-40 U/L
GGT	14	5–35 U/L
IL-6	< 0.5 ng/Ml[a]	

Abbreviations: *LDH* lactate dehydrogenase, *CRP* C-reactive protein, *ESR* erythrocyte sedimentation rate, *AST* aspartate transaminase, *ALT* alanine transaminase, *GGT* gamma-glutamyl transferase, *Il* Interleukin
[a]Level drawn 6 days after initial presentation and 4 days after a IV dose of methylprednisolone

Table 2 Differential diagnosis

Rheumatologic/ hematologic	Neoplastic	Infectious	Cardiac
Polyarteritis nodosa	Paraneoplastic vasculitis	Septic emboli	Cardiac myxoma
Leukocytoclastic vasculitis, inflammatory		Leukocytoclastic vasculitis	
Coagulopathy (i.e., antiphospholipid syndrome, cryoglobulinemia, other inherited disorder)			
Henoch-Schonlein purpura			

atrium (LA), Fig. 2. Cardiac magnetic resonance was performed for tissue characterization of the LA mass [7] and showed a 2.7 × 2.3 cm lobulated and mobile mass within the left atrium adherent to the septum (Fig. 2), consistent with a left atrial myxoma.

The patient's rash and constitutional symptoms were attributed to the myxoma. Purpura and pain in the right toe was felt to be secondary to either micro-embolic phenomenon or vasospasm. The decision was made to proceed with surgical excision of the cardiac mass. She was observed off anticoagulation given the lack of any concerning neurologic symptoms until surgery, which followed shortly thereafter.

The patient underwent an uncomplicated surgical resection and the diagnosis of cardiac myxoma was confirmed histologically (Fig. 3). She had an uncomplicated post-operative course with resolution of fevers and systemic symptoms in the immediate post-operative period. At 3-week follow-up she continued to be afebrile with near complete resolution of her skin findings (Fig. 4). She had no concerning symptoms at her 8-month follow up.

Discussion and conclusions

Cardiac tumors are rare in children with an incidence of 0.17–0.2% [8, 9]. The most common pediatric cardiac tumors are rhabdomyomas [1, 4, 5, 10–12], 10% of which are familial and associated with Carney complex [6]. Cardiac myxomas have been diagnosed more frequently with the advent of echocardiography [3] and are most commonly located in the left atrium [5]. In children, the mean age of diagnosis is 9–10 years [5, 13]. Delayed or undiagnosed cardiac myxomas can result in severe or fatal complications due to embolization of these friable tumors or cardiac obstruction [14, 15].

As illustrated by our patient's recurrent fevers, fatigue, skin findings and elevated inflammatory markers, cardiac myxomas can present with variable clinical symptoms that mimic other conditions (Table 2). Extracardiac manifestations are often caused by embolic phenomena and inflammation due to the intrinsic secretion of cytokines. In a series of 112 cases in adults, 34% of patients presented with systemic or constitutional symptoms and 16% presented with embolic manifestations [3]. However, review of the literature reveals only 6 reported cases of pediatric cardiac myxomas presenting with systemic symptoms without cardiac manifestations [15–21] and no cases of distal emboli without concurrent neurologic symptoms from cerebral emboli. Our case's unique presentation with both systemic symptoms and vasculopathy (possibly due to emboli or vasospasm) highlights the importance of early recognition of the many features of these tumors to prevent to morbidity and mortality related to emboli.

A case series of children with cardiac myxomas causing cerebral emboli emphasizes the need for expedient diagnosis of cardiac myxomas; 6 out of 9 of these children had residual neurologic deficits and 1 died post-operatively [22]. Several of these children had distal extremity skin lesions noted before their neurologic events, demonstrating that earlier diagnosis

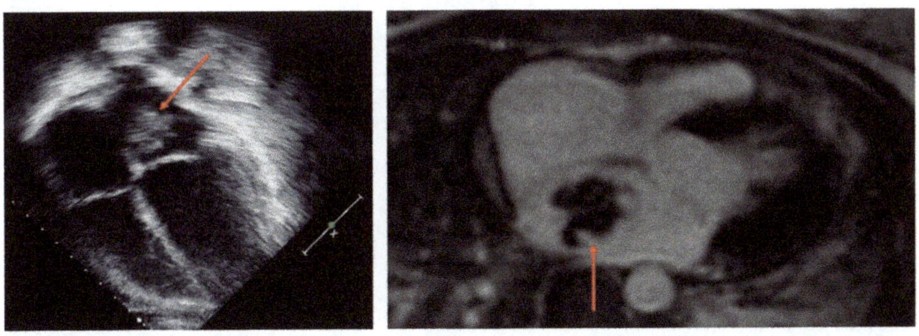

Fig. 2 Echocardiographic image in the apical four chamber view shows a pedunculated mass attached to the atrial septum, red arrow. Cardiac magnetic resonance imaging stud, the axial four-chamber view shows the left atrial mass. Tissue characterization with T1 and T2 weighted images, first pass gadolinium perfusion and delayed enhancement sequences was highly suggestive of a myxoma

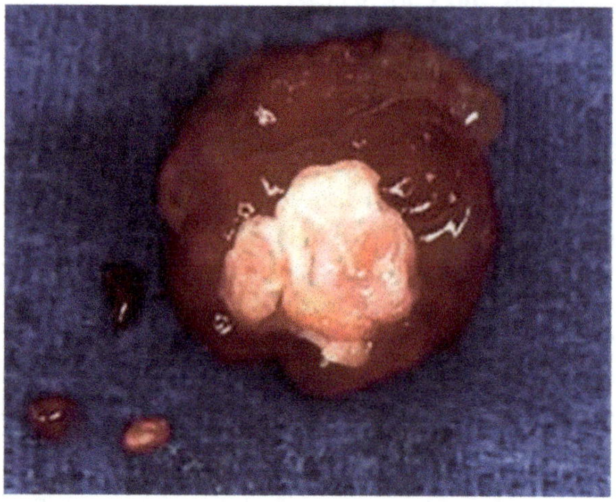

Fig. 3 3.5 X 3.5 X 2.5 lobular, gelatinous, myxomatous mass following resection from left atrium in the operating room. Microscopic examination substantiated the diagnosis of a myxoma

is possible with an elevated index of suspicion. Interestingly, none of these cases had associated systemic symptoms or significantly elevated inflammatory markers as our patient did, indicating that we cannot attribute all of her symptoms to embolic phenomena and consider inflammation intrinsic to the myxoma as well (Table 3).

Cardiac myxoma is known to secrete pro-inflammatory cytokine interleukin 6 (IL-6) and serum IL-6 plasma level is correlated with constitutional symptoms [23]. Serum IL-6 level was normal in our case but this was examined after IV methylprednisolone was initiated. A previous report demonstrated that 11 out of 12 patients (92%) with cardiac myxoma related vasculitis experienced improvement of symptoms with steroid administration, thus her normal IL-6 level likely reflected prior steroid therapy [2] .

Paraneoplastic vasculitis is an under recognized diagnosis, occurring in 5.2% of vasculitis cases [24]. Given the rarity of the concurrent conditions, diagnosis of malignancy is often delayed and the mean interval before diagnosis of malignancy is reported to be 11.9 months. A diagnosis of vasculitis requires rheumatological and infectious investigation, but search for malignancy is mandatory when clinical course becomes chronic and refractory to conventional therapy. While there have been several case series of cardiac myxomas mimicking vasculitis in adults and 2 reports in children nd 2 reports in children [2], our patient did not have any evidence of vasculitis on biopsy, making it unlikely that systemic inflammation was the etiology of our patient's distal skin findings.

In our case, systemic vasculitis and vasculopathy were the initial diagnostic considerations given our patient's systemic symptoms and distal purpura. An echocardiogram quickly

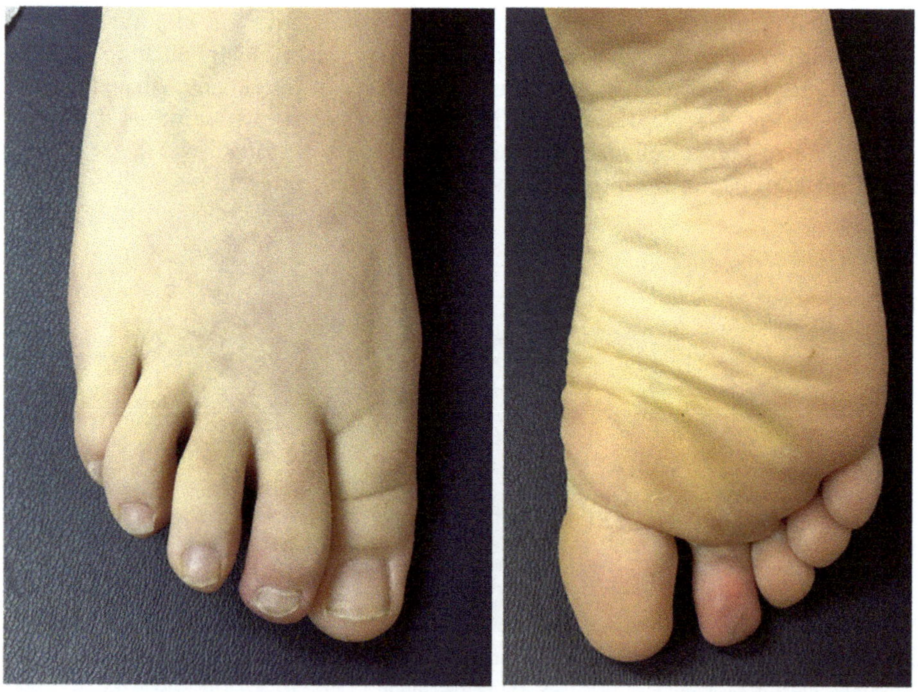

Fig. 4 Resolution of purpura with minimal residual erythema at the right second toe 3 weeks after resection

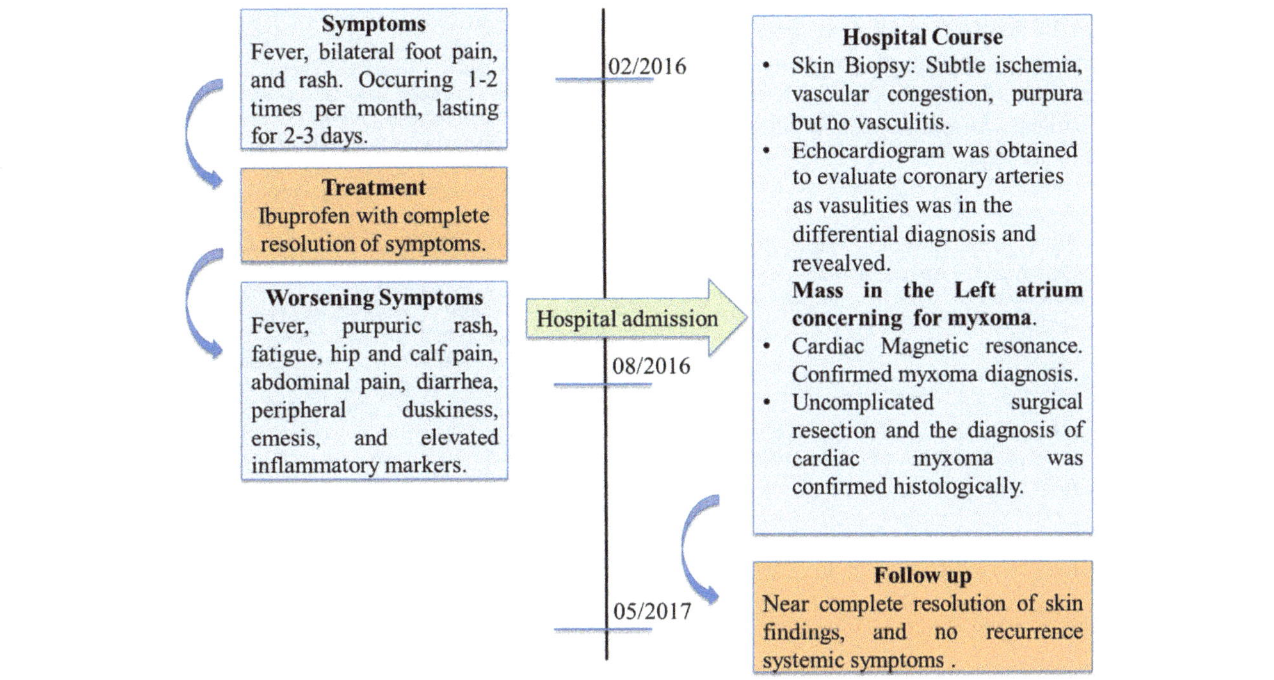

Fig. 5 Timeline

Table 3 Review of non-cardiac presentations of cardiac myxomas in the pediatric literature

Reference	Number of patients; age (years)/ Gender	Systemic symptoms	Embolic signs	Elevated IL-6
Xu [25]	1;13/F	None	Headache	NA
Goldberg [15]	1; 3/M	None	Right hemiparesis, red spots on foot; died	NA
Omeroglu [26]	2; 4/F, 6/F	None	Stroke	NA
Al-Mateen [22]	2; 11/F, 10/M	None	Acute hemiplegia, transient ischemic attack, red spots	NA
Hovels [16]	1; 6/F	Fever, arthralgia	None	yes
Park [17]	1; 5/M	Vasculitis	None	NA
Shiraishi [18]	1	Fever	none	NA
Patel [20]	1;17 /M	Fatigue; rash	none	NA
Kaminsky [21]	1;14/M	Arthropathy	None	NA
Saji [19]	1	NA	NA	NA
Domanski [27]	1; 8/M	None	Stroke	NA
Tipton [28]	1; 17/M	None	Right hemiparesis, lethargy	NA
Bobo [29]	1; 15/F	None	Right hemiparesis, headache	NA
Tonz [30]	1; 8/M	None	Right hemiparesis, seizures, aphasia, red spots, retinal artery occlusion	NA
Hung [31]	1; 10/F	None	Right hemiparesis, retinal artery occlusion	NA
Bayir [32]	1; 14/F	None	Right hemiparesis, aphasia, slurred speech, cool right leg	NA
Landers [33]	1; 8/F	None	Right hemiparesis, expressive aphasia, pulmonary embolus	NA
Macias	1:13/F	Fever, fatigue	Purpura/distal emboli	No

Embolic signs include stoke, purpura, retinal artery occlusion. Systemic symptoms include fever, arthralgia, and fatigue. *NA* not applicable as not evaluated or not mentioned in work up

raised high suspicion for cardiac myxoma, supported by tissue characterization by MRI. This allowed for expedient tumor resection and improvement of symptoms (Fig. 5). This case emphasizes the importance of considering a cardiac myxoma in a patient with both systemic inflammation and vasculopathic phenomena.

Abbreviations

ALT: Alanine transaminase; AST: Aspartate transaminase; CRP: C-reactive protein; ESR: Erythrocyte sedimentation rate; GGT: Gamma-glutamyl transferase; IL: Interleukin; LDH: Lactate dehydrogenase

Acknowledgements

The authors wish to acknowledge Dr. Carrie Coughlin, Washington University in St. Louis, School of Medicine, Division of Dermatology for her expert consultation and advice on this case report.

Funding

None.

Authors' contributions

SA conceptualized and designed the case report, reviewed and revised the manuscript, and approvedthe final manuscript as submitted. EM developed initial draft, reviewed and revised the manuscript, and approved the final manuscript as submitted. EN developed initial draft, revised the manuscript, and approved the final manuscript as submitted. KY developed initial draft, revised the manuscript, and approved the final manuscript as submitted. OP developed initial draft, revised the manuscript, and approved the final manuscript as submitted. CJ developed initial draft, revised the manuscript, and approved the final manuscript as submitted. KB developed initial draft, revised the manuscript, and approved the final manuscript as submitted.

Competing interests

The authors declare that they have no competing interests.

Author details

[1]Division of Cardiology, Department of Pediatrics, Washington University School of Medicine in St. Louis, One Children's Place, Campus Box 8116-NWT, St. Louis, MO 63110, USA. [2]Division of Dermatology, Department of Medicine, Washington University School of Medicine, St. Louis, MO, USA. [3]Division of Rheumatology, Department of Pediatrics, Washington University School of Medicine, St. Louis, MO, USA. [4]Division of Cardiothoracic Surgery, Department of Surgery, Washington University School of Medicine, St. Louis, MO, USA. [5]Mallinckrodt Institute of Radiology, Washington University School of Medicine, St. Louis, MO, USA.

References

1. Linnemeier L, Benneyworth BD, Turrentine M, et al. Pediatric cardiac tumors: a 45-year, single-institution review. World J Pediatr Congenit Heart Surg. 2015;6(2):215–9. https://doi.org/10.1177/2150135114563938.
2. Moreno M, Ortiz-Santamaria V, Deudero Infante A, et al. A classic mimicker of systemic vasculitis. Reumatol Clin. 2016;12(2):103–6. https://doi.org/10.1016/j.reuma.2015.03.006.
3. Pinede L, Duhaut P, Loire R. Clinical presentation of left atrial cardiac myxoma. A series of 112 consecutive cases. Medicine (Baltimore). 2001;80(3):159–72.
4. Marx GR, Moran AM. Cardiac Tumors. In: Allen HD, editor. Moss & Adams' Heart Disease in Infants, Children, and Adolescents, Including the Fetus and Young Adult. 9th ed. Philadelphia: Wolters Kluwer; 2016. p. 1669–79.
5. Shi L, Wu L, Fang H, et al. Identification and clinical course of 166 pediatric cardiac tumors. Eur J Pediatr. 2017;176(2):253–60. https://doi.org/10.1007/s00431-016-2833-4.
6. Jain S, Maleszewski J, Stephenson C, et al. Current diagnosis and management of cardiac myxomas. Expert Rev Cardiovasc Ther. 2015;13(4):369–75. https://doi.org/10.1586/14779072.2015.1024108.
7. Beroukhim RS, Prakash A, Buechel ER, et al. Characterization of cardiac tumors in children by cardiovascular magnetic resonance imaging: a multicenter experience. J Am Coll Cardiol. 2011;58(10):1044–54.
8. Freedom RM, Lee KJ, MacDonald C, et al. Selected aspects of cardiac tumors in infancy and childhood. Pediatr Cardiol. 2000;21(4):299–316.
9. Sallee D, Spector ML, Van Heeckeren DW, et al. Primary pediatric cardiac tumors: a 17 year experience. Cardiol Young. 1999;9(2):155–62.
10. Yadava O. Cardiac tumors in infancy. Indian Heart J. 2012;64(5):492–6. https://doi.org/10.1016/j.ihj.2012.05.004.
11. Barnes H, Conaglen P, Russell P, et al. Clinicopathological and surgical experience with primary cardiac tumors. Asian Cardiovasc Thorac Ann. 2014;22(9):1054–8. https://doi.org/10.1177/0218492314528922.
12. Delmo Walter EM, Javier MF, Sander F, et al. Primary Cardiac Tumors in Infants and Children: Surgical Strategy and Long-Term Outcome. Ann Thorac Surg. 2016;102(6):2062–9. https://doi.org/10.1016/j.athoracsur.2016.04.057.
13. Bielefeld KJ, Moller JH. Cardiac tumors in infants and children: study of 120 operated patients. Pediatr Cardiol. 2013;34:125. https://doi.org/10.1007/s00246-012-0399-034.
14. Animasahun AB, Kushimo OY, Fajuyile FA, et al. Atrial myxoma in 2 nigerian children: case reports and review of the literatura. World J Pediatr Congenit Heart Surg. 2010;1(3):397–9. https://doi.org/10.1177/2150135110381390.
15. Goldberg HP, Glenn F, Dotter CT, et al. Myxoma of the left atrium: diagnosis made during life with operative and post-mortem findings. Circulation. 1952;6:762–7.
16. Hövels-Gürich HH, Seghaye MC, Amo-Takyi BK, et al. Cardiac myxoma in a 6-year-old child--constitutional symptoms mimicking rheumatic disease and the role of interleukin-6. Acta Paediatr. 1999;88(7):786–8.
17. Park JM, Garcia RR, Patrick JK, et al. Right atrial myxoma with a nonembolic intestinal manifestation. Pediatr Cardiol. 1990;11(3):164–6.
18. Shiraishi I, Yamagishi M, Kato R, et al. A case in a child of giant left-atrial myxoma associated with recurrent high fever and myxoma cells expressing interleukin-6. Eur J Pediatr. 2006;165(5):346–7.
19. Saji T, Matsuo N, Shiono N, et al. Serum/tissue interleukin-6 concentrations and constitutional abnormalities in 4 patients with cardiac myxoma. Kokyu To Junkan. 1993;41(9):891–5 [Article in Japanese].
20. Patel R, Lynn KC. Masquerading myxoma. Am J Med Sci. 2009;338:161–3.
21. Kaminsky ME, Ehlers KH, Engle MA, et al. Atrial myxoma mimicking a collagen disorder. Chest. 1979;75(1):93–5.
22. Al-Mateen M, Hood M, Trippel D, et al. Cerebral embolism from atrial myxoma in pediatric patients. Pediatrics. 2003;112(2):e162–7.
23. Parissis JT, Mentzikof D, Georgopoulou M, et al. Correlation of interleukin-6 gene expression to immunologic features in patients with cardiac myxomas. J Interf Cytokine Res. 1996;16(8):589–93.
24. Fain O, Hamidou M, Cacoub P, et al. Vasculitides associated with malignancies: analysis of sixty patients. Arthritis Rheum. 2007;57(8):1473–80.
25. Xu J, Gao Y, Li Y, et al. Left Atrial Myoxma Presenting as Headache in the Pediatric Patient. J Emerg Med. 2015;48(2):161–4.
26. Omeroglu RE, Olgar S, Nisli K, et al. Recurrent Hemiparesis Due to Anterior Mitral Leaflet Myxomas. Pediatr Neurol. 2006;34(6):490–4.
27. Domanski O, Dubois R, Jegou B. Ischemic Stroke due to a Cardiac Myxoma. Pediatr Neurol. 2006;65:94–5.
28. Tipton K, Robertson JT, Robertson JH. Embolism to the central nervous system from cardiac myxoma. Report of two cases. J Neurosurg. 1977;47(6):937–40.
29. Bobo H, Evans OB. Intracranial aneurysms in a child with recurrent atrial myxoma. Pediatr Neurol. 1987;3(4):230–2.
30. Tönz M, Laske A, Carrel T, et al. Convulsions, hemiparesis and central retinal artery occlusion due to left atrial myxoma in child. Eur J Pediatr. 1992;151(9):652–4.
31. Hung PC, Wang HS, Chou ML, et al. Multiple cerebral aneurysms in a child with cardiac myxoma. J Formos Med Assoc. 1992;91(8):818–21.
32. Bayir H, Morelli PJ, Smith TH, et al. A left atrial myxoma presenting as a cerebrovascular accident. Pediatr Neurol. 1999;21(2):569–72.
33. Landers C, Baumann R, Cottrill MC, et al. Embolic strokes in an 8-year-old girl. Neurology. 2000;55(1):146. https://doi.org/10.1212/WNL.55.1.146.

23

Insulin metabolism markers are predictors of subclinical atherosclerosis among overweight and obese children and adolescents

Golaleh Asghari[1], Pooneh Dehghan[2], Parvin Mirmiran[3*], Emad Yuzbashian[4], Maryam Mahdavi[5], Maryam Tohidi[6], Tirang R. Neyestani[7], Farhad Hosseinpanah[8*] and Fereidoun Azizi[9]

Abstract

Background: To investigate the association between markers of insulin metabolism and carotid intima-media thickness(cIMT) among overweight and obese children and adolescents.

Methods: A total of 378 children and adolescents aged from 6 to 13 years, with WHO body mass index Z-Scores ≥2 were enrolled in this study. We measured fasting serum insulin and glucose, conducted a homeostatic model assessment of insulin resistance(HOMA-IR), and calculated the quantitative insulin sensitivity check index(QUICKI). Carotid intima-media thickness was measured in the common carotid artery with high-resolution ultrasonography.

Results: The study participants consisted of 198 boys and 180 girls with a mean(±SD) age of 9.3 ± 1.7 years, 18.3% being pre-pubertal. In boys, after controlling for confounders, a one-SD increase in fasting insulin and HOMA-IR were associated with 0.351 mm($P < 0.001$) and 0.350 mm($P < 0.001$) increases in cIMT, respectively. However, a one-SD increase in QUICKI was associated with a – 0.305 mm($P = 0.001$) decrease in cIMT. When categorizing into tertiles, a one-SD increase in fasting insulin and HOMA-IR were associated with 87 and 81% increases in the odds of higher categories of cIMT(both $P < 0.05$). However, a one-SD increase in QUICKI was associated with 37% lower odds of higher categories of cIMT($P = 0.022$). No significant associations were found among girls.

Conclusion: This study demonstrated that insulin resistance and sensitivity markers were independent predictors of cIMT in overweight and obese boys, but not in girls, highlighting the importance of chronically elevated insulin levels for predisposing these boys to alterations in their vascular structure.

Keywords: Insulin resistance, Atherosclerosis, Children, Adolescents, obesity

Background

Obesity-related insulin resistance and chronically elevated insulin concentrations that begin in childhood can induce atherothrombotic mechanisms, reduce fibrinolytic balance, and impair endothelial function, which independently contributes to future cardiovascular events in adulthood [1, 2]. Atherosclerosis develops gradually, over the course of a lifetime, and a long crucial phase of the process consists of several silent dysfunctional changes of the endothelium [3]. The increased mortality associated with atherosclerosis is related to the duration and intensity of risk factors presenting throughout a lifetime. Therefore, to prevent cardiovascular disease from manifesting and known factors leading to clinical events, it is important to unravel which factors play a role in the earlier and later stages of the atherosclerotic disease.

In recent years, high-resolution B mode ultrasonography has been frequently used in children and adolescents to measure carotid intima-media thickness (cIMT)

* Correspondence: mirmiran@endocrine.ac.ir; parvin.mirmiran@gmail.com; fhospanah@endocrine.ac.ir
[3]Nutrition and Endocrine Research Center, Research Institute for Endocrine Sciences, Shahid Beheshti University of Medical Sciences, P.O. Box: 19395-4763, Tehran, Iran
[8]Obesity Research Center, Research Institute for Endocrine Sciences, Shahid Beheshti University of Medical Sciences, P.O. Box: 19395-4763, Tehran, Iran
Full list of author information is available at the end of the article

for the purpose of assessing the presence of subclinical atherosclerosis. Atherosclerotic monitoring with IMT is both sensitive and reproducible, providing a surrogate measure of atherosclerotic burden and cardiovascular risk which may, in turn, serve as possible predictors of future cardiovascular events [4, 5]. Previous observational studies indicated that IMT in children and adolescents elevated with familial hypercholesterolemia [6], type 1 diabetes mellitus [7], and hypertension [8]. Measuring cIMT in children and adolescents with obesity has been recommended by the Association for European Paediatric Cardiology (AEPC), as it is capable of recognizing early vascular alterations and thus prevent myocardial infarction and stroke [9].

With regard to a possible relationship between IMT and insulin resistance/hyperinsulinemia in children and adolescents, the results remain inconsistent, with some studies reporting an adverse relation between insulin resistance and vascular measures [10, 11], while others observed no significant relations at all [12–14]. The studies in question did not look for differences based on gender or pubertal status.

By studying possible associations between insulin resistance and measures of vascular structure, while considering gender and pubertal maturation status, we may gain some insight on and advance our understanding of the complex gender-specific relations between obesity and vascular structure in response to insulin level. The present study has addressed this question by investigating possible associations between markers of insulin metabolism and cIMT among children and adolescents with either overweight or obesity.

Methods

Study population

This study was conducted during the baseline (cross-sectional) phase of a randomized, double-blind trial, aimed at investigating the effect of different doses of one-year vitamin D supplementation on cIMT and other bone and cardiovascular variables in children and adolescents with an age- and sex-specific body mass index (BMI) Z-score ≥ 1 (according to the criteria established by the World Health Organization). Participants, aged 6 to 13 years, were recruited from primary schools located in three Tehran (Iran) districts. The baseline screening took place between June 2016 and March 2017. Individuals were eligible for inclusion if they had no known medical illnesses such as diabetes, liver, or kidney diseases, were not taking any dietary supplements, or using pharmaceutical agents that affect glucose and lipid metabolism. A total of 378 participants met these selection criteria and were enrolled at the baseline. The sample size for the trial was determined by a sample size calculation designed to achieve 80% power to detect a 0.02 mm difference in cIMT with a 0.05 standard deviation (95% confidence interval) between different groups of the original trial.

Measurements

Fat and soft lean mass were assessed by portable bioelectrical impedance analyzer GAIA 359 PLUS 8-contact electrode bioelectrical impedance (BIA) system (Jawon Medical Co. Ltd., Shinsang, Korea). During the measurement, all participants removed their shoes and socks, wore light clothing, and stood with the soles of their feet making contact with the foot electrodes, while holding the hand electrodes in their bare hands. All necessary variables including sex, height, and age, were input into the instrument. The BIA system measured the impedance via a tetra-polar multi-frequency (5, 50, 250 kHz) electrode method. Resistance to the 500 μA current was measured while the participants stood motionless on the analyzer's platform, their arms raised about 30°, while lightly holding onto the hand electrodes. For the data interpretation, we used the manufacturer's software in its "standard" setting.

Body weight was measured using the scale function of the GAIA 359 PLUS (100-g accuracy) while the subjects were standing barefoot and wearing light clothing. Height was measured while participants were standing without shoes and shoulders in normal alignment, using a stadiometer with an accuracy of 0.5 cm. Body mass index (BMI) was calculated as weight (in kilograms) divided by height (in meters) squared (kg/m^2). Waist circumference (WC) was measured down to the nearest 0.5 cm at the level of the umbilicus, over light clothing, and without any pressure, using a tape meter.

Blood pressure was measured twice, at least 1 min apart, using a mercury sphygmomanometer and the Korotkoff sound technique, with an accuracy of 2 mmHg, after participants had been resting for 15 min on a chair; the average of both measurements served as the participant's final pressure; systolic/diastolic blood pressures (SBP/DBP) were determined from the first onset/disappearance of sound.

Blood samples were collected from all study participants between 8:00 and 10:00 AM, after 10–12 h of overnight fasting. All the blood analyses were carried out at the RIES research laboratory. Fasting blood glucose (FBG) was measured by enzymatic colorimetric method using glucose oxidase (Pars Azmoon, Tehran, Iran) and the Selectra 2 auto-analyzer (Vital Scientific, Spankeren, Netherlands) with intra- and inter-assay coefficients of variation (CVs) of 1.1 and 1.4%, respectively. Fasting serum insulin was determined by the electrochemiluminescence immunoassay (ECLIA) method, using Roche Diagnostics kits and the Roche/Hitachi Cobas e-411 analyzer (Roche Diagnostics, GmbH, Mannheim, Germany). Intra- and inter-assay

CVs were 1.3 and 2.5%, respectively. To monitor the quality of measurements, assayed serum controls in different concentrations were used for the glucose (Pars Azmoon, Tehran, Iran) and insulin assays (Lyphochek Immunoassay Plus Control, Bio-Rad Laboratories).

Physical activity was assessed using the Modifiable Activity Questionnaire (MAQ) to calculate metabolic equivalent task minutes per week; the high reliability (97%) and moderate validity (49%) of the Persian translated MAQ in adolescents have been ascertained previously [15].

Pubertal status was classified according to the Tanner scale by a well-trained endocrinologist, dividing the participants into 2 groups based on breast and genital stages: pre-pubertal (boys at genital stage I, girls at breast stage I) and pubertal (boys at genital stage ≥II, girls at breast stage ≥II).

Carotid intima-media thickness was measured by a well-trained radiologist (P.D.). Participants were examined in the supine position with the head slightly extended and rotated away from the examiner. The carotid arteries were interrogated using a high-resolution Samsung ultrasound machine (model UGEO WS80A) with a linear-array transducer operating at a frequency of at least 7 MHz. Depth, gain, and focus was adjusted for each participant individually so that the arterial lumen was completely anechoic and in the center of the image. Common cIMT was measured from longitudinal B-mode images of the distal 1 cm of the far wall of each common carotid artery (CCA), between the intimal-luminal and the medial-adventitial interfaces of the carotid artery wall, represented as a double-line density on the ultrasound image. In rare cases where appropriate images of the distal CCA could not be obtained, proximal or mid-CCA images were used for IMT measurement. Measurements were performed using the automated edge-tracking software (automated IMT calculator) which obviated the need to perform manual measurements.

Definitions

Insulin resistance/sensitivity was calculated as follows:

Homeostatic model assessment of insulin resistance (HOMA-IR) = [fasting insulin (μU/ml) × fasting glucose (mmol/l)]/22.5;

Quantitative insulin sensitivity check index (QUICKI) = 1/[log fasting insulin (μU/ml) + log fasting glucose (mg/dl)].

Abdominal obesity was defined as waist circumference (WC) ≥ 90th percentile for age and sex, according to national reference curves [16].

Statistical analysis

Quantitative variables were expressed as the mean ± SD or median (interquartile range) while categorical variables were expressed as percentages. Continuous and categorical variables were compared according to sex using a t-test and a Chi square-test, respectively. Multiple linear regression analysis was used to evaluate the association of markers of insulin metabolism and cIMT. A proportional odds model (POM) was used to test for a possible association between an insulin metabolism marker increase of approximately 1 SD and tertiles of cIMT using the ranges: cIMT< 0.38, 0.38 ≤ cIMT< 0.42, and cIMT≥0.42 mm. The proportional odds assumption was assessed through a chi-squared score test for each covariate to examine whether the assumption was violated. Proportional odds assumptions were generally appropriate. To test whether pubertal stage or gender could affect the contribution of fasting insulin, the interaction terms for [female × fasting insulin] and [pre--pubertal × fasting insulin] were used as separate inputs in our multivariable linear regression models. The likelihood ratio test for interaction terms was not significant. Nevertheless, the interaction term for gender was of biological importance which is why each model was performed in the subset specified by gender. Waist circumference, body fat percentage, physical activity, and Tanner stages were considered as confounding variables. Collinearity was assessed using Pearson's rank correlation coefficient and variance inflation factor. No collinearity was found between body fat percentage and WC. All analyses were performed using IBM SPSS for Windows, version 20 (SPSS, Chicago, IL, USA) with the significance level set at $P < 0{\cdot}05$ (two-tailed).

Results

The study consisted of 378 participants (198 boys and 180 girls) with a mean (±SD) age of 9.3 ± 1.7 years and 18.3% in the pre-pubertal stage. Compared to girls, boys had a higher physical activity, more hours of TV watching, a greater BMI, WC, soft lean mass, prevalence of obesity, a lower fat mass and HOMA-IR ($P < 0.05$, Table 1).

In boys, but not girls, both fasting insulin and HOMA-IR were positively, and QUICCKI negatively correlated with cIMT (Fig. 1). In boys, after controlling for body fat mass percentage, WC, physical activity, and Tanner stage, a one-SD increase in fasting insulin and HOMA-IR were associated with 0.351 mm ($P < 0.001$) and 0.350 mm ($P < 0.001$) increases in cIMT, respectively. However, a one-SD increase in QUICKI was associated with a − 0.305 mm ($P = 0.001$) decrease in cIMT. When categorizing into tertiles, a one-SD increase in fasting insulin and HOMA-IR were associated with 87 and 81% increases in the odds of higher categories of cIMT (both $P < 0.05$). However, a one-SD increase in QUICKI was associated with a 37% lower odds of higher categories of cIMT ($P = 0.022$). No significant associations were found among girls (Table 2).

Table 1 Characteristics of 378 overweight and obese children and adolescents

	Total (*n* = 378)	Girls (*n* = 180)	Boys (*n* = 198)	*P*-value
Age (years)	9.3 ± 1.7	9.2 ± 1.7	9.4 ± 1.8	0.326
Pre-pubertal (%)	18.3	15.0	21.3	0.113
Physical activity (MET/hr./wk)	13.3 (5.1–31.7)	8.9 (3.3–17.9)	20.1 (7.9–41.2)	< 0.001
Watching TV (hour/d)				
≤ 1	14.1	14.2	13.9	0.024
2–3	38.6	45.5	32.5	
≥ 4	47.3	40.3	53.6	
Height (cm)	139.7 ± 11.0	138.9 ± 10.9	140.5 ± 11.0	0.142
Z-Score Height	0.86 ± 1.00	0.80 ± 1.07	0.91 ± 0.93	0.291
BMI (kg/m^2)	23.3 ± 3.4	22.8 ± 3.2	23.8 ± 3.4	0.004
Z-Score BMI	2.55 ± 0.73	2.34 ± 0.83	2.74 ± 0.83	< 0.001
Obese (%)	68.8	55.6	80.8	< 0.001
Waist circumference (cm)	80.8 ± 9.5	79.4 ± 8.9	82.0 ± 10.0	0.009
Abdominal obesity (%)	92.6	93.1	92.1	0.705
Fat mass (%)	26.3 ± 6.9	28.6 ± 4.2	24.2 ± 8.1	< 0.001
Soft-lean mass (kg)	30.7 ± 7.2	29.1 ± 6.6	32.2 ± 7.3	< 0.001
Fasting glucose (mg/dl)	90.7 ± 9.3	91.5 ± 8.6	89.9 ± 9.9	0.103
Fasting insulin (μU/ml)	12.4 (8.5–19.0)	12.9 (9.3–20.6)	11.9 (7.9–18.2)	0.085
HOMA-IR	2.80 (1.92–4.34)	3.00 (2.02–4.56)	2.66 (1.67–4.13)	0.048
QUICKI	0.333 ± 0.040	0.328 ± 0.031	0.338 ± 0.046	0.023
Carotid intima media thickness (mm)	0.40 ± 0.057	0.40 ± 0.004	0.41 ± 0.060	0.100

BMI body mass index, *HOMA-IR* homeostatic model assessment of insulin resistance, *QUICKI* quantitative insulin sensitivity check index
Quantitative variables were expressed as the mean ± SD or median (interquartile range) and categorical ones as percentages
Abdominal obesity was defined based on national age- and sex-specific 90th percentile (1)

Discussion

This study demonstrated that markers of insulin metabolism were independent predictors of cIMT in overweight and obese boys, but not in girls. Both fasting insulin and HOMA-IR were positively, and QUICKI negatively associated with cIMT. This relationship remained significant even after adjusting for obesity features such as body fat percentage and WC, or pubertal status (Tanner stages). This result not only highlights the robustness of the link between insulin resistance and cIMT as an independent risk factor for the development of atherosclerosis, but it clearly underscores how arterial abnormalities are demonstrable already at a very early age in overweight and obese boys.

A number of observational studies among adults have shown adverse structural changes in cIMT in the presence of cardiovascular (CVD) risk factors [17, 18]. However, data regarding subclinical CVD using imaging such as cIMT in pediatrics with overweight and obesity is limited and inconsistent. While some studies reported that increased cIMT was mediated in part by obesity [19], insulin sensitivity [20], type 2 diabetes [21], DBP [22], SBP, inflammatory markers [23], epicardial adipose tissue thickness [24], WC [22, 25], others found no associations between cIMT and insulin resistance [14, 26], prediabetes state [27], polycystic ovary syndrome [28], and inflammatory chemokines [29].

Our findings are in agreement with results of recent investigations where higher insulin levels and the presence of insulin resistance were adversely associated with carotid wall thickness among children and adolescents. Ryder et al. (2016) conducted a cross-sectional study on 252 children, aged between 8 and 20 years and in Tanner stages ranging from 2 to 5, and observed that cIMT was positively related to insulin resistance (measured by hyperinsulinemic euglycemic clamp) [10]. In addition, type 2 diabetes, a state of insulin resistance, was associated with higher cIMT in youth aged 10–24 years [21]. Furthermore, Atabek et al. observed in obese children aged between 8 and 18 years that QUICKI was independently associated with cIMT, but not HOMA-IR [30]. However, Reinehr et al. did not find any significant correlation between insulin level and cIMT among 96 obese children with a mean age of 11 years, after controlling for pubertal status and body fat mass [23]. Besides, there was no significant difference with regard to IMT between obese insulin resistant and obese not insulin resistant children aged 12 to 18 years, a fact that

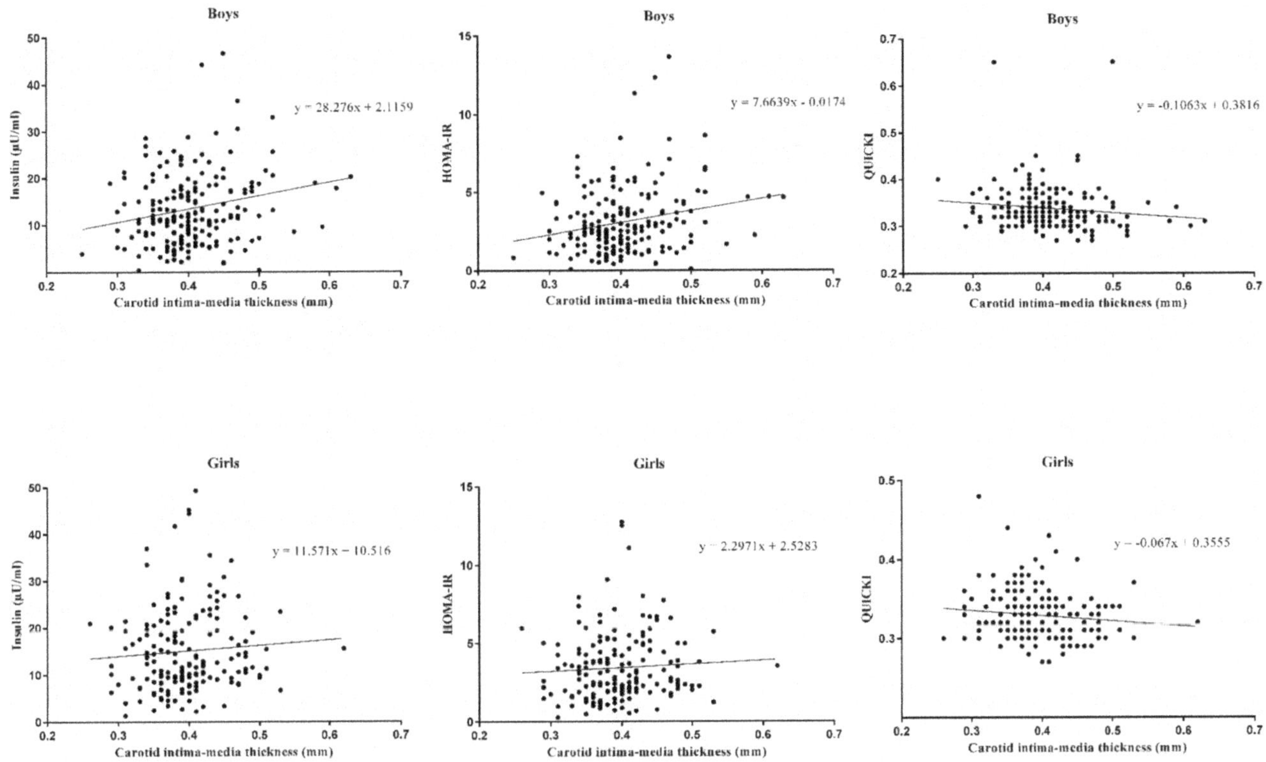

Fig. 1 Gender-specific correlations of fasting insulin, homeostatic model assessment of insulin resistance (HOMA-IR), and quantitative insulin sensitivity check index (QUICKI) with carotid intima-media thickness among 378 overweight and obese children and adolescents

could be due to the β-error associated with the sample size [14]. Compared to most previous studies, our study had a larger sample size, narrower age range, and accounted for potential confounding variables (physical activity, body fat percentage, WC, and pubertal status). In contrast to these studies, our findings clearly indicate how markers of insulin metabolism are associated with carotid atherosclerosis, and we found this association to be independent of adiposity. These differences may be due to the fact that we considered an overweight to an obese pediatric population with a narrower BMI than most other studies. In addition, these differences may also be partly due to differences in the protocol used for measuring cIMT.

Another difference compared to previous studies is that we separated our participants by gender. This yielded the somewhat surprising result that the association between insulin-related variables and cIMT exists only among boys but not among girls. The reason for this finding is not clear; there is a difference between girls and boys regarding weight status and WC values. Lower obesity prevalence and WC among girls compared to these among boys may be an explanation to justify lack of association between insulin resistance and IMT in girls. It might also explain the higher susceptibility of boys to developing CVD and the fact that CVD events occur approximately 10 years earlier in life for men that for women [31]. Increased adiposity, in combination with higher glucose and insulin levels during childhood, has been linked to a higher carotid thickness in later life [12, 30]. The Bogalusa Heart Study found that the cumulative levels of high BMI in childhood was associated with adult cIMT in both sexes, even after controlling for adult BMI [32]. Increased body weight may interact with insulin level and sensitivity by affecting atherosclerosis.

Several studies illustrated an association between obesity and thicker cIMT among children and adolescents. The significance of this relation became marginal once the model applied to 100 children with BMI >95th percentile was adjusted for glucose [19]. Besides, Reinehr et al. revealed that impaired fasting glucose, along with BMI, was an independent determinant of cIMT in obese children. Their results indicate the importance of impaired glucose hemostasis for the arterial structure during childhood and even adulthood [12]. Furthermore, the linkage of insulin resistance and increased cIMT may be explained by the atherogenic pattern of lipoprotein particles and higher endothelial-derived ICAM, which are both present among obese insulin-resistant adolescents [14].

By surveying a large number of children and adolescents, we could observe associations with regard to

Table 2 Associations of insulin metabolism markers with carotid intima media thickness according to sex

	Multiple linear regression		Multiple ordinal regression*	
	Standardized β	*P*-value	OR (95% CI)	*P*-value
Fasting insulin (μU/ml)				
Boys				
Unadjusted	0.299	< 0.001	1.49 (1.10–2.01)	0.009
Model 1†	0.351	< 0.001	1.87 (1.24–2.81)	0.003
Model 2‡	0.344	< 0.001	1.84 (1.22–2.79)	0.004
Girls				
Unadjusted	0.010	0.911	1.21 (0.93–1.58)	0.154
Model 1†	−0.090	0.344	0.93 (0.67–1.29)	0.672
Model 2‡	−0.116	0.242	0.89 (0.63–1.25)	0.506
HOMA-IR				
Boys				
Unadjusted	0.308	< 0.001	1.51 (1.12–2.04)	0.006
Model 1†	0.350	< 0.001	1.81 (1.22–2.70)	0.003
Model 2‡	0.343	< 0.001	1.80 (1.20–2.68)	0.004
Girls				
Unadjusted	−0.006	0.951	1.18 (0.91–1.55)	0.215
Model 1†	−0.096	0.314	0.91 (0.66–1.27)	0.601
Model 2‡	−0.122	0.217	0.87 (0.61–1.23)	0.425
QUICKI				
Boys				
Unadjusted	−0.288	< 0.001	0.82 (0.63–1.06)	0.126
Model 1†	−0.305	0.001	0.63 (0.42–0.93)	0.022
Model 2‡	−0.298	0.001	0.64 (0.43–0.95)	0.027
Girls				
Unadjusted	−0.034	0.704	0.70 (0.49–1.00)	0.051
Model 1†	0.051	0.581	0.96 (0.60–1.54)	0.859
Model 2‡	0.077	0.430	1.00 (0.61–1.64)	0.994

HOMA-IR homeostatic model assessment of insulin resistance, *QUICKI* quantitative insulin sensitivity check index
*Multiple ordinal regression was used with carotid intima media thickness as response with three ordered categories
†Adjusted for body fat mass percent, waist circumference, and physical activity
‡Additionally adjusted for Tanner stages

gender. BIA measurements allowed us to adjust for adiposity (body fat percentage) instead of only BMI. Despite these strengths, our study also has some inherent limitations: the participants came from a narrowly localized geographic region (the southern districts of Tehran), which may limit generalizability; due to this study having been strictly observational, causality could be established; despite measurement of a number of confounders, residual confounding could not be ruled out. Assessing breast development among overweight and obese girls may be overestimated because of difficulties in distinguishing between glandular breast tissue and subcutaneous fat; however, in the current study, a well-trained woman endocrinologist was used to visual assessment of breast budding (Tanner stage 2 development) which minimized measurement error. And lastly, our interpretation of insulin resistance is predominantly based on the HOMA-IR and not on euglycaemic clamp studies, which was simply not possible given our study parameters.

Conclusion

In conclusion, the current study showed that HOMA-IR and QUICKI, as a markers of insulin resistance and sensitivity, may serve as independent predictors of cIMT in overweight and obese boys, but not in girls. Our study provides biologically important information and further work is recommended to translate these findings into clinical practice for identifying high-risk children.

Abbreviations

BIA: bioelectrical impedance; BMI: body mass index; CCA: common carotid artery; cIMT: Carotid intima media thickness; DBP: diastolic blood pressure; FBG: fasting blood glucose; HOMA-IR: homeostatic model assessment of insulin resistance; POM: proportional odds model; QUICKI: quantitative insulin sensitivity check index; SBP: systolic blood pressure; SD: standard deviation; WC: waist circumference

Acknowledgments

We would like to acknowledge Ms. Niloofar Shiva for a critical edition of English grammar and syntax of the manuscript.

Funding

This work was funded by a grant from the Faculty of Nutrition Sciences and Food Technology, National Nutrition and Food Technology Research Institute, in addition to the Research Institute for Endocrine Sciences, Shahid Beheshti University of Medical Sciences, Tehran, Iran. The funder were not involved in the design of the study and collection, analysis, and interpretation of data and in writing the manuscript.

Authors' contributions

All authors have read and approved the final manuscript. Overall P. M., F. H., and F. A. supervised the project and approved the final version of the manuscript to be submitted. F. H., G. A. and E. Y. designed the research; M. T. and T. N. assessed the laboratory and biochemical parameters; P. D. measured carotid intima-media thickness; P. M., M. M. and G. A., analyzed and interpreted the data, and G. A., E.Y., and F. H. drafted the initial manuscript; F. A. critically revised the manuscript.

Competing interests

The authors declare that they have no competing interests.

Author details

[1]Department of Clinical Nutrition and Dietetics, Faculty of Nutrition Sciences and Food Technology, National Nutrition and Food Technology Research Institute, Shahid Beheshti University of Medical Sciences, Tehran, Iran. [2]Department of Imaging, Research Development Center, Taleghani Hospital, Shahid Beheshti University of Medical Sciences, Tehran, Iran. [3]Nutrition and Endocrine Research Center, Research Institute for Endocrine Sciences, Shahid Beheshti University of Medical Sciences, P.O. Box: 19395-4763, Tehran, Iran. [4]Nutrition and Endocrine Research Center, Research Institute for Endocrine Sciences, Shahid Beheshti University of Medical Sciences, Tehran, Iran. [5]Obesity Research Center, Research Institute for Endocrine Sciences, Shahid Beheshti University of Medical Sciences, Tehran, Iran. [6]Prevention of Metabolic Disorders Research Center, Research Institute for Endocrine Sciences, Shahid Beheshti University of Medical Sciences, Tehran, Iran. [7]Laboratory of Nutrition Research, National Nutrition and Food Technology Research Institute, Faculty of Nutrition Sciences and Food Technology, Shahid Beheshti University of Medical Sciences, Tehran, Iran. [8]Obesity Research Center, Research Institute for Endocrine Sciences, Shahid Beheshti University of Medical Sciences, P.O. Box: 19395-4763, Tehran, Iran. [9]Endocrine Research Center, Research Institute for Endocrine Sciences, Shahid Beheshti University of Medical Sciences, Tehran, Iran.

References

1. Sinaiko AR, Caprio S. Insulin resistance. J Pediatr. 2012;161(1):11–5.
2. Perkins JM, Joy NG, Tate DB, Davis SN. Acute effects of hyperinsulinemia and hyperglycemia on vascular inflammatory biomarkers and endothelial function in overweight and obese humans. American Journal of Physiology-Endocrinology and Metabolism. 2015;309(2):E168–76.
3. Rosvall M, Persson M, Östling G, Nilsson P, Melander O, Hedblad B, Engström G. Risk factors for the progression of carotid intima-media thickness over a 16-year follow-up period: the Malmö diet and Cancer study. Atherosclerosis. 2015;239(2):615–21.
4. Kuller L, Borthani N, Furberg C, Gardin J, Manolio T, O'leary D, Psaty B, Robbins J. Prevalence of subclinical atherosclerosis and cardiovascular disease and association with risk factors in the cardiovascular health study. Am J Epidemiol. 1994;139(12):1164–79.
5. Rahman TJ, Walker EA, Mayosi BM, Hall DH, Avery PJ, Connell JM, Watkins H, Stewart PM, Keavney B. Genotype at the P554L variant of the hexose-6 phosphate dehydrogenase gene is associated with carotid intima-medial thickness. PLoS One. 2011;6(8):e23248.
6. Tonstad S, Joakimsen O, Stensland-Bugge E, Leren TP, Ose L, Russell D, Bønaa KH. Risk factors related to carotid intima-media thickness and plaque in children with familial hypercholesterolemia and control subjects. Arterioscler Thromb Vasc Biol. 1996;16(8):984–91.
7. Järvisalo MJ, Putto-Laurila A, Jartti L, Lehtimäki T, Solakivi T, Rönnemaa T, Raitakari OT. Carotid artery intima-media thickness in children with type 1 diabetes. Diabetes. 2002;51(2):493–8.
8. Lande MB, Carson NL, Roy J, Meagher CC. Effects of childhood primary hypertension on carotid intima media thickness. Hypertension. 2006; 48(1):40–4.
9. Dalla Pozza R, Ehringer-Schetitska D, Fritsch P, Jokinen E, Petropoulos A, Oberhoffer R. Intima media thickness measurement in children: a statement from the Association for European Paediatric Cardiology (AEPC) working group on cardiovascular prevention endorsed by the Association for European Paediatric Cardiology. Atherosclerosis. 2015;238(2):380–7.
10. Ryder JR, Dengel DR, Jacobs DR Jr, Sinaiko AR, Kelly AS, Steinberger J. Relations among adiposity and insulin resistance with flow-mediated dilation, carotid intima-media thickness, and arterial stiffness in children. J Pediatr. 2016;168:205–11.
11. Woo KS, Chook P, Yu CW, Sung RY, Qiao M, Leung SS, Lam CW, Metreweli C, Celermajer DS. Overweight in children is associated with arterial endothelial dysfunction and intima-media thickening. Int J Obes Relat Metab Disord. 2004;28(7):852–7.
12. Yajnik CS, Katre PA, Joshi SM, Kumaran K, Bhat DS, Lubree HG, Memane N, Kinare AS, Pandit AN, Bhave SA, et al. Higher glucose, insulin and insulin resistance (HOMA-IR) in childhood predict adverse cardiovascular risk in early adulthood: the Pune Children's study. Diabetologia. 2015; 58(7):1626–36.
13. Gazolla FM, Neves Bordallo MA, Madeira IR, de Miranda Carvalho CN, Vieira Monteiro AM, Pinheiro Rodrigues NC, Borges MA, Collett-Solberg PF, Muniz BM, de Oliveira CL. Association between cardiovascular risk factors and carotid intima-media thickness in prepubertal Brazilian children. J Pediatr Endocrinol Metab. 2015;28(5–6):579–87.
14. Brar PC, Patel P, Katz S. The relationship between insulin resistance and endothelial dysfunction in obese adolescents. J Pediatr Endocrinol Metab. 2017;30(6):635–42.
15. Delshad M, Ghanbarian A, Ghaleh NR, Amirshekari G, Askari S, Azizi F. Reliability and validity of the modifiable activity questionnaire for an Iranian urban adolescent population. Int J Prev Med. 2015;6:3.
16. Kelishadi R, Gouya MM, Ardalan G, Hosseini M, Motaghian M, Delavari A, Majdzadeh R, Heidarzadeh A, Mahmoud-Arabi MS, Riazi MM. First reference curves of waist and hip circumferences in an Asian population of youths: CASPIAN study. J Trop Pediatr. 2007;53(3):158–64.
17. O'Leary DH, Polak JF, Kronmal RA, Manolio TA, Burke GL, Wolfson SK Jr. Carotid-artery intima and media thickness as a risk factor for myocardial infarction and stroke in older adults. N Engl J Med. 1999;340(1):14–22.
18. Simon A, Megnien J-L, Chironi G. The value of carotid intima-media thickness for predicting cardiovascular risk. Arterioscler Thromb Vasc Biol. 2010;30(2):182–5.
19. Iannuzzi A, Licenziati MR, Acampora C, Salvatore V, Auriemma L, Romano ML, Panico S, Rubba P, Trevisan M. Increased carotid intima-media thickness and stiffness in obese children. Diabetes Care. 2004;27(10):2506 8.
20. Rathsman B, Rosfors S, Sjoholm A, Nystrom T. Early signs of atherosclerosis are associated with insulin resistance in non-obese adolescent and young adults with type 1 diabetes. Cardiovasc Diabetol. 2012;11:145. –
21. Urbina EM, Kimball TR, McCoy CE, Khoury PR, Daniels SR, Dolan LM. Youth with obesity and obesity-related type 2 diabetes mellitus

demonstrate abnormalities in carotid structure and function. Circulation. 2009;119(22):2913–9.
22. Elkiran O, Yilmaz E, Koc M, Kamanli A, Ustundag B, Ilhan N. The association between intima media thickness, central obesity and diastolic blood pressure in obese and overweight children: a cross-sectional school-based study. Int J Cardiol. 2013;165(3):528–32.
23. Reinehr T, Kiess W, de Sousa G, Stoffel-Wagner B, Wunsch R. Intima media thickness in childhood obesity: relations to inflammatory marker, glucose metabolism, and blood pressure. *Metabolism*. 2006;55(1):113–8.
24. Elshorbagy HH, Fouda ER, Kamal NM, Bassiouny MM, Fathi WM. Evaluation oF Epicardial fat and carotid intima-media thickness in obese children. Iran J Pediatr. 2016;26(1):e2968.
25. Melo X, Santa-Clara H, Pimenta NM, Carrolo M, Martins SS, Minderico CS, Fernhall B, Sardinha LB. Body composition phenotypes and carotid intima-media thickness in 11-13-year-old children. Eur J Pediatr. 2014;173(3):345–52.
26. Miniello VL, Faienza MF, Scicchitano P, Cortese F, Gesualdo M, Zito A, Basile M, Recchia P, Leogrande D, Viola D, et al. Insulin resistance and endothelial function in children and adolescents. Int J Cardiol. 2014;174(2):343–7.
27. Shah AS, Gao Z, Urbina EM, Kimball TR, Dolan LM. Prediabetes: the effects on arterial thickness and stiffness in obese youth. J Clin Endocrinol Metab. 2014;99(3):1037–43.
28. Hughan KS, Tfayli H, Warren-Ulanch JG, Barinas-Mitchell E, Arslanian SA. Early biomarkers of subclinical atherosclerosis in obese adolescent girls with polycystic ovary syndrome. J Pediatr. 2016;168:104–111.e101.
29. Eikendal AL, Evelein AM, Uiterwaal CS, van der Ent CK, Visseren FL, Bots ML, Hoefer IE, den Ruijter HM, Dalmeijer GW. Relation between circulating inflammatory chemokines and vascular characteristics in healthy, young children. J Am Heart Assoc. 2015;4(12).
30. Atabek ME, Pirgon O, Kivrak AS. Evidence for association between insulin resistance and premature carotid atherosclerosis in childhood obesity. Pediatr Res. 2007;61(3):345–9.
31. Marmot MG, Elliott P: Coronary heart disease epidemiology: from aetiology to public health: Oxford Medical Publications; 2005.
32. Freedman DS, Patel DA, Srinivasan SR, Chen W, Tang R, Bond MG, Berenson GS. The contribution of childhood obesity to adult carotid intima-media thickness: the Bogalusa heart study. Int J Obes. 2008;32(5):749–56.

24

Early features of Kawasaki disease with pyuria in febrile infants younger than 6 months

Seo Hee Yoon, Dong Soo Kim and Jong Gyun Ahn*

Abstract

Background: Children with Kawasaki disease (KD) and pyuria have been misdiagnosed with urinary tract infection (UTI). We compared clinical and laboratory features at admission between two groups of infants under 6 months of age who showed initial pyuria, to identify the initial clues suggestive of KD.

Methods: We retrospectively reviewed the medical records of children with fever who were under 6 months of age with pyuria, over a 10-year period (2007–2017). We included infants with sterile pyuria who were finally diagnosed with KD and those with UTI.

Results: During the period investigated, 12 (9.9%) KD patients with sterile pyuria and 378 infants with UTI were included in this study. Older age ($P < 0.01$), a longer duration of fever; total and before admission ($P < 0.01$), more negative nitrite test ($P < 0.01$), higher platelet count ($P = 0.04$), increased C-reactive protein (CRP) ($P < 0.01$) and erythrocyte sedimentation rate (ESR) ($P < 0.01$), were identified as initial features of infants finally diagnosed with KD. In the receiver operating characteristic analysis, optimal cut-off values of 509 k/μL for platelet count, 60 mg/L for CRP, and 68 mm/H for ESR were selected. Patients with ESR > 68 mm/hr had a ninefold higher odds of KD compared to those with lower ESR levels (odds ratio: 8.963, 95% confidence intervals: 1.936–41.493, $P = 0.005$), whereas CRP and platelet count could not significantly increase in the odds of KD at a cut-off point.

Conclusion: Persistent fever, elevated ESR, and negative urine nitrite test can serve as early clues to suspect KD in febrile infants with pyuria.

Keywords: Differential diagnosis, Fever, Infant, Kawasaki disease, Urinary tract infection

Background

Kawasaki disease (KD) is an acute systemic vasculitis of unknown aetiology that affects infants and young children [1]. KD is characterized by inflammation of all the medium-sized arteries and multisystem involvement including the kidney [2]. Renal symptoms in KD include pyuria, prerenal acute kidney injury, haemolytic uremic syndrome, acute nephritic syndrome, nephrotic syndrome, and renal tubular abnormalities [3]. Among them, pyuria is the most frequent renal feature of KD occurring in 30–80% of the patients [4].

Some KD children with pyuria have been mistakenly attributed to urinary tract infection (UTI) [5, 6]. In particular, as infants under the age of 6 months with KD showed higher rate of incomplete presentation as well as pyuria [2, 7–9] that is a significant laboratory marker of UTI with high occurrence rate in these ages [10], it is a diagnostic challenge to distinguish between UTI and KD with pyuria in infants aged < 6 month. Considering that patients with KD younger than 6 months are also known to have a higher risk of developing coronary complications [11, 12], it is necessary that clinicians, who evaluate febrile infant under 6 months of age with pyuria, do not miss the diagnostic potential of KD.

Therefore, it is crucial to find the initial differences among patients with UTI and KD with pyuria to identify KD in febrile infants with pyuria during the early phase

* Correspondence: JGAHN@yuhs.ac
Department of Pediatrics, Severance Children's Hospital, Yonsei University College of Medicine, 50-1 Yonsei-ro, Seodaemun-gu, Seoul 03722, South Korea

of the disease. We studied the clinical and laboratory parameters of infants under 6 months of age who showed fever and pyuria at admission, in order to find initial clues for the early detection of KD that would allow timely initiation of therapy.

Methods

We retrospectively reviewed medical records of patients under 180 days of age with fever and pyuria who were admitted to Severance Children's Hospital between January 2007 and January 2017. Among these patients, we included infants who were finally diagnosed as KD or UTI. Diagnosis of KD was based on American Heart Association guidelines [13]. We also included incomplete KD, which showed prolonged unexplained fever, fewer than four of the major clinical manifestations, and compatible laboratory or echocardiographic findings [2]. The definition of pyuria was based on urinary white blood cell (WBC) count > 5 cells/high power field (HPF) and sterile pyuria is defined as pyuria with a negative urine culture [14, 15]. The diagnosis of UTI was based on the culture of a single organism from a catheterized urine culture with a colony count greater than 10,000 or from a clean-catch midstream urine culture with greater than 100,000 colonies [15, 16]. Two or more bacterial species isolated by culture were excluded. We only included patients with KD and with sterile pyuria in the analysis. This study was approved by the Institutional Review Board of our institution (Severance Hospital, IRB number: 4–2017-1199).

Statistics

Demographic and clinical data are presented as median (range) or frequency. Initial laboratory test data at admission were analysed. Categorical variables were compared using chi-squared test or Fisher's exact test, and continuous variables were compared by Mann-Whitney test. To compare the predictive capacity of various laboratory tests for diagnosis of KD, receiver operating characteristic (ROC) curves were analysed by estimating the area under the curve (AUC). Optimal cut-off values in the diagnosis of KD were determined according to Youden index [17]. Patients were stratified into two groups according to optimal cut-off values for analyses. Logistic regression analyses were conducted using these groups (higher vs. lower than cut-off value) to estimate odds ratios and 95% confidence intervals. Statistical analyses were performed using SPSS version 23.0 for Windows (SPSS Inc., Chicago, IL, USA) and MedCalc Statistical Software version 18.6 (MedCalc Software, Ostend, Belgium). $P < 0.05$ was considered statistically significant.

Results

A total of 121 patients under 6 months of age were diagnosed with KD over the study period. Forty-one (33.9%) of the 121 KD children had pyuria. Of the 41 pyuria patients, 12 had sterile pyuria, 7 had concomitant UTI, and 16 had combined bacterial growth which had to be excluded. The other 6 patients were unidentified because they did not perform the urine culture tests. The clinical presentations of the 12 KD infants with sterile pyuria are summarized in Table 1. Two patients satisfied the diagnostic criteria of complete Kawasaki disease, whereas the others were diagnosed with incomplete Kawasaki disease.

During the same period, 378 infants under 6 months of age were diagnosed with UTI. Clinical and laboratory findings between KD infants with sterile pyuria and UTI infants were compared (Table 2). Median age of KD group (5.2 months; range, 2.5–5.9 months) was older than that of UTI group (median 3.6 months; range, 0.9–6 months) ($P = 0.002$). Male-to-female ratios in KD and UTI infants were 1.4 (7/5) and 2.8 (277/101), respectively.

KD group showed longer duration of fever (before admission and total) compared to UTI group ($P < 0.01$). KD group also showed a significantly higher platelet count ($P = 0.04$), C-reactive protein (CRP) level ($P < 0.01$), and erythrocyte sedimentation rate (ESR) ($P < 0.01$) than UTI group.

UTI group showed higher presence of positive urine nitrite test ($P < 0.01$). There were no significant differences in white blood cell count, absolute neutrophil count, haemoglobin, aspartate aminotransferase, alanine aminotransaminase, albumin, sodium, total bilirubin, and urine β2-microglobulin (β2-MG) (Table 2).

Table 1 Clinical characteristics of patients with Kawasaki disease with sterile pyuria

Variables	*n* (%) or median (range)
Typical KD/Atypical KD	2/10 (16.7%/83.3%)
Female/male	7/5 (36.1%/63.9%)
Age (months)	5.2 (2.5–5.9)
Total duration of fever (days)	5.5 (3–13)
Duration of fever before admission (days)	4.5 (2–9)
IVIG usage (times)	
1	11 (91.7%)
≥2	1 (8.3%)
Presence of coronary artery lesion (CAL)[a]	3 (25%)
Bilateral coronary ectasia	1 (8.3%)
Left main artery dilatation	1 (8.3%)
LAD dilatation	1 (8.3%)

KD Kawasaki disease, *IVIG* intravenous immunoglobulin, *LAD* left anterior descending coronary artery, Data are presented as case number, percentages or median (range)

[a]CAL is defined according to the Japanese Ministry of Health and Welfare guidelines

Table 2 Comparison between patients with Kawasaki disease and patients with urinary tract infection at admission

Parameter (Median, Range)	KD with Sterile Pyuria (n = 12)	UTI (n = 378)	P-value
Age (months)	5.2 (2.5–5.9)	3.6 (0.9–6)	.002
Male/Female	7/5	277/101	.321
Duration of fever (days)			
Before admission	4.5 (2–9)	2 (1–8)	.000
Total duration	5.5 (3–13)	2 (1–16)	.000
WBC (/μL)	17,620 (7180–26,820)	15,130 (3390–33,480)	.232
ANC (/μL)	9390 (4010–15,490)	8035 (100–25,150)	.159
Hb (g/dL)	10.8 (9.5–11.7)	10.9 (8.0–13.3)	.293
Platelet count (k/μL)	532.5 (315–772)	442.0 (162–1492)	.040
CRP (mg/L)	74.6 (31.6–294.5)	33.7 (0.3–191.9)	.001
ESR(mm/hr)	80.0 (27–101)	31.0 (2–120)	.000
Na (mmol/L)	137 (135–141)	138 (114–142)	.352
AST (IU/L)	30 (18–178)	28 (13–507)	.642
ALT (IU/L)	21 (7–53)	22 (7–460)	.658
Albumin (g/dL)	3.9 (3.2–4.7)	3.9 (3.0–4.9)	.903
Total bilirubin (mg/dL)	0.3 (0.3–1.5)	0.4 (0.1–7.1)	.546
Urine β2-MG (mg/L)	0.2 (0.14–0.98)	0.2 (0.01–40.06)	.484
Urine nitrite test (+)	0 (0%)	201 (53.2%)	.000

KD Kawasaki disease, *UTI* urinary tract infection, *WBC* white blood cell, *Hb* haemoglobin, *ANC* absolute neutrophil count, *CRP* C-reactive protein, *ESR* erythrocyte sedimentation rate, *Na* sodium, *AST* aspartate aminotransferase, *ALT* alanine aminotransaminase, β2-MG, β2-microglobulin. Data are presented as case number, percentages or median (range)

We calculated the optimal cut-off values of platelet count, CRP, and ESR for differentiating KD with pyuria from UTI, by drawing ROC curves (Fig. 1). The cut-off value of platelet count to predict KD with pyuria was 509 k/μL with 58.3% sensitivity, 76.5% specificity, 98.3% negative predictive value, and 7.3% positive predictive value (P = 0.064). The cut-off value of CRP was 60 mg/L with 66.7% sensitivity, 76.1% specificity, 98.6% negative predictive value, and 8.2% positive predictive value ($P < 0.001$). The cut-off value of ESR was 68 mm/H with 72.7% sensitivity, 85.3% specificity, 99.0% negative predictive value, and 13.8% positive predictive value ($P < 0.001$). The area under the curve (AUC) was 0.674 (95% confidence interval [CI]: 0.625–0.720, $P = 0.064$) for platelet count, 0.749 (95% CI: 0.703–0.791, $P < 0.001$) for CRP, and 0.846 (95% CI: 0.804–0.882, $P < 0.001$) for ESR. Subjects with ESR > 68 mm/hr had a nine-folds higher odds of KD compared to those with lower ESR level (odds ratio: 8.963, 95% confidence intervals: 1.936–41.493, $P = 0.005$) (Table 3).

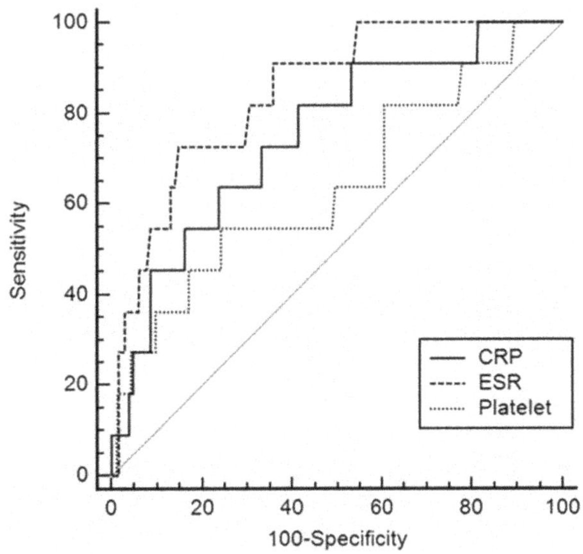

Fig. 1 Receiver operating characteristic (ROC) curves for C-reactive protein (CRP), erythrocyte sedimentation rate (ESR) and platelet count for discriminating Kawasaki disease with pyuria (n = 12) from urinary tract infection (n = 378). The area under the curve (AUC) was 0.674 (95% confidence interval [CI]: 0.625–0.720, $P = 0.064$) for platelet count, 0.749 (95% CI: 0.703–0.791, $P < 0.001$) for CRP, and 0.846 (95% CI: 0.804–0.882, $P < 0.001$) for ESR

Discussion

This study demonstrates that there are different initial features at admission between KD and UTI groups. Older age, longer duration of fever, higher platelet count, higher level of CRP and ESR, and more urine negative nitrite test were observed in KD group compared to UTI

Table 3 Odds ratios for diagnosis of Kawasaki disease using cut-off levels in febrile infants with pyuria

Variables	OR* (95% CI)	*P*-value
Platelet count (> 509 k μ/L)	2.299 (0.633–8.349)	.206
CRP (> 60 mg/L)	2.169 (0.523–8.998)	.286
ESR (> 68 mm/hr)	8.963 (1.936–41.493)	.005

OR odds ratio, *CI* confidence interval, *CRP* C-reactive protein, *ESR* erythrocyte sedimentation rate. Odds ratio, 95% confidence interval and *P* value were calculated by binary logistic regression analysis
*Higher vs. lower than cut off value

group. Our findings can provide early indicators for the early detection of KD in febrile infants with pyuria.

In the present study, the median age of KD group (5.2 months; range, 2.5–5.9 months) was older than that of UTI group (3.6 months; range, 0.9–6 months) ($P =$ 0.002). The age difference could be attributed to the fact that neonatal KD is extremely rare [18]. In a previous study, authors examined patients with KD younger than 6 months and reported that the median age was 5 months (range, 2–6) [12], or a mean age was 4.6 ± 3.5 months (range, 2–6) [7]. This is similar to the age range of the KD group in our results. Alternatively, the pooled prevalence rates of febrile UTI aged under 3 months ranges 7.5% (female) to 20.1% (uncircumcised males) [10]. Therefore, pyuria occurring in a febrile infant less than at least 2 months is more likely to be caused by UTI.

The diagnosis of KD is based on clinical criteria, but it could appear and progress in several days after onset of fever. Wu et al. [6] reported two cases of persistent fever and pyuria which were the initial presentation without signs suggestive of KD, and coronary artery abnormalities were noted in both cases. In our study, KD group showed longer fever duration of total and before admission compared to UTI group. In the infants under aged 6 months, prolonged fever might be the only clinical symptom of KD [2]. Thus, early suspicion of KD should be considered in any infant with prolonged fever and culture-negative pyuria.

The CRP, ESR, and platelet count were also higher in KD group than in UTI group in this study. Elevation of acute phase reactants such as CRP and ESR is characteristic laboratory findings of KD [2]. However, they are general indicators of an acute inflammatory process and also increased in UTI, especially upper UTI [19]. Thrombocytosis, classified as a secondary thrombocytosis, is also seen in the upper UTI as well as in KD [2, 20]. Gofrit et al. [21] reported thrombocytosis in a patient with upper UTI is not a random phenomenon, but a marker of kidney obstruction or perinephric abscess. Moreover, ESR > 68 mm/hr showed statistically significant increase in the odds of KD, whereas CRP and platelet count could not significantly increase in the odds of KD at a cut-off point in our study. Therefore, increased ESR itself could also be a good diagnostic marker for KD. However, the laboratory markers should be interpreted cautiously and used as a supportive method to diagnose patients KD using pyuria, in consideration of nonspecificity.

In urinalysis findings except for pyuria, urine nitrite test is helpful for diagnosis of UTI for its high specificity [22]. In this study, UTI group showed higher presence of positive urine nitrite test than KD group ($P < 0.01$). Among UTI patients, 53.2% had positive nitrite test but none in the KD infant. The findings suggest that urine nitrite test could be a useful marker to exclude KD if it is positive.

Sterile pyuria in KD was thought to be due to urethritis caused by a non-specific vasculitis of the urethra and/or the kidney as a result of mild and sub-clinical renal injuries [4, 23]. Urinary β2-MG is being used as a useful indicator to check the function of the renal-urinary tract. In our study, urinary β2-MG is not statistically different in KD and UTI groups. Choi et al. [24] reported that urine β2-MG was elevated in patients with KD and showed no difference between KD with pyuria and without pyuria groups. This result indicates the damage on renal function in most patients with KD.

A major limitation of our study is the small population size, which may have affected our statistical results. Future analysis, with a large sample size, is needed to verify the results of this study. Despite such shortcomings, our data can still provide information regarding initial indicators of KD in febrile infants with pyuria, which will be useful for clinicians.

Conclusions

Prolonged fever duration, elevated ESR, and negative urine nitrite test can serve as early clues to suspect KD in febrile infants with pyuria. Therefore, in patients presenting with these features as well as persistent fever despite appropriate antibiotic treatment for UTI, echocardiography is warranted to identify the possible presence of KD.

Abbreviations

AUC: Area under the curve; CI: Confidence interval; CRP: C-reactive protein; ESR: Erythrocyte sedimentation rate; HPF: High power field; KD: Kawasaki disease; OR: Odds ratio; ROC: Receiver operating characteristic; UTI: Urinary tract infection; WBC: White blood cell; β2-MG: β2-microglobulin

Acknowledgements

Not applicable.

Funding

This study has not been funded.

Authors' contributions
SHY primary responsibility for data collection, preliminary data analysis and writing the manuscript. DSK participated in the study design and data evaluation. JGA supervised the design and execution of the study, performed the final data interpretation and contributed the writing of the manuscript. All authors have read and approved the final manuscript.

Competing interests
The authors declare that they have no competing interests.

References

1. Burns JC, Glode MP. Kawasaki syndrome. Lancet. 2004;364(9433):533–44.
2. McCrindle BW, Rowley AH, Newburger JW, Burns JC, Bolger AF, Gewitz M, et al. Diagnosis, treatment, and long-term Management of Kawasaki Disease: a scientific statement for health professionals from the American Heart Association. Circulation. 2017;135(17):e927–e99.
3. Watanabe T. Kidney and urinary tract involvement in Kawasaki disease. Int J Pediatr. 2013;2013:831834.
4. Watanabe T. Pyuria in patients with Kawasaki disease. World J Clin Pediatr. 2015;4(2):25–9.
5. Ristoska-Bojkovska N, Stavric K, Tasic V. Kawasaki disease misdiagnosed as acute pyelonephritis. Pediatr Nephrol. 2003;18(8):851–2.
6. Wu CY, Hsieh KS, Chiou YH, Wang RS, Huang IF, Lee WY, et al. Prolonged fever and pyuria: a urinary tract infection presentation of incomplete Kawasaki disease. Acta Paediatr. 2005;94(3):375–7.
7. Chang FY, Hwang B, Chen SJ, Lee PC, Meng CC, Lu JH. Characteristics of Kawasaki disease in infants younger than six months of age. Pediatr Infect Dis J. 2006;25(3):241–4.
8. Yeom JS, Park JS, Seo JH, Park ES, Lim JY, Park CH, et al. Initial characteristics of Kawasaki disease with cerebrospinal fluid pleocytosis in febrile infants. Pediatr Neurol. 2012;47(4):259–62.
9. Liu HC, Lo CW, Hwang B, Lee PC. Clinical manifestations vary with different age spectrums in infants with Kawasaki disease. ScientificWorldJournal. 2012;2012:210382.
10. Shaikh N, Morone NE, Bost JE, Farrell MH. Prevalence of urinary tract infection in childhood: a meta-analysis. Pediatr Infect Dis J. 2008;27(4):302–8.
11. Rosenfeld EA, Corydon KE, Shulman ST. Kawasaki disease in infants less than one year of age. J Pediatr. 1995;126(4):524–9.
12. Yoon YM, Yun HW, Kim SH. Clinical characteristics of Kawasaki disease in infants younger than six months: a single-center study. Korean Circ J. 2016; 46(4):550–5.
13. Newburger JW, Takahashi M, Gerber MA, Gewitz MH, Tani LY, Burns JC, et al. Diagnosis, treatment, and long-term management of Kawasaki disease: a statement for health professionals from the committee on rheumatic fever, endocarditis, and Kawasaki disease, council on cardiovascular disease in the young, American Heart Association. Pediatrics. 2004;114(6):1708–33.
14. Hooker JB, Mold JW, Kumar S. Sterile pyuria in patients admitted to the hospital with infections outside of the urinary tract. J Am Board Fam Med. 2014;27(1):97–103.
15. Jan SL, Wu MC, Lin MC, Fu YC, Chan SC, Lin SJ. Pyuria is not always sterile in children with Kawasaki disease. Pediatr Int. 2010;52(1):113–7.
16. Robinson JL, Finlay JC, Lang ME, Bortolussi R. Urinary tract infections in infants and children: diagnosis and management. Paediatr Child Health. 2014;19(6):315–9.
17. Youden WJ. Index for rating diagnostic tests. Cancer. 1950;3(1):32–5.
18. Hangai M, Kubota Y, Kagawa J, Yashiro M, Uehara R, Nakamura Y, et al. Neonatal Kawasaki disease: case report and data from nationwide survey in Japan. Eur J Pediatr. 2014;173(11):1533–6.
19. Ayazi P, Mahyar A, Daneshi MM, Jahani Hashemi H, Pirouzi M, Esmailzadehha N. Diagnostic accuracy of the quantitative C-reactive protein, erythrocyte sedimentation rate and white blood cell count in urinary tract infections among infants and children. Malays J Med Sci. 2013;20(5):40–6.
20. Garoufi A, Voutsioti A, Getsi VC, Zeis P, Karpathios T. Platelet changes in urinary tract infections. Pediatr Res. 1999;45:903.
21. Gofrit ON, Shapiro A, Rund D, Verstandig AG, Landau EH, Katz R, et al. Thrombocytosis accompanying urinary tract infection suggests obstruction or abscess. Am J Emerg Med. 2006;24(1):118–21.
22. Roberts KB. Urinary tract infection: clinical practice guideline for the diagnosis and management of the initial UTI in febrile infants and children 2 to 24 months. Pediatrics. 2011;128(3):595–610.
23. Watanabe T, Abe Y, Sato S, Uehara Y, Ikeno K, Abe T. Sterile pyuria in patients with Kawasaki disease originates from both the urethra and the kidney. Pediatr Nephrol. 2007;22(7):987–91.
24. Choi JY, Park SY, Choi KH, Park YH, Lee YH. Clinical characteristics of Kawasaki disease with sterile pyuria. Korean J Pediatr. 2013;56(1):13–8.

25

A case of incomplete Kawasaki disease with extremely high serum ferritin and interleukin-18 levels

Takanori Noto[1,2], Hiroki Seto[1,2], Junji Fukuhara[1,2], Masao Murabayashi[1,2], Akihiro Yachie[3], Mamoru Ayusawa[2] and Ichiro Morioka[2*]

Abstract

Background: The clinical features and laboratory parameters of patients with Kawasaki disease (KD) and systemic juvenile idiopathic arthritis (sJIA) occasionally overlap. Therefore, serum levels of cytokine and ferritin are used as markers to distinguish between KD and sJIA. KD patients have a high level of interleukin (IL)-6, low level of IL-18, and no elevation of the level of serum ferritin. Conversely, sJIA patients have a low level of IL-6 and high levels of IL-18 and ferritin in the serum. However, to the best of our knowledge, no case report of KD with a low serum level of IL-6 and extremely high levels of IL-18 and ferritin is found.

Case presentation: A 6-year-old boy presented with a history of fever for 9 days and a rash that appeared 7 days from the onset. He was diagnosed with incomplete KD because of fever, skin rash, oral cavity erythematous changes, and erythema and edema of the hands with laboratory findings of serum albumin level < 3.0 g/dL, elevated alanine aminotransferase level and leukocyturia. Intravenous immunoglobulin and prednisolone and oral aspirin were introduced on the 10th day. Fever subsided 1 day after initiating the treatment, but arthritis of both knees appeared in addition to hepatosplenomegaly. We suspected sJIA, as the serum level of ferritin was 19,740 ng/mL, IL-6 was < 3 pg/mL, and IL-18 was 132,000 pg/mL. Skin desquamation of the fingertips was observed 18 days from the onset; thus, he was finally diagnosed with incomplete KD with arthritis. At 32 days from the onset, we stopped the prednisolone therapy and no symptoms of relapse were observed afterwards. In the follow-up at 16 months from the onset, he had neither signs of active joint or skin involvement, nor cardiac involvement.

Conclusions: Although patients with sJIA generally have high serum levels of IL-18 and ferritin, this was a case of incomplete KD with extremely high serum levels of IL-18 and ferritin. Serum cytokine and ferritin are often used for the differential diagnosis of KD and sJIA. We need to recognize the existence of KD with high serum levels of IL-18 and ferritin.

Keywords: Ferritin, Interleukin-6, Interleukin-18, Kawasaki disease, Systemic juvenile idiopathic arthritis

Background

Classic Kawasaki disease (KD) is clinically diagnosed based on the five following symptoms: the continuity of fever for at least 5 days, oral cavity erythematous changes (cracked lips, strawberry tongue), bilateral bulbar conjunctival injection, skin rash (maculopapular, diffuse erythroderma, or erythema multiforme-like), erythema and edema of the hands and feet, and cervical lymphadenopathy (usually unilateral) [1]. Incomplete KD has also been known as one type of KD, which is diagnosed based on fever more than 5 days with two or three of the five aforementioned symptoms or fever for ≥7 days without other explanations, and compatible laboratory or echocardiographic findings [1, 2]. Desquamation of the periungual region in the fingers usually begins in 2 to 3 weeks after the onset of fever. Some patients with KD develop arthritis, and the frequency of this condition is reported as 7.5–16% [2–4]. Systemic juvenile idiopathic arthritis (sJIA) is characterized by

* Correspondence: morioka.ichiro@nihon-u.ac.jp
[2]Department of Pediatrics and Child Health, Nihon University School of Medicine, 30-1, Oyaguchi, Kami-cho, Itabashi-ku, Tokyo 173-8610, Japan
Full list of author information is available at the end of the article

remitting fever, a typical skin rash, and arthritis. Diagnosis of sJIA is often challenging, particularly before patients have the symptoms for 6 weeks as shown by the International League of Associations for Rheumatology and American College of Rheumatology criteria [5]. Given that the clinical features, especially in arthritis, in patients with incomplete KD and sJIA sometimes overlap, cytokines [6–10] and ferritin [11] in serum are used as markers to distinguish KD from sJIA. KD patients have a high interleukin (IL)-6 level and low IL-18 and ferritin levels in their serum. Conversely, sJIA patients have a low IL-6 level and high IL-18 and ferritin levels [6–11]. Contrary to these facts, however, we report for the first time a case of incomplete KD with a low serum IL-6 level and extremely high serum IL-18 and ferritin levels with written informed consent from the parents of the patient.

Case presentation

A 6-year-old boy was referred to our hospital due to a 9-day history of fever. On day 3 of illness, a diffuse maculopapular rash appeared. He was orally treated with cefcapene pivoxil prescribed by his family pediatrician. On admission, his weight and height were 24 kg and 124 cm, respectively. He had a temperature of 38.9 °C and had a diffuse maculopapular rash. His lips, hands, and feet were erythematous. In addition, he also developed hepatosplenomegaly and had pitting edema in his feet. There was no history or findings of conjunctival injection and cervical lymphadenopathy.

His clinical course is shown in Fig. 1. Blood examination revealed the following: white blood cell count of 12,800/μL (neutrophils, lymphocytes, and monocytes were 88, 9, and 3%, respectively). C-reactive protein of 5.85 mg/dL; hemoglobin level of 11.7 g/dL; and platelet count of 26.6×10^4/μL. Other blood findings were as follows: serum albumin of 2.7 g/dL, total bilirubin of 0.7 mg/dL, sodium of 131 mEq/L, potassium of 3.1 mEq/L, aspartate aminotransferase of 100 IU/L, alanine aminotransferase of 87 IU/L, lactate dehydrogenase of 613 IU/L, and ferritin of 19,740 ng/mL. His urinalysis showed leukocyturia without any bacteria (10–14 white blood cells/high power field). His chest radiograph showed normal findings. Echocardiography revealed a normal ejection fraction, but perivascular echo brightness of the coronary arteries was found.

Given that his clinical symptoms did not fulfill the diagnostic criteria for classic KD, he was diagnosed with an incomplete KD according to the American Heart Association guideline [2]. Therefore, intravenous immunoglobulin (IVIG, 2 g/kg/dose), intravenous prednisolone (PSL, 2 mg/kg/day), and oral aspirin (30 mg/kg/day) were administered on the 10th day of illness. In addition to IVIG, PSL was used for his treatments to prevent coronary artery abnormalities based on the result of RAISE study [12]. His temperature returned to normal soon after the first IVIG therapy was completed. On the 12th day of illness, however, he showed symptoms of arthritis in both knee joints, which led to a gait disturbance. sJIA was suspected based on the appearance of arthritis and an extremely high level of serum ferritin. To distinguish KD from sJIA, serum IL-6 and IL-18 levels were examined during that time. The serum levels of IL-6 and IL-18 were extremely low and high, respectively (Fig. 1 and Table 1). Given the markedly elevated serum ferritin

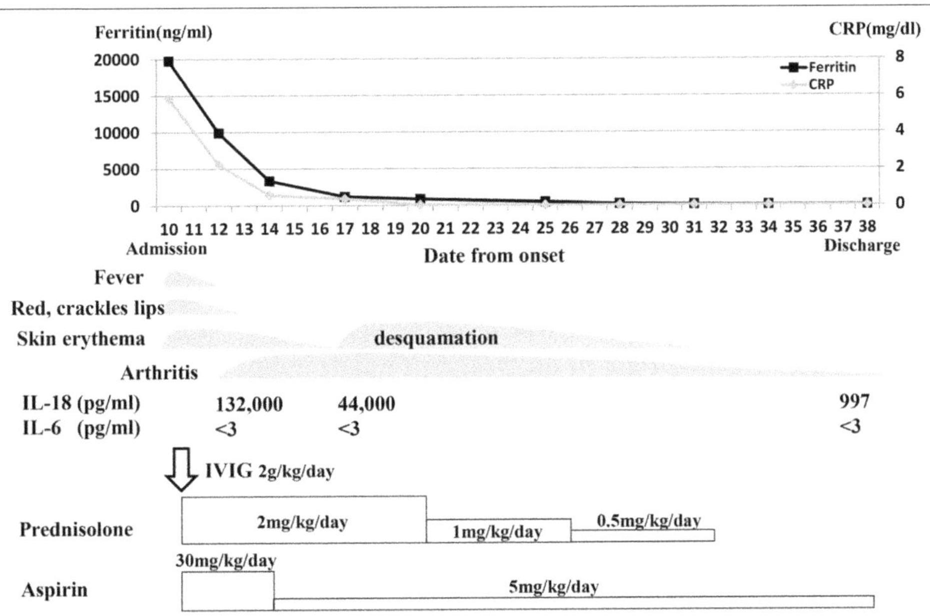

Fig. 1 Clinical course. CRP, C-reactive protein; IL, interleukin; IVIG, intravenous immunoglobulin

Table 1 Serum ferritin, IL-18, and IL-6 levels of our case and the reference levels

	Our case	KD	sJIA
Ferritin, ng/mL	19,740	14–2376	63–68,310
IL-18, pg/mL	132,000	260–660	10,860–330,000
IL-6, pg/mL	< 3	106–1200	7–580

The reference values of ferritin in KD and sJIA are from Mizuta et al. [11] and those of IL-18 and IL-6 are from Takahara et al. [7]
IL interleukin, *KD* Kawasaki disease, *sJIA* systemic juvenile idiopathic arthritis

and IL-18 levels, we suspected sJIA rather than incomplete KD. However, his rheumatoid factor and anti-nuclear antibody were negative. On the 17th day of illness, the elevated serum IL-18 level persisted (44,000 pg/mL) and his arthritis worsened. On the 18th day of illness, because skin desquamation of the fingertips occurred, he was diagnosed with incomplete KD. After the PSL treatment of 2 mg/kg/day for 11 days, PSL was tapered to 1 mg/kg/day for 5 days and then 0.5 mg/kg/day for 5 days. On the 32nd day of illness, the PSL treatment was discontinued, as his joint symptoms were markedly improved. After the aspirin treatment of 30 mg/kg/day for 5 days, aspirin of 5 mg/kg/day was discontinued after 2 months of the disease onset. On the 116th day of illness, serum IL-18 level returned to normal. At 16 months after the disease onset, he had never shown any signs of joint or skin involvement and cardiac abnormalities including coronary arteries.

Discussion and conclusions

The clinical features and laboratory findings in some patients with incomplete KD and other systemic inflammatory diseases such as macrophage activation syndrome or sJIA overlap. No cytopenia, hypertriglyceridemia and hypofibrinogenemia were found in his clinical course (serum triglyceride level of 217 mg/dL and plasma fibrinogen level of 323 mg/dL). There was no elevation of serum soluble interleukin-2 receptor level (344 U/mL). Based on these findings, because hemophagocytic lymphohistiocytosis was not suspected, a bone marrow examination was not performed for him. However, it has been reported that the patients who were considered as having refractory KD were finally diagnosed with sJIA [13]. Therefore, some serum markers have been proposed to distinguish KD from sJIA. Mizuta et al. reported that the serum ferritin level was significantly higher in sJIA patients than in KD patients, for which the cutoff value was 368.6 ng/mL [11]. In cytokines, the characteristics of serum markers in sJIA patients include significantly higher levels of IL-18 and lower levels of IL-6 than those in KD patients [6, 7, 9, 10]. In our case, because extremely high serum ferritin and IL-18 levels, unelevated IL-6 levels, and arthritic symptoms were observed during the clinical course (Table 1), sJIA was suspected. However, we finally diagnosed the patient with incomplete KD accompanied with arthritis, because of the following reasons. First, perivascular echo brightness of the coronary arteries was found. Second, a periungual desquamation was observed during the recovery phase (Fig. 1). Third, his arthritis improved within 6 weeks, and the sJIA criteria were not completely fulfilled [14]. Fourth, the IVIG treatment was effective. Fifth, the disease improved during PSL treatment, and no relapse was found after the dose of PSL was tapered. Finally, his clinical symptoms were different from those of sJIA, such as flares of clinical signs and intermittent fever with rash. He looked so sick and agitated during the disease period, although patients with sJIA look almost normal during the intermittent afebrile period.

In conclusion, patients with sJIA generally have high serum IL-18 and ferritin levels [6–11]. This was a case of incomplete KD with extremely high serum levels of IL-18 and ferritin, although KD patients with coronary artery lesions have been reported to have mild IL-18 elevations [15]. Serum cytokines and ferritin are often used for the differential diagnosis of KD and sJIA. However, we should need to recognize the existence of KD in patients with high serum IL-18 and ferritin levels. Further studies are needed about the novel biomarkers to clearly distinguish sJIA from KD at an early phase of the disease progression.

Abbreviations

IL: Interleukin; IVIG: Intravenous immunoglobulin; KD: Kawasaki disease; PSL: Prednisolone; sJIA: systemic juvenile idiopathic arthritis

Acknowledgments

This research is supported by Japan Agency for Medical Research and Development, AMED (grant number: 18kk0205014s2103) and the Kawano Masanori Memorial Foundation for Promotion of Pediatrics.

Funding

Not applicable.

Authors' contributions

All authors contributed to the intellectual content of this manuscript and approved the final manuscript as submitted. TN and IM drafted the initial manuscript. TN, HS, JF, and MM cared the patient and collected the clinical samples or data. AY measured serum cytokine levels for this patient. TN, MM, AY, MA, and IM interpreted the data. MA revised the article critically for important intellectual content.

Consent for publication

We obtained the written consent for publication from the guardian of the patient.

Competing interests

All authors have no conflicts of interest to declare for this work. Outside the submitted work, I.M. has received grants from Japan Blood Product

Organization, Daiichi Sankyo Co., Ltd., MSD Co., Ltd., AbbVie LLC, Taisho Toyama Pharmaceutical Co., Ltd., and Air Water Inc.; lecture fees from MSD Co., Ltd., Pfizer Japan, Inc., Novo Nordisk Pharma Ltd., Shionogi Co., Ltd., AbbVie LLC, Japan Vaccine Co., Ltd., Asahikasei Medical Co., Ltd., and Atom Medical Corp.; manuscript fees from Atom Medical Corp., Sanofi K.K., Asahikasei Medical Co., Ltd., and Japan Blood Product Organization,; and honoraria from Sanofi K.K.

Author details

[1]Department of Pediatrics, Numazu City Hospital, 550, Harunoki, Higashi-Shiroji, Numazu 4100302, Japan. [2]Department of Pediatrics and Child Health, Nihon University School of Medicine, 30-1, Oyaguchi, Kami-cho, Itabashi-ku, Tokyo 173-8610, Japan. [3]Department of Pediatrics, School of Medicine, Institute of Medical, Pharmaceutical and Health Sciences, Kanazawa University, 13-1, Takaramachi, Kanazawa 9208641, Japan.

References

1. McCrindle BW, Rowley AH, Newburger JW, Burns JC, Bolger AF, Gewitz M, et al. Diagnosis, treatment, and long-term management of Kawasaki disease: a scientific statement for health professionals from the American Heart Association. Circulation. 2017;135:e927–99.
2. Baker AL, Lu M, Minich LL, Atz AM, Klein GL, Korsin R, et al. Associated symptoms in the ten days before diagnosis of Kawasaki disease. J Pediatr. 2009;154:592–5.
3. Gong GW, McCrindlc BW, Ching JC, Yeung RS. Arthritis presenting during the acute phase of Kawasaki disease. J Pediatr. 2006;148:800–5.
4. Álvarez EP, Rey F, Peña SC, Rubio A, Calvo C, Collado P. Has articular involvement lessened in Kawasaki disease? Rheumatol Clin. 2017;13:145–9.
5. Stabile A, Avallone L, Compagnone A, Ansuini V, Bertoni B, Rigante D. Focus on juvenile idiopathic arthritis according to the 2001 revised Edmonton classification from the international league of associations for rheumatology. Eur Rev Med Pharmacol Sci. 2006;10:229–34.
6. Shimizu M, Yokoyama T, Yamada K, Kaneda H, Wada H, Wada T, et al. Distinct cytokine profiles of systemic-onset juvenile idiopathic arthritis-associated macrophage activation syndrome with particular emphasis on the role of interleukin-18 in its pathogenesis. Rheumatology. 2010;49:1645–53.
7. Takahara T, Shimizu M, Nakagishi Y, Kinjo N, Yachie A. Serum IL-18 as a potential specific marker for differentiating systemic juvenile idiopathic arthritis from incomplete Kawasaki disease. Rheumatol Int. 2015;35:81–4.
8. Xia Y, Cui P, Li Q, Liang F, Li C, Yang J. Extremely elevated IL-18 levels may help distinguish systemic-onset juvenile idiopathic arthritis from other febrile diseases. Braz J Med Biol Res. 2017;50:1414–31.
9. Nomura Y, Masuda K, Maeno N, Yoshinaga M, Kawano Y. Serum levels of interleukin-18 are elevated in the subacute phase of Kawasaki syndrome. Int Arch Allergy Immunol. 2004;135:161–5.
10. Maeno N, Takei S, Nomura Y, Imanaka H, Hokonohara M, Miyata K. Highly elevated serum levels of interleukin-18 in systemic juvenile idiopathic arthritis but not in other juvenile idiopathic arthritis subtypes or in Kawasaki disease. Arthritis Rheum. 2002;46:2539–41.
11. Mizuta M, Shimizu M, Inoue N, Kasai K, Nakagishi Y, Takahara T, et al. Serum ferritin levels as useful diagnostic marker for the distinction of systemic juvenile idiopathic arthritis and Kawasaki disease. Mod Rheumatol. 2016;26:929–32.
12. Kobayashi T, Saji T, Otani T, et al. Efficacy of immunoglobulin plus prednisolone for prevention of coronary artery abnormalities in severe Kawasaki disease (RAISE sturdy) : a randomized, open-label, blined-endpoints trial. Lancet. 2012;379:1613–20.
13. Rigante D, Valentini P, Onesimo R, Angelone DF, De Nisco A, Bersani G, et al. Incomplete Kawasaki syndrome followed by systemic onset juvenile idiopathic arthritis mimicking Kawasaki syndrome. Rheumatol Int. 2010;30:535–9.
14. Petty RE, Southwood TR, Manners P, Baum J, Glass DN, Goldenberg J, et al. International league of associations for rheumatology classification of juvenile idiopathic arthritis: second revision, Edmonton, 2001. J Rheumatol. 2004;31:390–2.
15. Wang KP, Hsieh KS, Huang SH, Ou SF, Lai TJ, Tang CW, et al. Interleukin-18 and coronary artery lesions in patients with Kawasaki disease. J Chin Med Assoc. 2013;76:438–45.

Parental anxiety related to referral of childhood heart murmur

Tonje Bårdsen[1*], Mari Hoven Sørbye[1], Håvard Trønnes[2,3], Gottfried Greve[1,4] and Ansgar Berg[1,3]

Abstract

Background: Detection of a heart murmur in healthy children is common, but may generate anxiety among parents. Many parents believe a heart murmur is a sign of heart disease, although the majority of heart murmurs are innocent. The purpose of this study was to assess anxiety and concerns in parents of children referred for evaluation of a heart murmur and to evaluate the effect of receiving a fact sheet about heart murmurs before the cardiologic consultation.

Methods: Parents of children referred for evaluation of a heart murmur responded to questionnaires assessing family and patient characteristics, parental concerns and anxiety. Anxiety was measured using the State Trait Anxiety Index (STAI) before and two weeks after the consultation. One third of the parents received a fact sheet before the consultation.

Results: Two hundred fifty-eight parents of 178 children participated. About 60 % of the parents had an increased level of anxiety before the consultation. The majority of the parents (71 %) had at least one major concern about heart murmurs in children, and having a concern was related to higher anxiety levels ($p = 0.02$). Anxious personality and lower education predicted an increased anxiety level. Before the consultation, parents who received a fact sheet presented a lower mean STAI state anxiety level (33.2) than those who did not (35.3), but the difference was not significant ($p = 0.09$). Fewer parents in the intervention group believed their child would have increased risk of heart disease later in life ($p = 0.04$) or that heart murmurs in children represents valvular-or congenital heart disease ($p = 0.02$). After the consultation, parental anxiety decreased from a mean STAI state of 34.9 to 30.6 ($p < 0.01$), and the mean STAI state scores were similar for the control and intervention group.

Conclusion: Parents with a child referred for a heart murmur presented a higher mean anxiety level than pre-school parents, and having an anxious personality, a major concern or low education predicted an increased anxiety level. After the consultation, parental anxiety decreased. Receiving a fact sheet about heart murmurs did not significantly reduce parental anxiety levels, but had a modest effect on concerns for the consequences of a heart murmur.

Keywords: Cardiology, Childhood, Heart murmur, Parental anxiety, Fact sheet

* Correspondence: tonje.bardsen@gmail.com
[1]Department of Clinical Science, University of Bergen, Bergen, Norway
Full list of author information is available at the end of the article

Background

Detection of a heart murmur in otherwise healthy children is common, but may generate parental anxiety. Many parents deem a heart murmur as a sign of structural heart abnormality despite the fact that most childhood heart murmurs are innocent and do not cause morbidity [1–7]. Previous studies have shown that parental concern is common and that parents may interpret a heart murmur as a condition that most likely implicates medication, surgery or restriction of physical activity [1, 2, 6]. We have in a previous study shown that only 10 % of Norwegian children referred to a paediatric cardiologist for evaluation of a heart murmur needed follow-up, medication or surgery [8]. Still, unwarranted parental anxiety may have consequences for the child. Bergman and Stamm [6] found that 40 % of healthy children whose parents at one point had perceived that their child had "something wrong with their heart" were restricted in some way.

Several studies have identified predictors for parental anxiety in general and parental anxiety related to referral for a heart murmur, including low education [3, 6, 9, 10], an anxious personality [1], being a mother [2, 9–11], not knowing what the term "heart murmur" means [7] and previous family history of heart disease [6], but few have assessed if parental concerns for the implications of a heart murmur (hereafter called "major concerns") predict anxiety [7].

It has been shown that examination and information by a paediatric cardiologist is an effective measure to ease anxiety and clarify misconceptions [1–4, 7], although some parents have persisting anxiety [1–5, 7]. A fact sheet with information about heart murmurs may contribute to ease parental anxiety as well as relieve major concerns, but to our knowledge, this has not previously been properly evaluated.

Our primary aims were to assess the level of anxiety among parents with a child referred for cardiologic examination of a heart murmur and to evaluate the effect of a fact sheet on anxiety levels. The secondary aims were to assess major concerns among the parents and to explore possible predictors for having an increased level of anxiety. We hypothesised that major concerns about heart murmurs increase anxiety and that parental concerns and anxiety levels would be reduced after receiving a written fact sheet about childhood heart murmurs compared to the control group.

Methods

Study design

The design of this study was part observational and part interventional. In the observational part, we explored anxiety levels using the State-Trait Anxiety Inventory (STAI), version X1, before and two weeks after the consultation. Parental concerns were assessed by different questions about the cause and consequences of heart murmurs in children. We also investigated possible predictors for increased anxiety levels and concerns. The intervention was a fact sheet on heart murmurs in children (Additional file 1), which was sent to the last one third of the parents (n = 70). Since all children underwent a cardiologic evaluation including an echocardiogram, this was not considered as an intervention.

Study population

All participants were recruited from the Outpatient Clinic at Haukeland University Hospital in Bergen, Norway in the period February 21st 2012 to October 29th 2013. The study subjects consisted of parents of children referred to a paediatric cardiologist for a first time evaluation of a heart murmur without other signs of cardiologic disease. Parents were invited to participate in the study if they were able to communicate and read Norwegian. If both parents were present at the consultation, both were included. We excluded parents who returned an incomplete questionnaire. Parents with more than one child referred for evaluation of a heart murmur were included only once. Inclusion of parents is shown in Fig. 1. All children were referred from a general practitioner or a paediatrician and were examined clinically and with echocardiography by an experienced paediatric cardiologist, to rule out the presence of a structural heart defect and to reassure the parents. All parents gave informed, written consent. The study was approved by the "Western Regional Ethics Committee, Norway", the regional committee for medical and health research ethics.

Data collection

Parental anxiety was assessed with the STAI in two questionnaires given to the parents before the consultation: one to complete prior to the consultation and the other 1–2 weeks later. In the first questionnaire we also assessed parental concern with different questions, and parents reported socio-demographic data and if they had a family history of heart murmurs or heart disease (Additional file 2).

Information on the children's demographic data and previous disease that caused hospitalisation was obtained from their hospital records. From this source, we also acquired the waiting time from referral to consultation, if the referring doctor was a general practitioner or paediatrician and the final diagnosis after the consultation.

The fact sheet was mailed to the last third of the recruited parents two weeks prior to the consultation. The fact sheet presented the most common causes of heart murmurs in children and emphasised the low risk of

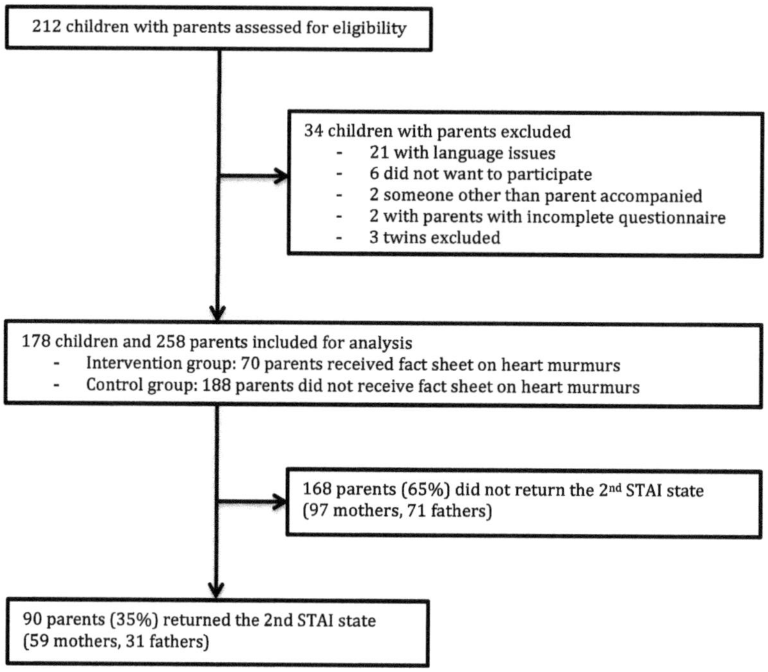

Fig. 1 Flow chart of inclusion of study group, intervention and response rate

having a serious heart condition with an isolated heart murmur (Additional file 1).

Outcomes

The primary outcomes of this study were anxiety levels measured by the STAI state [12], including anxiety levels before and after the consultation as well as with or without intervention. The STAI is a self-reporting questionnaire consisting of two parts: the STAI state and the STAI trait. The STAI state assesses anxiety at a particular moment in time and therefore it will vary depending on the situation. The STAI trait assesses general anxiety in a person and therefore it will be relatively stable over time, and independent of the situation. It is a validated and acknowledged tool for assessing anxiety in different populations and languages [12] and has been used in several studies on parental anxiety related to childhood heart murmurs and other health conditions in children [1, 7, 9–11, 13]. Each questionnaire consists of 20 statements with a scale ranging from 1 to 4. The level of anxiety is measured with scores ranging from 20 to 80 with higher scores correlating with higher levels of anxiety. We used a Norwegian version of the STAI, translated and validated by K. Håseth [14]. We assessed the STAI state level before and two weeks after the consultation. We also compared the STAI state levels between the control group who did not receive a fact sheet and the intervention group who did.

The secondary outcomes of this study were parent's major concerns on heart murmurs and what parents believed to be the most common cause of heart murmurs in children. We assessed parental concerns about heart murmurs with different questions regarding the relation between childhood heart murmurs and heart disease (Additional file 2). The questions were similar to statements used in previous studies [1–3], but they have not been validated. The questions were the following:

1. *What impact do you believe the heart murmur will have on your child's activity?*
2. *How serious is it to have a physiologic heart murmur?*
3. *To what degree do you believe your child has increased risk of heart disease later in life?*

The parents were asked to grade the different questions from 1 to 5 on a Visual Analogue Scale (VAS) with anchors (not at all-very much). The cut-off point for having a major concern was set to a score higher than 1.5 on the VAS, this point being measured with a ruler. The parents were also asked what they thought was the most common cause of heart murmurs in children, with the options being "natural phenomenon", "valvular heart disease", "heart attack", or "congenital heart disease". If the parent responded other than "natural phenomenon", it was also considered a major concern.

We considered socio-demographic factors, low education (12 years of education or less), previous hospitalisation of the child, family history of heart murmur or heart disease, major concerns about heart murmurs, long wait time and being referred by a general practitioner as opposed to a specialist as potential predictors for having an increased level of anxiety. We wanted to investigate the effect of seeking information on heart murmurs beforehand and how that would influence anxiety levels, and if there was a difference on the effect depending on the source (internet, friends/family, encyclopaedias or newspapers).

Data analysis

When comparing STAI state scores of different groups we used the variable as continuous. Comparisons of STAI state scores between mothers and fathers, responders and non-responders and control and intervention group, were carried out with Mann–Whitney *U* test. We used Wilcoxon signed-rank test to evaluate the parents' STAI scores before and after the cardiologic consultation. Comparisons of concerns in the control group and in the intervention group were performed with Chi-square tests.

We used a binary logistic regression model to identify potential predictors for increased anxiety levels. The STAI state scores were not normally distributed (Shapiro-Wilk statistic =0.952, *P* value <0.01), and were therefore used as a binary variable for this analysis. To our knowledge, there is no STAI state norm for parents of young children. However, a previous study reported a mean STAI state score of 31 for Norwegian parents of preschool children [11]. Since this study group was relatively comparable to ours, we defined a STAI state score of 31 as a cut-off point. Parents with a STAI state score less than or equal to 31 were defined as having a decreased level of anxiety and those with a score over 31 were defined as having an increased level.

Since more than one parent per child were included in the study group, some observations were not entirely independent. Therefore, we repeated all analyses with inclusion of only one parent per child. All statistical tests were two-sided with a significance level of 5 % and were performed with the use of SPSS statistics, version 20.

Results

Study population

Of 212 children who met with their parents for evaluation of an isolated heart murmur, a total of 258 parents of 178 children were included (Fig. 1). Of these, 90 parents (35 %) returned the second STAI questionnaire. Among the 70 parents who received a fact sheet about heart murmurs in children before the appointment, 27 parents (39 %) returned the second questionnaire. Characteristics of the study population are outlined in Table 1. The children were almost equally divided between boys and girls. The mean age was 3.5 years with an age range from 3 months to 15 years. There were no large

Table 1 Characteristics of parents and children participating in the study

Characteristics	Numbers (percent)
Parents *n* = 258	
Female gender	156 (61 %)
Both parents live with child	227 (88 %)
More than 12 years of education	148 (59 %)
Parent with more than one child	192 (74 %)
Family history of HD	64 (25 %)
Family history of HM	64 (25 %)
Looked up information on HM	113 (44 %)
Children *n* = 178	
Age (years, mean ± SD)	3.50 ± 3.03
Previous hospitalisation	55 (31 %)
General info	
Waiting time for consultation (months, mean ± SD)	2.50 ± 0.98
Referred by a specialist	40 (16 %)
Returned the second STAI questionnaire	90 (35 %)
Received informational sheet	70 (27 %)

Abbreviations: HD Heart disease, *HM* Heart murmur, *SD* Standard deviation, *STAI* State trait anxiety inventory

differences in parent and child characteristics, STAI scores between those who returned the second STAI questionnaire and those who did not (Additional file 3) or between the control and the intervention group (Additional file 4).

Anxiety level

The final STAI state and trait scores were obtained following the STAI manual [12]. Before the consultation, 42 % of the parents were in the decreased anxiety group (STAI state score ≤31) and 58 % in the increased anxiety group (STAI state score >31). The mean STAI trait and STAI state score of all parents before the appointment were 37.6 and 34.7, respectively. The mothers had a significantly higher mean STAI state score than the fathers (36.0 and 32.8, respectively, $p = 0.03$). The mean STAI trait score of the mothers (38.8) was also significantly higher than the fathers' (35.8) ($p = 0.01$). After restricting the analysis to include only one parent per child, the gender difference in mean STAI state score diminished, while the difference in STAI trait score remained unchanged.

Parents who received a fact sheet before the consultation had a lower level of anxiety (mean 33.2) than the control group (mean 35.3), but the difference was not significant ($p = 0.09$). Overall parental anxiety was significantly lower after the cardiologic examination, with a decrease in mean STAI state score from 34.9 to 30.7 ($p < 0.01$, Table 2). The post-consultation STAI scores were similar for those who received or did not receive

Table 2 Parental STAI state scores of responders (n = 90) before and after the consultation, Wilcoxon signed rank test

STAI State (mean ± SD)	Before consultation	After consultation	*P*-value
All n = 90	34.93 ± 9.57	30.67 ± 9.03	<0.01
Control n = 63	34.76 ± 9.84	30.75 ± 9.28	<0.01
Intervention n = 27	35.33 ± 9.23	30.48 ± 8.58	0.01

Abbreviations: SD Standard deviation, *STAI* State trait anxiety inventory

a fact sheet (Table 2). Restricting the analysis to only one parent per child did not substantially change the overall STAI state scores, and the comparison of the control and the intervention group was not meaningful due to small numbers.

Variables associated with increased anxiety

Predictors for an increased level of anxiety are displayed in Table 3. Parents who had major concerns about the implications of a heart murmur, with increased STAI trait scores or low education were more likely to have an increased STAI state score. Seeking information on heart murmurs beforehand, regardless the source, presented neither a lower nor a higher anxiety level than the others'. Furthermore, a family history of heart murmurs or heart disease, or previous hospitalisation of the child did not affect the anxiety level. Parental anxiety was not influenced by the wait time or if the referring doctor was a specialist. The estimates were practically similar after restricting the analyses to only one parent per child.

Table 3 Risk factors for an increased level of anxiety in parents (STAI score >31)

Characteristics	Odds ratio	95 % CI for OR	*P*-value
Parent			
STAI trait	1.24[a]	1.18–1.31	<0.01
Female gender	1.25	0.75–2.06	0.39
12 years education or less	2.53	1.49–4.32	<0.01
Parents live separately	1.87	0.79–4.41	0.16
Parent with only one child	1.17	0.64–2.12	0.61
Family history of HD	1.03	0.58–1.83	0.93
Family history of HM	0.92	0.54–1.56	0.75
Sought information on HM	1.49	0.90–2.46	0.12
Child			
Age over 2 years	0.96	0.58–1.58	0.86
Previous hospitalisation	1.13	0.65–1.96	0.66
General info			
Waiting time for consultation >2 months	1.02	0.62–1.67	0.95
Referred by a specialist	0.75	0.38–1.49	0.42
Did not received a fact sheet	1.46	0.84–2.53	0.18
Returned STAI after appointment	1.13	0.67–1.89	0.66
Concerns			
It is serious to have a physiological HM	2.72	1.59–4.65	<0.01
HM will restrict the Child's activity	3.13	1.65–5.91	<0.01
HM will increase risk of HD later in life	2.72	1.60–4.63	<0.01
Most likely cause of HM in children is CDH	1.75	1.01–3.03	0.05
Has a major concern	2.54	1.47–4.38	<0.01

Abbreviations: CHD Congenital Heart disease, *HD* Heart disease, *HM* Heart murmur, *SD* Standard deviation, *STAI* State trait anxiety inventory
[a]Odds ratio with increment of 1 STAI-trait score

Major concerns

Most parents (71 %) in our study had at least one major concern about their child's heart murmur. The most common concern was that this finding probably represented serious illness (57 %). Half of the parents (50 %) believed that their child would be at increased risk of heart disease later in life. Approximately one third (34 %) of the parents answered that a heart murmur is most likely caused by valvular-or congenital heart disease, and 26 % thought that the presence of a heart murmur would result in restriction of their child's physical activity. Analysis with only one parent per child showed similar results.

A comparison of the level of major concerns between the control and intervention group is presented in Table 4. Generally, the total level of major concerns was slightly lower in the intervention group (64 %) than in the control group (73 %), but the difference was not significant (p = 0.18). However, fewer parents in the intervention group believed that their child would have increased risk of heart disease later in life (p = 0.04) or that the most probable cause of heart murmur in children was valvular-or congenital heart disease (p = 0.02). Again, analysis of subgroups with restrictions of one parent per child provided no meaningful results.

A total of 18 (10 %) children were in need of a follow-up appointment and 14 children (8 %) were diagnosed with a congenital heart disease.

Discussion

The present study is the largest study that has assessed anxiety and concerns in parents of children referred for heart murmurs and the first to evaluate if a fact sheet about heart murmurs reduces anxiety and concerns in parents of children with a heart murmur.

We found that parents with a child referred for evaluation of a heart murmur presented an overall higher mean level of anxiety than previously reported for Norwegian parents of preschool children [11]. The parents who received an informational fact sheet on childhood heart murmurs had slightly, but not significantly, less concerns compared to the control group. There was no difference in anxiety levels. After the

Table 4 Comparing concerns in control group vs. intervention group. Parents have a major concern if score > 1.5 on VAS scale

Major concerns	Control group	Intervention group	*P* value
	n = 188	*n* = 70	
It is serious to have a physiological heart murmur	111 (59 %)	36 (51 %)	0.12
The heart murmur will restrict the child's activity	48 (26 %)	18 (26 %)	0.85
The child has increased risk of heart disease later in life	101 (54 %)	28 (40 %)	0.04
Most likely cause of heart murmur in children is structural heart disease	71 (38 %)	16 (23 %)	0.02
Total			
Has a major concern	137 (73 %)	45 (64 %)	0.18

cardiologic consultation, anxiety levels were similar in both groups and significantly lower than before the consultation. This suggests that thorough examination of the child and oral information from a cardiologist is reassuring for parents of a child with a heart murmur, as previous studies have showed [1–4, 7], whereas a fact sheet does not provide an additional benefit.

Predictors of increased anxiety levels were having major concerns about paediatric heart murmurs, an anxious personality, and low education. The association between low education and increased STAI state score has also been found in other studies [3, 9, 10]. In line with the STAI manual, an increased STAI trait score predicted an increased STAI state score [12]. A possible explanation is that people with anxious personalities are prone to respond to a stressful situation with anxiety. Unexpectedly, having a family history of heart disease or heart murmur did not influence the level of anxiety. We expected to find higher anxiety levels among parents with a family history of heart disease as shown by Bergman and Stamm [6], and lower anxiety levels among parents with family history of heart murmurs. Previous studies have reported that mothers have a significantly higher level of anxiety than fathers [2, 9–11], which is in accordance with our findings.

In our study, only 56 % of the parents could identify that the most common cause of heart murmur in children is a natural phenomenon. In accordance with our hypothesis major concerns and misconceptions among parents were predictors for an increased anxiety level. Parents who sought information about heart murmurs before the consultation had the same anxiety levels and rate of major concerns as other parents, which may indicate that self-attained information may be difficult to interpret and does not offer reassurance. It is thus possible that providing reliable information about heart murmurs to parents would reduce misconceptions and thereby decrease parental anxiety. Scanlon [15] tested if a fact sheet about innocent heart murmurs could be educative towards a group of parents of healthy children. The intervention group showed significant decrease in the number of parents with "harmful understanding" and "anxious" responses concerning innocent heart murmurs compared to the control group [15]. In the present study, however, a fact sheet did not significantly reduce anxiety and only had a modest effect on the parents' concerns.

Strengths of this study are a large sample size and an unselected study group. Our findings mostly correspond with previous studies from different countries [1–5, 15] and this suggests that the results may be generalised to different cultures and social groups. Our study group was quite evenly distributed regarding parental sex and education, whereas previous studies tend to have an overrepresentation of mothers [1, 2, 5, 7, 13]. Anxiety was assessed using the STAI-X1, which is a well-validated psychometric instrument that has been used in different populations, cultures and languages as well as in other studies measuring anxiety parental anxiety [1, 7, 9–14]. Our study was, to our knowledge, the first to evaluate the effect a fact sheet has on anxiety and concerns of parents with a child with a heart murmur.

An important weakness is the overall low response rate on the second STAI questionnaire (35 %). This has most likely hampered the power of the study, which may have led to a type II error. It is also possible that parents who were reassured were more likely to respond, resulting in a selection bias. If so, the observed reduction in STAI state score after the consultation may have been exaggerated. However, there were no substantial differences in characteristics or pre-consultation STAI-scores between responders and non-responders, suggesting that selection bias was less likely to be present. A weakness is also that the distribution of the fact sheets was not randomised, which theoretically could cause additional selection bias. Still, there was no reason to believe that parents of children referred in a specific period of time would differ from the control group. The selection of the intervention group may therefore be regarded as a proxy to randomisation. This notion is supported by the findings of similar characteristics in the two groups.

Another limitation is that more than one parent per child participated in almost half of the cases. This could have biased the results, since parents of the same child may present the same view. We pursued this possibility by restricting the analysis to one parent per child and found no large impact on the results. The statements regarding heart murmurs have not been validated, although variants of these have been used in previous studies [1–3]. Because of the lack of validation, the results concerning these statements must be interpreted with caution.

Setting a cut-off point of the STAI score also poses a challenge. The STAI score is a continuous variable, and it is therefore impossible to find an exact cut-off point that divides the population in two homogenous groups, as anxiety levels will vary in both groups. It is important to keep in mind that the STAI state score ranges from 20–80, and that a score >31 represents a higher score than the mean of parents of preschool children [11], and not necessarily a high level of anxiety. A certain level of anxiety may also be reasonable, since 8 % of the children in our study and 10 % in our previous study [8] were diagnosed with congenital heart disease.

Conclusion

Parents with a child referred for a heart murmur presented a higher mean anxiety level than previously reported for pre-school parents, and having a major concern, an anxious personality and a low educational level predicted an increased anxiety level. Receiving a fact sheet on heart murmurs had a modest impact on parental concerns, but the overall anxiety level was not significantly reduced. In contrast, parental anxiety was significantly reduced after the cardiologic consultation. This confirms that cardiologic evaluation and information is an important measure for reassuring these parents and suggests that receiving a fact sheet provides no substantial benefit.

Additional files

Additional file 1: Translated fact sheet: A translated version of the fact sheet that was distributed to 1/3 of the parents before the consultation.

Additional file 2: Translated questionnaire: the distributed questionnaire, translated from Norwegian.

Additional file 3: Comparison of characteristics between responders (*n* = 90) and non-responders (*n* = 168) of the second STAI questionnaire, table.

Additional file 4: Comparison of characteristics between control group (did not receive a fact sheet) and intervention group (received a fact sheet), table.

Abbreviations

STAI: State trait anxiety index; VAS: Visual analogue scale.

Competing interests

The authors declare that they have no competing interests.

Authors' contributions

TB participated in study design and conception, collected and analysed the data, interpreted the results and drafted the manuscript. MHS participated in study design and conception, collected and analysed data, interpreted the results and contributed to the manuscript draft. HT supervised the statistical analyses and revised the manuscript. GG participated in study design and conception, assisted with data collection and revised the manuscript. AB participated in study design and conception, assisted with data collection and revised the manuscript. All authors read and approved the final manuscript.

Acknowledgements

First of all we would like to express our gratitude to all the parents who participated in the study. We would also like to thank Stein and Kimberly Sorbye for valuable input on language editing. The study was funded by University of Bergen, Department of clinical science. No external funding was received.

Author details

2Department of Clinical Science, University of Bergen, Bergen, Norway. Department of Global Public Health and Primary Care, University of Bergen, Bergen, Norway. [3]Department of Paediatrics, Haukeland University Hospital, Bergen, Norway. [4]Department of Heart Disease, Haukeland University Hospital, Bergen, Norway.

References

1. Geggel RL, Horowitz LM, Brown EA, Parsons M, Wang PS, Fulton DR. Parental anxiety associated with referral of a child to a pediatric cardiologist for evaluation of a Still's murmur. J Pediatr. 2002;140(6):747–52.
2. Simunovic N, Roncevic Z. Innocent murmurs: parental viewpoint, what are the most common misconceptions and how to avoid them. Coll Antropol. 2010;34 Suppl 1:89–92.
3. McCrindle BW, Shaffer KM, Kan JS, Zahka KG, Rowe SA, Kidd L. An evaluation of parental concerns and misperceptions about heart murmurs. Clin Pediatr (Phila). 1995;34(1):25–31.
4. Advani N, Menahem S, Wilkinson JL. Innocent murmurs: the perception of the parents versus that of the child. Cardiol Young. 2002;12(6):587–8.
5. Young PC. The morbidity of cardiac nondisease revisited. Is there lingering concern associated with an innocent murmur? Am J Dis Child. 1993;147(9):975–7.
6. Bergman AB, Stamm SJ. The morbidity of cardiac nondisease in schoolchildren. N Engl J Med. 1967;276(18):1008–13.
7. Giuffre RM, Walker I, Vaillancourt S, Gupta S. Opening Pandora's box: parental anxiety and the assessment of childhood murmurs. Can J Cardiol. 2002;18(4):406–14.
8. Norgard G, Greve G, Rosland GA, Berg A. Referral practice and clinical assessment of heart murmurs in children. Tidsskr Nor Laegeforen. 2005; 125(8):996–8.
9. Skreden M, Skari H, Malt UF, Haugen G, Pripp AH, Faugli A, et al. Long-term parental psychological distress among parents of children with a malformation–a prospective longitudinal study. Am J Med Genet. 2010; 152A(9):2193–202.
10. Skreden M, Skari H, Bjork MD, Malt UF, Veenstra M, Faugli A, et al. Psychological distress in mothers and fathers of preschool children: a 5-year follow-up study after birth. BJOG-Int J Obstet Gy. 2008;115(4):462–71.
11. Skreden M, Skari H, Malt UF, Pripp AH, Bjork MD, Faugli A, et al. Parenting stress and emotional wellbeing in mothers and fathers of preschool children. Scand J Public Healt. 2012;40(7):596–604.
12. Spielberger CD. Manual for the State-Trait Anxiety Inventory STAI. Inc: Consulting Psychologists Press; 1983.
13. Botngard A, Skranes LP, Skranes J, Dollner H. Multimedia based health information to parents in a pediatric acute ward: a randomized controlled trial. Patient Educ Couns. 2013;93(3):389–93.

27

Universal screening for cardiovascular disease risk factors in adolescents to identify high-risk families

Michael Khoury[1], Cedric Manlhiot[1], Don Gibson[2], Nita Chahal[1], Karen Stearne[2], Stafford Dobbin[2] and Brian W. McCrindle[1*]

Abstract

Background: Universal screening of children for dyslipidemia and other cardiovascular risk factors has been recommended. Given the clustering of cardiovascular risk factors within families, one benefit of screening adolescents may be to identify "at-risk" families in which adult members might also be at elevated risk and potentially benefit from medical evaluation.

Methods: Cross-sectional study of grade 9 students evaluating adiposity, lipids and blood pressure. Data collected by Heart Niagara Inc. through the Healthy Heart Schools' Program. Parents completed questionnaires, evaluating family history of dyslipidemia, hypertension, diabetes and early cardiovascular disease events in parents and siblings (first-degree relatives), and grandparents (second-degree relatives). Associations between positive risk factor findings in adolescents and presence of a positive family history were assessed in logistic regression models.

Results: $N = 4014$ adolescents ages 14–15 years were screened; 3467 (86 %) provided family medical history. Amongst adolescents, 4.7 % had dyslipidemia, 9.5 % had obesity, and 3.5 % had elevated blood pressure. Central adiposity (waist-to-height ratio ≥0.5) in the adolescent was associated with increased odds of diabetes in first- (OR:2.0 (1.6–2.6), $p < 0.001$) and second-degree relatives (OR:1.3 (1.1–1.6), $p = 0.002$). Dyslipidemia was associated with increased odds of diabetes (OR:1.6 (1.1–2.3), $p < 0.001$), hypertension (OR:2.2 (1.5–3.2), $p < 0.001$) and dyslipidemia (OR:2.2 (1.5–3.2),$p < 0.001$) in first degree relatives. Elevated blood pressure did not identify increased odds of a positive family history.

Conclusions: Presence of obesity and/or dyslipidemia in adolescents identified through a universal school-based screening program is associated with risk factor clustering within families. Universal pediatric cardiometabolic screening may be an effective entry into reverse cascade screening.

Keywords: Obesity, Cardiovascular disease, Adolescent, Cardiometabolic risk factors, Cholesterol, Cross-sectional study

* Correspondence: brian.mccrindle@sickkids.ca
[1]Labatt Family Heart Centre, Department of Pediatrics, The Hospital for Sick Children, University of Toronto, 555 University Avenue, Toronto, ON M5G 1X8, Canada
Full list of author information is available at the end of the article

Background

Landmark autopsy studies have shown that, in children who died accidentally, there was an exponential increase in the extent of their atherosclerotic burden as the number of cardiovascular risk factors increased [1–4]. Many of these risk factors are modifiable, such as obesity, dyslipidemia, hypertension, and abnormal glucose metabolism including increased insulin resistance and diabetes. It has been well established that the presence of these risk factors in childhood increases the incidence of cardiometabolic disease in adulthood [5–7]. In addition, cardiovascular risk factors often cluster within members of families, with both genetic and common environmental/behavioral determinants [8, 9].

Amongst adults, those between 18 and 44 years old have the lowest health-care utilization [10], creating the potential for delayed identification and management of cardiometabolic risk factors and disease. Children, however, typically receive continuous medical care, and recent integrated guidelines have recommended universal lipid screening of pre-pubertal children [11]. Therefore, screening children for dyslipidemia and other cardiovascular risk factors may serve as an entry point to identifying at-risk family members. We sought to evaluate the association between pediatric cardiometabolic risk factors identified through universal school-based cardiometabolic screening and the presence of elevated cardiometabolic risk factors and cardiovascular disease (CVD) in family members.

Methods

We conducted a population-based cross-sectional study of grade 9 students (14–15 years old) in the Niagara Region of Ontario, Canada during the 2009–2010 school year. The study was undertaken in co-operation with Heart Niagara Inc. Healthy Heart Schools' Program. This curriculum enrichment program is designed to provide personalized education regarding cardiometabolic risk and healthy lifestyle behaviours, as well as individualized testing, to students in a classroom setting. The program annually targets the entire grade 9 population through their mandatory physical education class (the last school grade where such a mandate exists) in the geographically and administratively defined Niagara Region, Ontario. No students were excluded from participating in the screening. During the 2009–2010 school year, 4104 students participated. All parents of students were provided with questionnaires (described below). Data analysis included all participants who had participated in the screening and had completed the questionnaires. Adolescents presenting with adverse cardiovascular risk profiles were referred back to their primary care provider, where the whole family is encouraged to undergo screening, thus potentially providing a reverse cascade screening tool. The detailed methods of the Healthy Heart Schools' Program have been previously described [12]. Adolescents provided informed assent and parents/guardians provided written consent to participate in the assessment; the consent included a statement that the participant's deidentified data may be used for research purposes. Formal ethics approval was obtained by Heart Niagara, Inc. from the research ethics committees of both the Niagara Catholic District School Board and the District School Board of Niagara. The Hospital for Sick Children investigators were approved by Heart Niagara, Inc. for secondary use of deidentified data through a negotiated data-sharing agreement between Heart Niagara, Inc. and The Hospital for Sick Children.

Data collection

Heart Niagara Inc. staff performed all physical measurements during a scheduled assessment day during usual class time. Height and weight measurements were obtained in a standardized manner. Body mass index (BMI) was calculated (weight in kilograms divided by height in meters squared) and age- and sex-specific percentiles and z scores were determined using the 2006 World Health Organization growth standards [13]. Overweight was defined as a BMI between the 85th and less than the 95th percentile, and obesity was defined as a BMI greater than or equal to the 95th percentile [13]. Waist circumference was measured in a standardized manner, with land marking at the top of the posterior iliac crest with the subject standing. The waist-to-height ratio (WHtR, waist circumference divided by height) was calculated and classified into 3 categories: <0.5, 0.5–< 0.6, and ≥0.6. Previous studies have suggested that a WHtR above 0.5 may be an effective indicator of increased cardiometabolic risk [14–16]. The two remaining categories were based on the methodology of previous studies [17, 18].

Finger stick capillary samples were used to obtain nonfasting levels of total cholesterol (TC) and high-density lipoprotein cholesterol (HDL-C). From this, non-high-density lipoprotein cholesterol was calculated (non-HDL-C, TC minus HDL-C).

Blood pressure was evaluated in a standardized manner as previously described [12]. Systolic and diastolic measurements were converted to age-, sex-, and height-specific percentiles [19]. These values were used to classify the subjects as normotensive (<90th percentile), prehypertensive (90th–< 95th percentile), stage 1 hypertensive (95th–< 99th percentile), or stage 2 hypertensive (≥99th percentile) [19]. If initial measurements were at or above the 95th percentile, the measurements were repeated. If the second measurement was less than the 95th percentile, that value was used and no further blood pressure measurements were performed. However, if the second measurement was at or above the 95th percentile, 6 automated readings were taken at 1-min intervals and the average was calculated.

Students were provided with a questionnaire aimed at reporting whether first degree (siblings and parents) and second-degree relatives (grandparents) had a medical history of dyslipidemia, hypertension, diabetes mellitus, and a history of premature CVD. Premature CVD was defined as any male relative with a heart attack or stroke before 55 years and any female relative before 65 years [12]. The questionnaires were completed at home by the students with help from their parents (for family history questions) and submitted prior to the assessment day.

Data analysis

Data were analyzed and displayed as means with standard deviations and frequencies, as appropriate. Odds ratios with confidence intervals were used to assess associations between identified cardiometabolic risk factor in adolescents and a positive family history for cardiometabolic risk or early CVD. Only subjects with all completed measurements and a completed questionnaire were included in the analysis. Statistical analyses were performed using SAS statistical software version 9.3 (The SAS Institute, Cary NC).

Results

Enrollment in the school program for the study period was 4104 adolescents, of which 3467 (85 % of all registered grade 9 students, 50 % male, average age 14.6 ± 0.5 years) adolescents had family history data available. Table 1 shows the descriptive data for the grade 9 participants. Significant differences between male and female students were noted with BMI classification and lipid values. Family history data are shown in Table 2.

Forest plots depicting the odds ratios with confidence intervals for a positive family history of diabetes, dyslipidemia, elevated blood pressure, and/or premature CVD in first and second degree family members (based on parental reporting) for a given identified cardiometabolic risk factor in the adolescents are shown in Fig. 1. Adolescents with increased adiposity (BMI ≥95th percentile or WHtR ≥0.5) had increased odds of having a first- or second-degree family member with diabetes. WHtR showed greater odds ratios than BMI. Adolescents with

Table 1 Characteristics of the study population

Variable	Number	Male	Female	p
	3467	1718 (50 %)	1749 (50 %)	
BMI classification (World Health Organization)	3382			0.002
Underweight (<5th percentile)		36 (2 %)	32 (2 %)	
Normal weight (≥5th–<85th percentile)		1042 (62 %)	1157 (68 %)	
Overweight (≥85th–<95th percentile)		251 (15 %)	239 (14 %)	
Obese (≥95th percentile)		349 (21 %)	276 (16 %)	
Waist-to-height ratio	3382			0.24
<0.5		1324 (79 %)	1379 (81 %)	
0.5–< 0.6		281 (17 %)	266 (16 %)	
≥0.6		73 (4 %)	59 (3 %)	
Elevated blood pressure (maximum systolic/diastolic blood pressure)	3359			
Normal (<90th percentile)		1526 (91 %)	1544 (91 %)	0.46
Pre-hypertension (90–< 95th percentile)		76 (5 %)	91 (5 %)	
Stage 1 hypertension (95th–< 99th percentile)		52 (3 %)	44 (3 %)	
Stage 2 hypertension (≥99th percentile)		15 (1 %)	11 (1 %)	
Total cholesterol classification	3061			<0.001
Normal (<4.4 mmol/L)		1282 (84 %)	1122 (73 %)	
Borderline high (4.4–< 5.2 mmol/L)		191 (13 %)	323 (21 %)	
High (≥5.2 mmol/L)		50 (3 %)	93 (6 %)	
Low high-density lipoprotein (HDL-C) (<1.03 mmol/L)	3005	572 (38 %)	279 (18 %)	<0.001
Non-high density lipoprotein (non-HDL-C) classification	3061			0.001
Normal		1224 (80 %)	1149 (75 %)	
Borderline high (≥3.10 to <3.75 mmol/L)		196 (13 %)	268 (17 %)	
High (≥3.75 mmol/L)		103 (7 %)	121 (8 %)	

P values correspond to differences between males and females regarding classification distribution or prevalence of abnormalities

Table 2 Family history

	Number	Positive history (%)
Diabetes mellitus-1st degree	3296	291 (9 %)
Diabetes mellitus-2nd degree	3311	1457 (44 %)
Hypertension-1st degree	3229	702 (22 %)
Hypertension-2nd degree	3240	1956 (60 %)
Hyperlipidemia-1st degree	3193	618 (19 %)
Hyperlipidemia-2nd degree	3206	1670 (52 %)
Early atherosclerotic event	3467	1127 (34 %)

an elevated TC had increased odds of having a first-degree family member with diabetes, dyslipidemia or hypertension. Adolescents with an elevated non-HDL-C had increased odds of having a first-degree family member with diabetes, dyslipidemia, or hypertension, and a second-degree family member with diabetes. Adolescents with elevated blood pressure did not have increased odds of having a family member with a positive family history. None of the measured cardiometabolic risk factors in adolescents were significantly associated with increased odds of having a positive family history of premature CVD.

Discussion

The findings of our study indicate that cardiometabolic risk factors identified through universal school-based screening of adolescents is associated with the presence of risk factors in family members. The presence of dyslipidemia was associated with a positive family history of diabetes, dyslipidemia, and hypertension while the presence of increased adiposity was associated with a positive family history of diabetes. Adolescents with increased blood pressure measurements did not have increased odds of having family members with increased cardiometabolic risk factors. It should be noted that the elevated blood pressure measurements identified in a universal screening setting are not indicative of a diagnosis of hypertension. This may partially explain why no associations were seen in these subjects. Future studies are required to evaluate this further. No cardiometabolic risk factors in adolescents were associated with increased odds of an early CVD event in a family member. However, obesity, elevated WHtR, and dyslipidemia showed trends towards increased odds.

A number of studies have assessed the association between pediatric cardiometabolic risk factors and the presence of cardiovascular risk factors and disease in

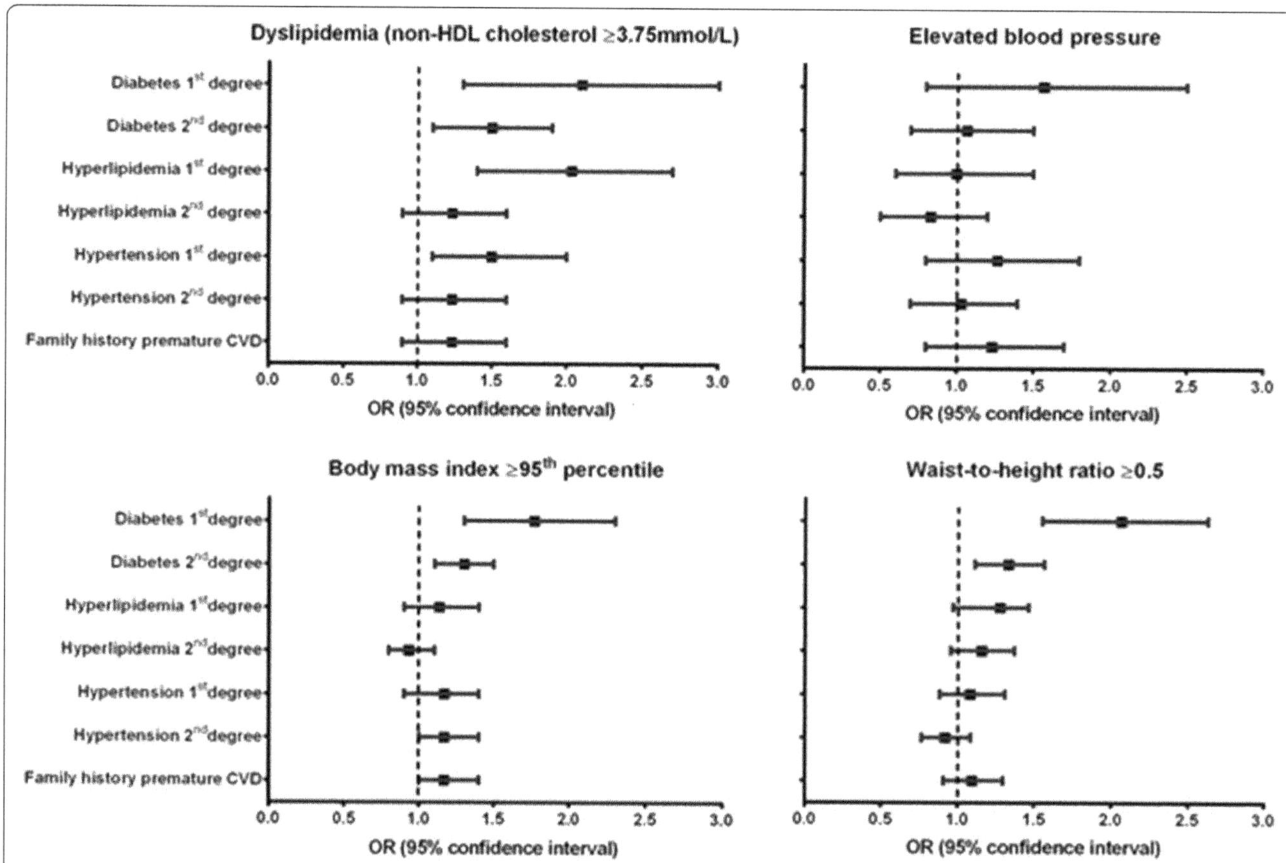

Fig. 1 Association between positive screening in the adolescent and odds of abnormalities in 1st and 2nd degree relatives

family members. Morrison et al.[20] recently evaluated the utility of risk factor screening in 5–19 year-old school children for predicting families at high risk for parental CVD, type 2 diabetes and high blood pressure 26 years later. They found the risk for CVD was greater if children had high TC (relative risk (RR) 1.30) or high low-density lipoprotein cholesterol (LDL-C) (RR 1.26) on screening. Risk for paternal type 2 diabetes was higher in families with pediatric high BMI (RR 1.53). Risk for parental high blood pressure was higher in children who were overweight (BMI ≥85th percentile, RR 1.23), had an elevated LDL-C (RR 1.15), or elevated blood pressure (RR 1.22). In addition, significant child-parent correlations for TC, HDL-C, LDL-C, and glucose were observed. This study concluded that identifying parents, initiated through screening of their children (reverse cascade screening), could possibly identify a cohort of young adults where interventions could be initiated to prevent later CVD, diabetes and hypertension. Our present study showed that parents of adolescents with cardiometabolic risk factors already have increased odds of silent (dyslipidemia and hypertension) and overt (diabetes) cardiometabolic disease. Therefore, not only are family members of children with cardiometabolic risk factors at increased risk of developing cardiometabolic disease in the future, they appear to be at increased risk of having cardiometabolic disease at the time of the school-based screening.

Reis et al.[21] found that parents of children who were obese or had an elevated waist circumference had about 6 times increased odds of having obesity or an increased waist circumference themselves, while children who had hypertension had 15 times increased odds of having a parent with hypertension. These are stronger associations than those observed in our study, possibly due to the small sample size (children and parents from 94 families) and a heterogeneous, high-risk population (52 % of subjects were overweight or obese, 33 % had an elevated waist circumference and 69 % were black). A German study [22] found that children with an elevated waist circumference had 2.55 times increased odds of having a parent with increased waist circumference, while children with elevated blood pressure did not have increased odds of having a parent with hypertension. A child with a raised non-HDL-C had 2.90 times increased odds of having a parent with an increased non-HDL-C. These results are generally similar to the findings in our study, with slightly greater odds ratio values. However, the results of this study may not be generalizable as it used a young (mean age 6.8 years), solely German population with a low incidence of obesity (4.5–4.9 % of children). In addition, similar to Reis et al.[21], this study focused on child-parent correlations for a given cardiometabolic risk factor, whereas our study assessed the odds of a positive family history of dyslipidemia, hypertension, diabetes, and premature CVD for each identified pediatric risk factor.

Muratova et al.[23] performed nonfasting lipid screening of 709 fifth grade children, with confirmation testing for those who screened positive. Of children with confirmed dyslipidemia, 66 % of their parents had confirmed dyslipidemia. The study may not be universally applicable as it took place in a high-risk area, with low education, low socioeconomic status, and low levels of cholesterol screening among adults. In addition, only 36 % of the children who screened positive had confirmatory testing due to logistical issues. Gidding et al.[24] and Polonsky et al.[25] have both shown that children with abnormal lipid levels have an increased incidence of having one or both parents with a lipid disorder. Two studies have shown an increased incidence of premature CVD in grandfathers of dyslipidemic children [26, 27].

Overall, our study shows similar trends to those noted in the literature outlined above, namely that children may be an effective proband for identifying parents and families at risk. However, there are some novel features and findings of the current study. First, our study was performed within an established universal screening program performed in a school-based setting with a large number of subjects. Second, our study assessed a self-reported history of established hypertension, dyslipidemia, and diabetes in family members, showing increased odds of manifest cardiometabolic disease in family members of children with cardiometabolic risk factors. Third, this study showed that children who screened positive for dyslipidemia had increased odds of having parents or siblings with dyslipidemia, hypertension, and diabetes. Identifying a raised risk profile of established cardiometabolic disease in parents and siblings of dyslipidemic children that is this broad is a significant finding. In addition, these results indicate that universal pediatric lipid screening may also identify family members with previously undiagnosed cardiometabolic disease, thus making it a potentially effective entry into reverse cascade screening. Further studies are needed to confirm this.

Recent guidelines [11] have recommended universal lipid screening of all pre-pubertal children between the ages of 9–11, with the aim of early identification of both dyslipidemia of obesity and genetic disorders of dyslipidemia, such as familial hypercholesterolemia (FH). This recommendation has been met with controversy and debate [28–30], with some concerns raised as to whether the available evidence justified the recommendation. The present study has shown a potential added benefit of universal lipid screening that may not have been considered previously: universal school-based lipid screening, when coupled with family history assessment, may identify risk factors clustering within families. Heterozygous FH is relatively common, with a prevalence of at least

1:500 in North America. If left untreated, approximately 25 % of females and 50 % of males will experience a CVD event by the age of 50 [31]. Lipid screening in children can potentially identify previously undetected FH, possibly creating the conditions for an effective and efficient public health initiative. As children typically have parents in an age cohort that typically does not partake in regular health-care visits, identifying children at risk may allow for early identification and intervention for both the child and the parents.

There are a number of limitations that should be considered when interpreting the results of this study. Given the cross-sectional design, only associations, but not causality, can be inferred. As data were collected within a universal screening program, family history data was obtained from questionnaires rather than direct detection of cardiovascular risk factors through measurement of family members. This does not allow for the detection of previously undiagnosed cardiometabolic risk factors or disease in family members. Given that previous studies have shown a large proportion of identified disease in family members to be previously undiagnosed [23, 24], the results of our study may be interpreted as conservative estimates of the true increased risk in family members. However, given that the family history information was obtained from a questionnaire, its accuracy cannot be ensured. In future studies it will be important to perform direct measurements on family members in order to detect previously undiagnosed cardiometabolic risk factors and disease. This will allow a stronger evaluation of the utility of universal pediatric screening as a reverse cascade-screening tool in the detection of cardiometabolic risk factors and disease in family members. Further, the ages of the parents, siblings, and grandparents were unfortunately not available. Ethnicity and pubertal staging data were unavailable. Morrison et al. had previously shown that pubertal status was not a significant explanatory variable for parental outcomes [20]. Finally, the Heart Niagara Inc. screening program currently screens grade 9 students. This is not in keeping with the current expert panel guidelines [11], which suggest the first screening in the pre-pubertal grade 5 population. Future school-based screening studies are needed in this younger population to help further validate the guidelines.

Conclusions

Adolescents who have cardiometabolic risk factors, identified through universal screening, have increased odds of having family members with diagnosed cardiometabolic risk factors and disease. This indicates that school-based cardiometabolic screening, along with family history assessment, may identify risk factor clustering within families. Future studies are needed to assess the effectiveness of screening pre-pubertal children to help validate recent expert panel guidelines. In addition, further studies are required to establish school-based cardiometabolic screening as an effective reverse cascade-screening tool to detect previously undiagnosed cardiometabolic disease in family members.

Abbreviations

BMI: body mass index; CVD: cardiovascular disease; HDL-C: high-density lipoprotein cholesterol; LDL-C: low-density lipoprotein cholesterol; non-HDL-C: non-high-density lipoprotein cholesterol; OR: odds ratio; RR: relative risk; TC: total cholesterol; WHtR: waist-to-height ratio.

Competing interests

The authors declare that they have no competing interests.

Authors' contributions

MK conceived the study, interpreted the data and drafted the manuscript. CM analyzed the data, interpreted the data and drafted the manuscript. DG conceived the study, collected the data and interpreted the data. NC and KS conceived the study, collected the data and interpreted the data. SD conceived the study, interpreted the data. BWM conceived the study, analyzed the data and interpreted the data. All authors read and approved the final manuscript.

Acknowledgements

This work was supported by the CIBC World Markets Children's Miracle Foundation Chair in Child Health Research and the Canadian Institute of Health Research Team Grant in Childhood Obesity.

Author details

[1]Labatt Family Heart Centre, Department of Pediatrics, The Hospital for Sick Children, University of Toronto, 555 University Avenue, Toronto, ON M5G 1X8, Canada. [2]Heart Niagara Inc., Niagara Falls, ON, Canada.

References

1. Newman 3rd WP, Freedman DS, Voors AW, Gard PD, Srinivasan SR, Cresanta JL, et al. Relation of serum lipoprotein levels and systolic blood pressure to early atherosclerosis. The Bogalusa heart study. N Engl J Med. 1986;314:138–44.
2. Berenson GS, Srinivasan SR, Bao W, Newman 3rd WP, Tracy RE, Wattigney WA. Association between multiple cardiovascular risk factors and atherosclerosis in children and young adults. The Bogalusa heart study. N Engl J Med. 1998;338:1650–6.
3. McMahan CA, McGill HC, Gidding SS, Malcom GT, Newman WP, Tracy RE, et al. PDAY risk score predicts advanced coronary artery atherosclerosis in middle-aged persons as well as youth. Atherosclerosis. 2007;190:370–7.
4. McMahan CA, Gidding SS, Malcom GT, Tracy RE, Strong JP, McGill Jr HC. Pathobiological determinants of atherosclerosis in youth risk scores are associated with early and advanced atherosclerosis. Pediatrics. 2006;118:1447–55.
5. Morrison JA, Friedman LA, Gray-McGuire C. Metabolic syndrome in childhood predicts adult cardiovascular disease 25 years later: the Princeton lipid research clinics follow-up study. Pediatrics. 2007;120:340–5.
6. Baker JL, Olsen LW, Sorensen TI. Childhood body-mass index and the risk of coronary heart disease in adulthood. N Engl J Med. 2007;357:2329–37.
7. Freedman DS, Khan LK, Serdula MK, Dietz WH, Srinivasan SR, Berenson GS. The relation of childhood BMI to adult adiposity: the Bogalusa heart study. Pediatrics. 2005;115:22–7.
8. Chen W, Srinivasan SR, Elkasabany A, Berenson GS. The association of cardiovascular risk factor clustering related to insulin resistance syndrome (syndrome X) between young parents and their offspring: the Bogalusa heart study. Atherosclerosis. 1999;145:197–205.
9. Chen W, Srinivasan SR, Bao W, Berenson GS. The magnitude of familial associations of cardiovascular risk factor variables between parents and offspring are influenced by age: the Bogalusa heart study. Ann Epidemiol. 2001;11:522–8.

10. Bernstein ABHE, Moss AJ, Allen KF, Siller AB, Tiggle RB. Health care in America: trends in utilization. National Center for Health Statistics: Hyattsville, Maryland; 2003.
11. Expert panel on integrated guidelines for cardiovascular health and risk reduction in children and adolescents. Summary report. Pediatrics 2011; 128(Suppl 5):S213-256.
12. McCrindle BW, Manlhiot C, Millar K, Gibson D, Stearne K, Kilty H, et al. Population trends toward increasing cardiovascular risk factors in Canadian adolescents. J Pediatr. 2010;157:837–43.
13. de Onis M, Onyango AW, Borghi E, Siyam A, Nishida C, Siekmann J. Development of a WHO growth reference for school-aged children and adolescents. Bull World Health Organ. 2007;85:660–7.
14. McCarthy HD, Ashwell M. A study of central fatness using waist-to-height ratios in UK children and adolescents over two decades supports the simple message–'keep your waist circumference to less than half your height'. Int J Obes. 2006;30:988–92.
15. Ashwell M, Hsieh SD. Six reasons why the waist-to-height ratio is a rapid and effective global indicator for health risks of obesity and how its use could simplify the international public health message on obesity. Int J Food Sci Nutr. 2005;56:303–7.
16. Hsieh SD, Muto T. The superiority of waist-to-height ratio as an anthropometric index to evaluate clustering of coronary risk factors among non-obese men and women. Prev Med. 2005;40:216–20.
17. Khoury M, Manlhiot C, McCrindle BW. Role of the waist/height ratio in the cardiometabolic risk assessment of children classified by body mass index. J Am Coll Cardiol. 2013;62:742–51.
18. Khoury M, Manlhiot C, Dobbin S, Gibson D, Chahal N, Wong H, et al. Role of waist measures in characterizing the lipid and blood pressure assessment of adolescents classified by body mass index. Arch Pediatr Adolesc Med. 2012;166:719–24.
19. National High Blood Pressure Education Program Working Group on High Blood Pressure in Children and Adolescents. The fourth report on the diagnosis, evaluation, and treatment of high blood pressure in children and adolescents. Pediatrics 2004; 114(2 Suppl):555–576.
20. Morrison JA, Glueck CJ, Wang P. The child as proband for future parental cardiometabolic disease: the 26-year prospective Princeton lipid research clinics follow-up study. J Pediatr. 2012;160:590–7. e593.
21. Reis EC, Kip KE, Marroquin OC, Kiesau M, Hipps Jr L, Peters RE, et al. Screening children to identify families at increased risk for cardiovascular disease. Pediatrics. 2006;118:e1789–97.
22. Schwandt P, Bischoff-Ferrari HA, Staehelin HB, Haas GM. Cardiovascular risk screening in school children predicts risk in parents. Atherosclerosis. 2009; 205:626–31.
23. Muratova VN, Islam SS, Demerath EW, Minor VE, Neal WA. Cholesterol screening among children and their parents. Prev Med. 2001;33:1–6.
24. Gidding SS, Whiteside P, Weaver S, Bookstein L, Rosenbaum D, Christoffel K. The child as proband. High prevalence of unrecognized and untreated hyperlipidemia in parents of hyperlipidemic children. Clin Pediatr. 1989;28:462–5.
25. Polonsky SM, Simbartl LA, Sprecher DL. Triglyceride and high-density lipoprotein cholesterol: predicting disorders in parents from their children. Pediatrics. 1994;94:824–31.
26. Moll PP, Sing CF, Weidman WH, Gordon H, Ellefson RD, Hodgson PA, et al. Total cholesterol and lipoproteins in school children: prediction of coronary heart disease in adult relatives. Circulation. 1983;67:127–34.
27. Schrott HG, Clarke WR, Wiebe DA, Connor WE, Lauer RM. Increased coronary mortality in relatives of hypercholesterolemic school children: the Muscatine study. Circulation. 1979;59:320–6.
28. Newman TB, Pletcher MJ, Hulley SB. Overly aggressive new guidelines for lipid screening in children: evidence of a broken process. Pediatrics. 2012; 130:349–52.
29. McCrindle BW, Kwiterovich PO, McBride PE, Daniels SR, Kavey RE. Guidelines for lipid screening in children and adolescents: bringing evidence to the debate. Pediatrics. 2012;130:353–6.
30. Gillman MW, Daniels SR. Is universal pediatric lipid screening justified? JAMA. 2012;307:259–60.
31. Kwiterovich Jr PO. Recognition and management of dyslipidemia in children and adolescents. J Clin Endocrinol Metab. 2008;93:4200–9.

28

Repeatability of echocardiographic parameters to evaluate the hemodynamic relevance of patent ductus arteriosus in preterm infants

Christoph E. Schwarz[1*], Antonio Preusche[1], Winfried Baden[2], Christian F. Poets[1] and Axel R. Franz[1,3]

Abstract

Background: The hemodynamically relevant patent ductus arteriosus in preterm infants is not well defined. Different clinical and echocardiographic parameters are used and the diagnostic accuracy is unknown because of the lack of a gold standard definition. Our study evaluates the inter-observer repeatability of echocardiographic and Doppler-ultrasound parameters.

Methods: This prospective observational study included 19 very low birth weight preterm infants (median [interquartile range]: gestational age 28.0 (28.0–29.0) weeks, birth weight 1130 (905–1321) g, postnatal age at measurement 8.7 (4.8–23.5) d) with a clinical suspicion of ductal patency in whom 27 repeated echocardiographic and Doppler-ultrasound examinations were performed within 30 min by 2 of 3 independent observers (54 measurements overall). The repeatability index (=2 times the standard deviation of the differences/mean of all measurements) according to Bland and Altman was used to assess repeatability of different parameters.

Results: The repeatability indices of the echocardiographic parameters (left Atrium-to-Aortic root-ratio, diameter of the patent ductus arteriosus at its narrowest part, the left-ventricular-preejection-period-to-ejection-time-ratio and the ratio of the velocity time integrals in the large vessels were 16, 21, 23 and 26 % respectively. The repeatability indices of Doppler-ultrasound measurements (resistance index in celiac artery and anterior cerebral artery) were 11 and 14 %, respectively.

Conclusions: The inter-observer repeatability of all echocardiographic parameters was poor compared to that of resistance indices in peripheral vessels. Therefore, interventions for ductal patency should be indicated based on averaged repeated rather than single measurements, especially when measured values are close to their cut-off value - both in clinical routine and for study purposes.

Keywords: Reproducibility, Doppler-ultrasound, Inter-observer

* Correspondence: c.schwarz@med.uni-tuebingen.de
[1]Department of Neonatology, University Children's Hospital of Tuebingen, University of Tuebingen, Calwerstr. 7, 72076 Tuebingen, Germany
Full list of author information is available at the end of the article

Background

The patent ductus arteriosus (PDA) in preterm infants is associated with increased mortality and morbidity [1–7]. However, there is little evidence as to which parameters define a PDA that requires treatment. Zonnenberg and de Waal showed that, besides clinical parameters, echocardiographic and Doppler-ultrasound measurements are used to evaluate the magnitude and clinical relevance of the left-to-right shunt through a PDA, and hence the need for treatment: In a systematic review of 67 randomised controlled trials (RCTs) they described the following most frequently used parameters and applied cut-off values: Left-atrium-to-aortic-root-ratio (LA/Ao-ratio) used in 34 trials, median cut-off >1.3 (range: 1.15–1.70); diastolic reverse flow in peripheral vessels (21 trials); and PDA-diameter (8 trials), cut-off >1.5 (1.5–2.0) mm [8]. McNamara and Sehgal suggested a scoring system including clinical and echocardiographic criteria to define hrPDA [9]. The echocardiographic part of this staging seems to be predictive for neonatal morbidity and can serve as a guide to clinical decisions [10], whereas the clinical criteria comprise unspecific respiratory signs. Prospective data suggesting that application of the echocardiographic parameters summarized by Zonnenberg and de Waal or the score by McNamara and Sehgal results in improved outcome is lacking. However, recent retrospective data suggest that echocardiographic screening for PDA within the first 3 postnatal days may reduce mortality in infants born at <29 weeks gestation [11].

To inform future studies and clinical guidelines on PDA treatment, this study aimed to evaluate the inter-observer repeatability of echocardiographic and Doppler-ultrasound parameters, which are frequently determined to assess the need for PDA treatment.

Methods

This prospective observational cohort study was approved by the research ethics committee at the facutly of medicine and the university hospital of the Eberhard Karls University Tuebingen and written informed parental consent obtained. To assess the repeatability of echocardiographic parameters commonly used to determine the magnitude of the left-to-right shunt, a convenience sample of preterm infants with suspected PDA was analysed. Inclusion criteria were: birth weight ≤1500 g and clinical suspicion of PDA such as cardiac murmur, bounding pulses, ventilator dependency and increased oxygen demand. Syndromal anomalies and congenital heart defects except persisting foramen ovale or atrial septal defect were exclusion criteria. The period of recruitment was between June 2012 and May 2013 at the Department of Neonatology, University Children's Hospital of Tuebingen, University of Tuebingen, Germany.

Within 30 min (to minimize fluctuations in hemodynamic status), 2 of 3 investigators (with more than 20, 10, or 3 years, respectively, of experience in neonatal echocardiography, everyday skills or every week, respectively, 2 were board certified paediatric cardiologists, one investigator is attending physician at the NICU) prospectively and independently performed repeated echocardiographic and Doppler-sonographic measurements including the following parameters:

LA/Ao-ratio [12]; resistance index (RI) in celiac artery (CA) [13] and anterior cerebral artery (ACA) [14]; diameter of the PDA at its narrowest part [15]; the left-ventricular-preejection-period-to-ejection-time-ratio, calculated by including 3–4 cardiac cycles (LVPEP/LVET) [16]; and the ratio of the velocity time integrals in the large vessels (VTI_Ao/VTI_Pa). The VTI_Ao was measured from an apical-5-chamber-view, the VTI_Pa was measured in a parasternal short axis calculated automatically with built-in software. We assumed that, in the absence of congenital heart defects, this ratio correlates with the ductal left-to-right shunt. The PDA-diameter was measured at its narrowest part (identified via colour Doppler) and measured in B-Mode to avoid the influence of gain-settings on the PDA-width if assessed on colour Doppler images.

All measurements were done with a Toshiba "Aplio" using a 6.5 MHz phased array transducer.

Statistical analyses involved repeatability coefficient (RepC = 2 times the standard deviation of the differences) and repeatability index (RepI = RepC/mean of all measurements) according to Bland and Altman [17] and a confidence-step-analysis (CSA) [18]. The RepC represents the upper limit of the 95 % confidence interval of the absolute differences between two measurements performed by two independent observers. The RepI describes the relation between RepC and the mean value of the measurements. This allows comparison of repeatability between different measures. A high CSA value (CSA = difference between lowest and highest value / RepC) indicates that differences between low and high values in this parameter observed in a given population are unlikely related to inter-/intra-observer variability, whereas a CSA of ≤1 indicates that observed differences between low and high values in this population are likely due to inter-/intra-observer variability.

For unexpected RepI differences, 95 % confidence intervals (CI) were exploratorily calculated post-hoc and differences between echo-parameters classified as 'significant' if these 95 %-CI did not overlap.

Data are shown as median (interquartile range).

Results

Twenty-seven repeated measurements were performed in 19 preterm infants. One infant with a birth weight of

1550 g was included inadvertently due to a weight at the time of measurement of 1465 g.

Gestational age at birth was 28.0 (28.0–29.0) weeks, birth weight 1130 (905–1321) g, postnatal age at measurement 8.7 (4.8–23.5) d and weight at the time of measurements 1243 (1024–1528) g. The mean difference in time between the first measurements of the repeated echocardiographic examinations was 12 min with a standard deviation (SD) of 4 min. The mean heart rate while recording left ventricular time intervals during all examinations was 167/min, and mean heart rate difference between repeated examinations was 2/min with a SD of 10/min. Arterial oxygen saturation was targeted at 90–95 % if on supplemental oxygen. Supplemental oxygen was necessary in 8 patients (respiratory support: 4 intubated and ventilated, 4 on binasal CPAP). Of 19 infants in room air, 5 were without respiratory support and 14 on binasal CPAP. No infant required catecholamines, and 3 had indomethacin within 24 h prior to measurements (0.1/0.2/0.4 mg/kg bodyweight/day, respectively).

A left-to-right shunt was identified by colour-Doppler-ultrasound in 15/27 measurements. PDA-diameter at the narrowest part could rarely be measured by both investigators ($n = 6$) because of difficulties visualizing the PDA in its complete course in B-mode (not colour Doppler-mode). The results are presented in Table 1.

Discussion

In general, a good diagnostic parameter can easily and quickly be determined and has high repeatability, sensitivity and specificity. Neonatal echocardiography can be performed easily and quickly to determine the need for treatment in preterm infants with PDA, however, the diagnostic accuracy is unknown because of the lack of a gold standard definition of a hrPDA.

Table 1 Repeatability Index (RepI), Repeatability Coefficient (RepC) and Confidence-Step-Analysis (CSA) values for Echocardiographic Parameters in Preterm Infants with Suspected Patent Ductus Arteriosus

Parameter	N	CSA	Repeatability Coefficient		Repeatability Index	
			RepC	95 % CI	RepI [%]	95 % CI
RI_CA	23	6.5	0.09	0.07–0.13	11	9–17*
RI_ACA	23	4.1	0.11	0.08–0.16	14	11–20**
LA/Ao	23	4.9	0.23	0.17–0.33	16	12–23
LVPEP/LVET	27	3.3	0.08	0.06–0.11	23	18–32
VTI_Ao/VTI_Pa	23	8.2	0.28	0.21–0.40	26	20–38
PDA - diameter	6	7.6	0.28	0.15–1.47	21	12–112

RI (resistance index) in CA (celiac artery) and ACA (anterior cerebral artery), LA/Ao-ratio (Left-atrium-to-aortic-root-ratio), LVPEP/LVET (left-ventricular-preejection-period-to-ejection-time-ratio), VTI_Ao/VTI_Pa (ratio of the velocity time integrals in the large vessels) and PDA diameter (patent ductus arteriosus); 95 % CI (95 % confidence interval) significantly smaller than RepI of LVPEP/LVET and VTI_Ao/VTI_Pa marked with " * ", "significantly" smaller than RepI of VTI_Ao/VTI_Pa marked with " ** "

This work on the largest cohort reported to date shows that repeatability of neonatal echocardiographic and Doppler-ultrasound parameters in preterm infants with suspected PDA is far from optimal. This is not due to a lack of expertise because our results are in the range of those few reports that previously addressed the issue of the repeatability of echocardiographic parameters in smaller cohorts (Table 2) [18–22]. However, as summarised in Table 2, of the parameters elected here, only the RI_ACA has previously been addressed in a repeatability study.

In fact, our protocol simulated a "best case scenario", as it evaluated repeated measurements by experienced investigators using the same ultrasound device within a short time interval on the same patient. Our study adds that the concerns regarding repeatability raised in the 1990s [18–22] are still relevant today despite improved ultrasound technology. Nevertheless, knowledge about the poor repeatability has not yet been taken into account in clinical treatment guidelines or current study protocols. The comparability and generalizability of results of data on echocardiography-guided PDA treatment are limited because of differences in the parameters applied and the poor reproducibility of all these parameters.

A large number of echocardiographic and Doppler-ultrasound parameters are used to quantify left-to-right shunt through, and hemodynamic relevance of, a PDA (summarised in [8]). These may include ductal flow pattern and velocity, absent or reverse diastolic flow in superior mesenteric artery, diastolic flow velocity in left pulmonary artery, reverse flow in descending aorta, and LVO/SVC-flow ratio (left ventricular output/superior vena cava-flow ratio). Some of these parameters may include redundant information [23], others, such as LVO/SVC-flow ratio, may not be trivial to measure, because of the complex cross sectional area of the SVC. Our selection of parameters reflects local preferences and was limited to reduce examination time and hence study-driven burden on the infants and subsequent fluctuations of their hemodynamic status in time.

In general, precision of a measurement with poor repeatability can be increased by averaging results of repeated measurements. In the context of this study, the effect of averaging measurements was cut-off dependent: Choosing, for example, cut-offs of >1.15, 1.3, 1.5, and 1.7 for the LA/Ao-ratio as the most frequently used parameter (i.e., cut-offs previously reported [8]) would result in $n = 22$, 16, 10 and 5, respectively, of the 27 episodes with at least one single-observer-measurement above the cut-off. In contrast, if only the mean of 2 measurements were considered, LA/Ao would

Table 2 Repeatability Index (RepI) of Echocardiographic Parameters in Paediatric Patients According to the Literature, [18–22]

author, year	N	Gestational age/Postnatal age		Birthweight		Parameter	RepI
		Mean (SD)/Median	Range	Mean (SD)/Median	Range		
Groves, 2008	9	28 w	27–30 w	1250 g	910–1900 g	diameter Aorta descendens	31 %
						VTI Aorta descendens	57 %
Skinner, 1996	26	34 w	26–40 w	2406 g	975–4480 g	PDA Vmax sys.	28 %
						PDA Vmean	36 %
Hudson, 1990	20	NR	27–43 w	NR	2380–4020 g	Ao Leading Edge to Leading Edge	10 %
Moorthy, 1990	12	"preterm"		NR		RI_ACA	20 %
van Dijk, 1996	44	8.4 (4.7) y		NR		RVPEP	17 %
						RVET	57 %

Abbreviations: *VTI* velocity time integral, *PDA* patent ductus arteriosus, *Ao* Diameter Aorta, *RI_ACA* resistance index in anterior cerebral artery, *RVPEP* right ventricular preejection period, *RVET* right ventricular ejection time, *w* weeks, *y* years, *NR* not reported

have been above the cut-off in 20, 15, 8 and 2 episodes, indicating that in 4–11 % of cases a treatment decision based on LA/Ao-ratio would have been changed by averaging results of only 2 repeated measurements.

Before embarking on this study, we assumed that the VTI_Ao/VTI_Pa-ratio might be another easily determined parameter suitable for quantifying ductal left-to-right shunt. Unfortunately, repeatability was similarly poor, presumably because this parameter required measurements in two different views (parasternal short axis and apical 5-chamber view) and VTI_PA was corrupted by the ductal jet (Fig. 1). It is also important to note that VTI_Ao/VTI_Pa-ratio may not accurately reflect the degree of shunt through a PDA because of inter-atrial shunting which is commonly observed in VLBW infants just like in our cohort (only 1 out of 19 infants had no inter-atrial shunting, no infant had a ventricular septal defect). This latter limitation also applies to more commonly used parameters such as the LA/Ao ratio. Furthermore, the assumption underlying the determination of VTI_Ao/VTI_Pa-ratio that the cross-sectional areas of P- and Ao-valve are similar may not applicable to all infants. However, despite poor repeatability, VTI_Ao/VTI_Pa had a high CSA-value, indicating a high potential in identifying inter-individual differences and consequently permitting accurate classification (Table 1). Similarly, determination of the PDA-diameter was challenging,

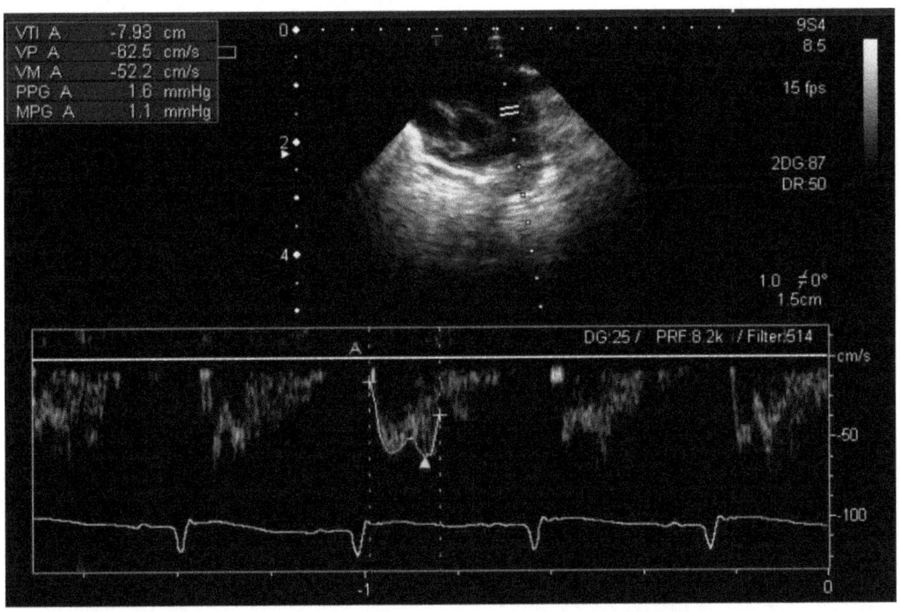

The pulsed-wave Doppler-sonographic measurement of VTI_Pa in a parasternal short axis view is corrupted by ductal jet extending to the pulmonary valve.

Fig. 1 Measurement of VTI_Pa in a parasternal short axis view. The pulsed-wave Doppler-sonographic measurement of VTI_Pa in a parasternal short axis view is corrupted by ductal jet extending to the pulmonary valve

because it requires visualisation of the PDA from the aorta to the pulmonary artery.

A limitation of our study is that extremely immature preterm infants with the highest risk of PDA are under-represented because we were hesitating to subject these most vulnerable infants during their first postnatal days to repeated measurements. Future studies need to assess intra-observer repeatability.

Conclusions

The repeatability of echocardiographic parameters to evaluate ductal left-to-right shunt is poor. The highest repeatability was achieved by RIs in ACA and CA. This has implications for clinical practice as well as the design of future studies on PDA treatment. In both settings, repeated measurements and averaging of results should be implemented, especially when measured values are close to their cut-off value.

Abbreviations

ACA: anterior cerebral artery; CA: celiac artery; CI: confidence interval; CPAP: continuous positive airway pressure; CSA: confidence-step-analysis; LA/Ao-ratio: left-atrium-to-aortic-root-ratio; LVO/SVC-flow: left -ventricular -output-to-superior -vena -cava-flow - ratio; LVPEP/LVET: left-ventricular-preejection-period-to-ejection-time-ratio; PDA: patent ductus arteriosus; RepC: repeatability coefficient; RepI: repeatability index; RI: resistance index; SD: standard deviation; VLBW: very low birth weight; VTI_Ao: velocity time integral ascending Aorta; VTI_Pa: velocity time integral pulmonary artery.

Competing interests

The authors declare that they have no competing interests.

Authors' contributions

CES has contributed to the design of the study, measurements, statistical analysis, has drafted the initial and the revised version of the manuscript. AP has contributed to the measurements, statistical analysis and writing of the manuscript. WB participated in the measurements and writing of the manuscript. CFP participated in the design of the study and critically reviewed the manuscript. ARF conceived of the study, and participated in its design, measurements, statistical analysis and coordination and helped to draft the manuscript. All authors read and approved the final manuscript.

Acknowledgements

We like to thank the "Else Kröner-Fresenius-Stiftung" for supporting this study.

Author details

[1]Department of Neonatology, University Children's Hospital of Tuebingen, University of Tuebingen, Calwerstr. 7, 72076 Tuebingen, Germany. [2]Department of Pediatric Cardiology, University Children's Hospital of Tuebingen, University of Tuebingen, Tuebingen, Germany. [3]Center for Pediatric Clinical Studies, University Children's Hospital of Tuebingen, University of Tuebingen, Tuebingen, Germany.

References

1. Cassady G, Crouse DT, Kirklin JW, Strange MJ, Joiner CH, Godoy G, et al. A randomized, controlled trial of very early prophylactic ligation of the ductus arteriosus in babies who weighed 1000 g or less at birth. N Engl J Med. 1989;320(23):1511–6.
2. Shortland DB, Gibson NA, Levene MI, Archer LN, Evans DH, Shaw DE. Patent ductus arteriosus and cerebral circulation in preterm infants. Dev Med Child Neurol. 1990;32(5):386–93.
3. Rojas MA, Gonzalez A, Bancalari E, Claure N, Poole C, Silva-Neto G. Changing trends in the epidemiology and pathogenesis of neonatal chronic lung disease. J Pediatr. 1995;126(4):605–10.
4. Evans N, Kluckow M. Early ductal shunting and intraventricular haemorrhage in ventilated preterm infants. Arch Dis Child Fetal Neonatal Ed. 1996;75(3): F183–6.
5. Kluckow M, Evans N. Ductal shunting, high pulmonary blood flow, and pulmonary hemorrhage. J Pediatr. 2000;137(1):68–72.
6. Oh W, Poindexter BB, Perritt R, Lemons JA, Bauer CR, Ehrenkranz RA, et al. Association between fluid intake and weight loss during the first ten days of life and risk of bronchopulmonary dysplasia in extremely low birth weight infants. J Pediatr. 2005;147(6):786–90.
7. Noori S, McCoy M, Friedlich P, Bright B, Gottipati V, Seri I, et al. Failure of ductus arteriosus closure is associated with increased mortality in preterm infants. Pediatrics. 2009;123(1):e138–44.
8. Zonnenberg I, de Waal K. The definition of a haemodynamic significant duct in randomized controlled trials: a systematic literature review. Acta Paediatr. 2012;101(3):247–51.
9. McNamara PJ, Sehgal A. Towards rational management of the patent ductus arteriosus: the need for disease staging. Arch Dis Child Fetal Neonatal Edition. 2007;92(6):F424–7.
10. Schena FFG, Cappelleri A, Picciolli I, Mayer A, Mosca F, Fumagalli M. Association between hemodynamically significant patent ductus arteriosus and bronchopulmonary dysplasia. J Pediatr. 2015;166(6):1488–92.
11. Rozé JC, Cambonie G, Marchand-Martin L, Gournay V, Durrmeyer X, Durox M, et al. Association between early screening for patent ductus arteriosus and in-hospital mortality among extremely preterm infants. JAMA. 2015; 313(24):2441–8.
12. Green TP, Thompson TR, Johnson DE, Lock JE. Furosemide promotes patent ductus arteriosus in premature infants with the respiratory-distress syndrome. N Engl J Med. 1983;308(13):743–8.
13. Shimada S, Kasai T, Konishi M, Fujiwara T. Effects of patent ductus arteriosus on left ventricular output and organ blood flows in preterm infants with respiratory distress syndrome treated with surfactant. J Pediatr. 1994;125(2): 270–7.
14. Martin CG, Snider AR, Katz SM, Peabody JL, Brady JP. Abnormal cerebral blood flow patterns in preterm infants with a large patent ductus arteriosus. J Pediatr. 1982;101(4):587–93.
15. Kluckow M, Evans N. Early echocardiographic prediction of symptomatic patent ductus arteriosus in preterm infants undergoing mechanical ventilation. J Pediatr. 1995;127(5):774–9.
16. Robel-Tillig E, Knupfer M, Pulzer F, Vogtmann C. Dopplersonographic findings in neonates with significant persistent ductus arteriosus. Z Geburtshilfe Neonatol. 2002;206(2):51–6.
17. Bland JM, Altman DG. Statistical methods for assessing agreement between two methods of clinical measurement. Lancet. 1986;1(8476):307–10.
18. Skinner JR, Boys RJ, Heads A, Hey EN, Hunter S. Estimation of pulmonary arterial pressure in the newborn: study of the repeatability of four Doppler echocardiographic techniques. Pediatr Cardiol. 1996;17(6):360–9.
19. Groves AM, Kuschel CA, Knight DB, Skinner JR. Echocardiographic assessment of blood flow volume in the superior vena cava and descending aorta in the newborn infant. Arch Dis Child Fetal Neonatal Ed. 2008;93(1):F24–8.
20. Hudson I, Houston A, Aitchison T, Holland B, Turner T. Reproducibility of measurements of cardiac output in newborn infants by Doppler ultrasound. Arch Dis Child. 1990;65(1 Spec No):15–9.
21. Moorthy B, Colditz PR, Ives KN, Rees DG, van't Hoff WG, Hope PL. Reproducibility of cerebral artery Doppler measurements. Arch Dis Child. 1990;65(7 Spec No):700–1.
22. van Dijk AP, Hopman JC, Klaessens JH, van der Werf T, Daniels O. Is noninvasive determination of pulmonary artery pressure feasible using deceleration phase Doppler flow velocity characteristics in mechanically ventilated children with congenital heart disease? Am J Cardiol. 1996;78(12): 1394–9.
23. Carmo KB, Evans N, Paradisis M. Duration of indomethacin treatment of the preterm patent ductus arteriosus as directed by echocardiography. J Pediatr. 2009;155:819–22.

29

Interrelationships between BMI, skinfold thicknesses, percent body fat, and cardiovascular disease risk factors among U.S. children and adolescents

David S. Freedman[1*], Cynthia L. Ogden[2] and Brian K. Kit[2]

Abstract

Background: Although the estimation of body fatness by Slaughter skinfold thickness equations ($PBF_{Slaughter}$) has been widely used, the accuracy of this method is uncertain. We have previously examined the interrelationships among the body mass index (BMI), $PBF_{Slaughter}$, percent body fat from dual energy X-ray absorptiometry (PBF_{DXA}) and CVD risk factor levels among children who were examined in the Bogalusa Heart Study and in the Pediatric Rosetta Body Composition Project. The current analyses examine these associations among 7599 8- to 19-year-olds who participated in the (U.S.) National Health and Nutrition Examination Survey from 1999 to 2004.

Methods: We analyzed (1) the agreement between (1) estimates of percent body fat calculated from the Slaughter skinfold thickness equations and from DXA, and (2) the relation of lipid, lipoprotein, and blood pressure levels to BMI, $PBF_{Slaughter}$ and PBF_{DXA}.

Results: $PBF_{Slaughter}$ was highly correlated ($r \sim 0.85$) with PBF_{DXA}. However, among children with a relatively low skinfold thicknesses sum (triceps + subscapular), $PBF_{Slaughter}$ underestimated PBF_{DXA} by 8 to 9 percentage points. In contrast, $PBF_{Slaughter}$ overestimated PBF_{DXA} by 10 points among boys with a skinfold thickness sum ≥ 50 mm. After adjustment for sex and age, lipid levels were related similarly to the body mass index, PBF_{DXA} and $PBF_{Slaughter}$. There were, however, small differences in associations with blood pressure levels: systolic blood pressure was more strongly associated with body mass index, but diastolic blood pressure was more strongly associated with percent body fat.

Conclusions: The Slaughter equations yield biased estimates of body fatness. In general, lipid and blood pressure levels are related similarly to levels of BMI (following adjustment for sex and age), $PBF_{Slaughter}$, and PBF_{DXA}.

Keywords: BMI, Skinfold thicknesses, Body fat, DXA, Children, NHANES

Background

The body mass index (BMI, kg/m^2) is widely used as a screening tool to identify obese children, and a high BMI in early life is associated with adverse levels of cardiovascular disease risk factors and the initial stages of atherosclerosis [1]. Although children and adolescents with a high BMI level also tend to have a high level of body fatness [2], BMI is composed of both fat mass and lean body mass, and it can be a poor indicator of fatness among those who have normal or relatively low levels of percent body fat [3, 4].

Despite the large measurement errors associated with skinfold thicknesses [5, 6], skinfold thicknesses are widely used among children and adolescents [7–9] to assess body fatness. Although several investigators have found the levels of percent body fat estimated from skinfold thickness equations [3, 10, 11] are more strongly correlated with more accurate estimates of body fatness than is BMI, this does not necessarily mean that skinfolds are better predictors of adverse levels of cardiovascular

* Correspondence: dxf1@cdc.gov
[1]Division of Nutrition, Physical Activity, and Obesity, Centers for Disease Control and Prevention, Atlanta, GA, USA
Full list of author information is available at the end of the article

disease (CVD) risk factors. Several studies of children and adults have found that BMI is as strongly associated with levels of lipids, blood pressure and insulin as are more accurate estimates of body fatness [12–20]. This similarity may result from the independent association of lean body mass to adverse levels of several CVD risk factors [15] or from the errors associated with either skinfold thickness measurements [5] or the equations that are used estimate body fatness [21].

We have previously reported that BMI and skinfold thicknesses were related similarly to levels of CVD risk factor levels among children and adolescents who in the Bogalusa Heart Study [19]. The objectives of the current study were to (1) assess the accuracy of the Slaughter skinfold thickness equations in the estimation of percent body fat ($PBF_{Slaughter}$) for levels of percent body fat calculated form dual energy X-ray absorptiometry (PBF_{DXA}), and (2) compare the magnitudes of the relations of levels of CVD risk factors to levels of PBF_{DXA}, $PBF_{Slaughter}$, and BMI levels among children and adolescents. These associations are examined among these 7599 8- to 19-year-olds who participated in the U.S. National Health and Nutrition Examination Survey (NHANES), 1999–2004.

Methods

Ethics statement

The procedures for NHANES were in accord with the ethical standards of CDC, and the protocols were approved by the National Center for Health Statistics Research Ethics Review Board. No approval was required for the current analyses, and the data are publicly available at http://www.cdc.gov/nchs/nhanes/nhanes_questionnaires.htm.

Study population

The 1999–2004 NHANES is a representative, cross-sectional sample of the U.S. civilian, non-institutionalized population. Parental permission was obtained for minors under the age of 18 years; 7- to 17-year-olds also provided documented assent. Consent was obtained for all adults, 18 years and older. Race and ethnicity were self-reported, and we classify subjects as non-Hispanic white, non-Hispanic black, Mexican American and other. The overall examination response rate for 6- to 19-year-olds in NHANES 1999–2004 was 85 % [22]. The current analyses included 7599 8- to 19-year-olds (see below).

DXA examinations

DXA scans were acquired in NHANES 1999–2004 for boys and non-pregnant girls who were at least 8 years of age using a Hologic QDR 4500A fan-beam densitometer (Hologic Inc., Bedford MA) [23, 24]. Scans were analyzed using Hologic Discovery software (version 12.1). Percentage body fat from DXA (PBF_{DXA}) was calculated as 100 × (DXA estimated total fat mass ÷ DXA estimated total mass).

We used the NHANES DXA Multiple Imputation Data Files [24] in the analyses. About 10 % of the children and adolescents in the current study were missing at least one DXA measurement, and because missingness was related to BMI and other characteristics, an analysis restricted to the non-missing values could be biased. The 1999–2000 DXA data for 8- to 17-year-old girls are available only in the Research Data Center, and these data are not used in the current analyses. We do, however, use the 1999–2000 data from 18- and 19-year-old girls. There were 7599 children and adolescents who had data for both PBF_{DXA} (either calculated or imputed) and BMI in the current study.

BMI and skinfold thicknesses

Body weight and height were measured using standardized techniques, and BMI (kg/m^2) was calculated as a measure of relative weight. BMI-for-age z-scores (SDs) and percentiles were calculated for each child based on the CDC Growth Charts [25]; these values express the BMIs of the examined 8- to 19-year-olds relative to their sex-age peers in the U.S. between 1963 and 1980. A child with a BMI-for-age ≥ 95th percentile of the CDC reference population is considered to be obese, and 120 % of the 95th percentile [26] is used as the cutoff for extreme obesity.

Because BMI z-scores based on the CDC growth charts have several limitations, including an upper limit of about 3.0 at most ages [27], several analyses are based on the residuals of regression models in which BMI was predicted by age (modeled using restricted cubic splines) within each sex. These residuals represent a child's BMI relative to other children of the same sex and age in the current study in kg/m^2 units (rather than as SD scores), and we refer to these values as 'adjusted BMI'. It has been shown [28] that BMI is preferable to BMI-for-age z-scores when examining longitudinal changes.

The thickness of the triceps and subscapular skinfolds were measured to the nearest 0.1 mm using Holtain skinfold calipers. These data were missing for about 7 % (subscapular) and 4 % (triceps) of children in the current study because of measurement difficulties. We used the *Amelia II* package in R [29, 30] to impute missing skinfold thicknesses from sex, race, age, BMI, PBF_{DXA}, and CVD risk factors. We used the logarithm of the skinfold thickness in the imputations to improve normality.

We estimated $PBF_{Slaughter}$ from equations in Slaughter et al. [31]. This set of equations incorporates linear and squared terms for the sum of the thicknesses of the subscapular and triceps skinfolds (SF sum), along with sex, maturation, and race (white/black) to estimate percent body fat. The intercepts and slopes of these equations differ by sex and SF sum; they also differ by maturation stage and race among boys who have a SF sum < 35 mm. As has been done in other investigations [7], we used the age of the child as a surrogate for sexual maturation: boys <12 y were considered pre-pubescent, those 12.0 to 13.9 y as pubescent, and those ≥ 14 y as post-pubescent. The equations for white boys were used to estimate percent body fat among all non-black boys.

Lipids and blood pressure

Serum levels of lipids and high-density lipoprotein (HDL) cholesterol were measured for NHANES participants aged ≥ 3 y [32, 33]. Fasting levels of triglycerides (TG) were available for participants aged ≥ 12 y who reported that they had fasted for 8.5 – 23 h before the morning examination [32]. For fasting TG levels <400 mg/dL, low-density-lipoprotein (LDL) cholesterol was calculated from the Friedewald equation [34]. Levels of TG were skewed and were log-transformed in all analyses.

Blood pressure measurements were taken in the mobile examination center after the participants rested quietly in a sitting position for 5 min. Three consecutive blood pressure readings were attempted, and if a measurement was interrupted or incomplete, a fourth attempt was made. The mean of these determinations was used to calculate blood pressure z-scores and percentiles relative to a child's sex, age and height [35].

Of the 7599 subjects who had data on BMI and PBF_{DXA}, 735 did not have a lipid measurement and 245 did not have a SBP or DBP. These subjects, along with an additional 153 children who reported being told that they had diabetes or were taking drugs that affect lipid or blood pressure levels, were excluded from the risk factor analyses. These exclusions resulted in the samples for the analyses of CVD risk factors consisting of 7311 (SBP and DBP), 6735 (TC), and 6733 (HDLC) subjects. Sample sizes for the analyses of fasting levels of TG and LDL-C were 2301 and 2291, respectively.

Statistical analyses

Analyses were performed using the *survey* and *mitools* packages in R [30, 36], and all analyses account for the sample weights, sample design and multiple imputations. NCHS provided 5 complete DXA Multiple Imputation Data Files [24], in which the missing DXA estimates were imputed using multiple imputation [37]. For the missing skinfold thickness data, we imputed 1 estimate in each of these 5 DXA datasets using information on sex, age, BMI, DXA measurements, non-missing skinfold values, sample weights and other characteristics; this yielded 5 datasets that had complete information for both the DXA and skinfold thickness measurements. We accounted for the uncertainty of the imputed values by analyzing each of the 5 datasets separately and then combining the results [38–41].

The agreement between levels of PBF_{DXA} and $PBF_{Slaughter}$ was assessed in Bland-Altman plots [42], in which the mean of the 2 estimates of percent body fat (x-axis) is plotted vs. the difference (y-axis: $PBF_{Slaughter}$ - PBF_{DXA}). We also examined levels of PBF_{DXA} and $PBF_{Slaughter}$ by sex and levels of the SF sum; 4 categories the SF sum (approximately the sex-specific 33rd, 67th and 90th percentiles) were used in these analyses. We used lowess which accounted for the sample weights, to graphically examine the relation of SF sum to levels of PBF_{DXA} and $PBF_{Slaughter}$. The y-axis of the lowess curves represents the mean of the estimated values over the 5 imputations.

We then examined the weighted correlations between BMI, $PBF_{Slaughter}$ and PBF_{DXA} with levels of the CVD risk factors. To control for the influence of age, these analyses used the residuals from sex-specific regression models in which each characteristic was regressed on age. The statistical significance of the observed differences (e.g., are levels of HDL cholesterol more strongly correlated with PBF_{DXA} than with adjusted BMI?) were based on jackknife replicate weights which were calculated using the 'withReplicates' function of the *survey* package [36]. Variances were then combined across the imputations.

Results

Various characteristics of the sample are shown among boys and girls in Table 1. About 18 % of the children were obese, with 6 % considered to be extremely obese (BMI ≥ 120 % of the CDC 95th percentile). Mean levels of the SF sum, PBF_{DXA} and $PBF_{Slaughter}$ were about 30 to 40 % higher among girls than boys ($p < 0.001$ for all comparisons). As seen in the final 2 rows of Table 1, the Slaughter estimate of percent body fat, however, substantially underestimated the mean PBF_{DXA} among both boys (by 4 percentage points) and girls (by 6 percentage points); $p < 0.001$ for both comparisons). Additional sex-specific analyses indicated that PBF_{DXA} was more strongly correlated with both $PBF_{Slaughter}$ and the SF sum ($r = 0.82$ to 0.86) than with BMI-for-age ($r = 0.75$ to 0.80). Whereas mean levels of PBF_{DXA} generally increased with age among girls, mean levels decreased among boys between the ages of 12 and 16 y (data not shown).

As seen in the Bland-Altman mean-difference plot (Fig. 1), the agreement between the Slaughter and DXA estimates of percent body fat varied substantially by the degree of body fatness. The largest underestimation of PBF_{DXA} occurred at low levels of body fatness. This underestimation decreased at higher levels of percent body fat, and at about 35 % (boys) and 45 % (girls) there

Table 1 Descriptive Characteristics of the Sample [a]

Characteristic	Boys ($n = 4493$)	Girls ($n = 3106$)
Race/Ethnicity		
Non-Hispanic White	61 %	62 %
Non-Hispanic Black	15 %	15 %
Mexican-American	11 %	11 %
Other	7 %	7 %
Age (y)	13.9 ± 0.1	13.9 ± 0.1
BMI (kg/m²)	21.8 ± 0.1	22.2 ± 0.2
BMI-for-age (z-score) [b]	0.46 ± 0.03	0.51 ± 0.04
Obese (%) [c]	18 ± 1	17 ± 1
Extreme Obesity (%) [c]	6 ± 1	6 ± 1
Subscapular skinfold thickness (mm)	9.1 ± 0.2	12.8 ± 0.3
Triceps skinfold thickness (mm)	11.2 ± 0.2	17.4 ± 0.3
Skinfold thickness sum (mm)	20.2 ± 0.5	30.8 ± 0.6
Slaughter estimated body fat (%)	21.1 ± 0.3	27.4 ± 0.3
DXA calculated body fat (%)	25.4 ± 0.2	33.3 ± 0.3

[a]Values represent prevalences or means (± SE). Because the skinfold thickness measures were skewed, values for these 3 variables represent estimates of the medians and their SEs
[b]Z-score (standard deviation score) of children relative to the 2000 CDC growth charts
[c]Obesity is defined as a BMI-for-age ≥ 95th percentile of the CDC reference population or a BMI ≥ 30 kg/m². Extreme obesity is defined as a BMI-for-age ≥ 120 % of the 95th percentile [26]

was little difference between the 2 estimates. Among children (particularly boys) who had higher levels of percent body fat, $PBF_{Slaughter}$ substantially overestimated PBF_{DXA}. Additional analyses, stratified by sex and age group (<12 y, 12 to 13.9 y, and ≥14 y) indicated that within each sex-age group, the overestimation of PBF_{DXA} by $PBF_{Slaughter}$ was most pronounce at low levels of body fatness, and the overestimation decreased as body fatness increased (data not shown).

We then examined differences between $PBF_{Slaughter}$ and PBF_{DXA} within strata of the SF sum (Table 2). At relatively low (below the 33rd percentile) levels of the SF sum (<17 mm, boys; <25 mm, girls), $PBF_{Slaughter}$ underestimated PBF_{DXA} by 8 to 9 percentage points. The magnitude of this difference decreased at higher SF sum levels, and for children in the highest SF sum category, $PBF_{Slaughter}$ overestimated PBF_{DXA} by about 10 percentage points among boys but only by 1.5 percentage points among girls.

Figure 2 shows the relation of the SF sum to levels of PBF_{DXA} for each child (points), along with the relation of the SF sum to both $PBF_{Slaughter}$ (dashed line) and PBF_{DXA} (solid line). As illustrated by the lowess curve (solid line), the association between SF sum and PBF_{DXA} was curvilinear, with the slope decreasing as the SF sum increased. In contrast, there were only small changes in the relation of SF sum to $PBF_{Slaughter}$ (dashed line), with the slope decreasing from 0.84 to 0.78 at a SF sum of 35 mm among white boys and from 0.78 to 0.55 among girls. These differences in the slopes of the 2 lines resulted in $PBF_{Slaughter}$ underestimating PBF_{DXA} among most children, but overestimating PBF_{DXA} among boys with a very high SF sum.

Table 3 shows mean levels of the CVD risk factors by sex and $PBF_{Slaughter}$ category. As $PBF_{Slaughter}$ increased, the prevalence of obesity varied from 0 to 58 % among boys and from 0 to 68 % among girls. Children in the highest $PBF_{Slaughter}$ group also had adverse levels of

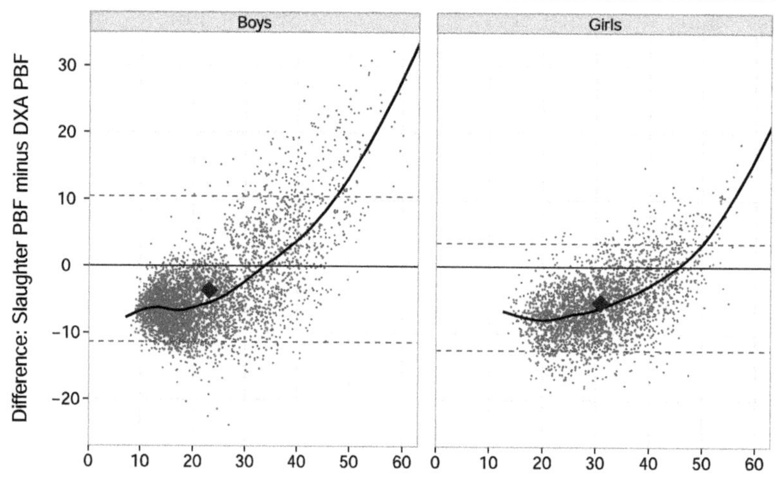

Fig. 1 Bland-Altman plot for the agreement between the DXA and Slaughter estimates of percent body fat. Eachpoint represents an individual children and the black line is the smoothed (lowess) curve. The overall medians are shown by the large diamonds, and the dashed lines represent the 95% CI for the agreement between the 2 methods; If the estimates for the 2 methods were identical, all points would fall along the y=0 line. The $PBF_{Slaughter}$ estimates appear to be biased, with $PBF_{Slaughter}$ underestimating PBF_{DXA} among most children, but overestimating PBF_{DXA} among the heaviest children, particularly among boys

Table 2 Levels of various characteristics within categories of the skinfold sum

Sex	SF Sum category (mm) [a]	N	Age[b]	% Obese	% Extreme Obesity	SF sum (mm)	$PBF_{Slaughter}$ [b]	PBF_{DXA} [b]	PBF Difference: Slaughter – DXA
Boys	<17	1548	13.3 ± 0.1	0	0	13.8 ± 0.1	11.2 ± 0.1	19.2 ± 0.1	−8.0
	17–27.4	1387	14.4 ± 0.1	2 ± 1	0	21.3 ± 0.2	17.8 ± 0.1	23.6 ± 0.2	−5.8
	27.5–49	1125	14.1 ± 1.5	38 ± 2	7 ± 1	36.6 ± 0.3	30.2 ± 0.2	32.2 ± 0.4	−2.0
	≥50	433	14.6 ± 0.2	92 ± 2	50 ± 4	60.1 ± 0.6	48.7 ± 0.6	38.9 ± 0.4	+9.7
Girls	<25	991	13.0 ± 0.1	0	0	18.9 ± 0.1	17.8 ± 0.1	26.6 ± 0.2	−8.8
	25–39	1090	14.6 ± 0.2	3 ± 1	0	31.9 ± 0.2	26.8 ± 0.1	33.3 ± 0.2	−6.4
	40–56	652	14.9 ± 0.2	38 ± 3	7 ± 2	47.1 ± 0.3	35.4 ± 0.2	39.3 ± 0.3	−3.9
	≥ 57	373	15.9 ± 0.3	87 ± 3	39 ± 4	67.1 ± 0.9	46.4 ± 0.5	44.8 ± 0.4	+1.5

[a]Cut-points for the SF sum categories approximately the 33rd, 67th, and 90th weighted percentiles within each sex
[b]Values are mean or prevalence ± SE within each SF sum category

PBF_{DXA} and the various CVD risk factors as compared to children in the lowest $PBF_{Slaughter}$ group. With the exception of DBP, all risk factor differences between the lowest and highest $PBF_{Slaughter}$ groups were statistically significant at the 0.01 level. Although the mean age of girls differed across the $PBF_{Slaughter}$ categories, additional adjustment for age substantially influenced only levels of DBP, reducing the magnitude of the difference from 3 to 1 mm Hg among girls.

Table 4 shows correlations between the levels of the various risk factors (columns) with levels of adjusted BMI, $PBF_{Slaughter}$, and PBF_{DXA}. (Regression models were used to adjust all characteristics for sex and age, and the values in the table represent the correlations between the residuals of these models.) With the exception of DBP, risk factor levels were significantly associated with the 3 body size measures. Furthermore, there was little difference in the relation of the 3 body size measures to levels of lipids and lipoproteins. For example, correlations with non-HDL cholesterol varied from $r = 0.31$ to 0.32 across the body size measure among boys and from $r = 0.19$ to 0.22 among girls.

There were, however, differences in the magnitudes of the associations with blood pressure levels. SBP levels were more strongly associated with adjusted BMI than with levels of $PBF_{Slaughter}$ or PBF_{DXA}; among boys, for example, the 3 correlations were $r = 0.32$ (BMI), 0.25 ($PBF_{Slaughter}$), and 0.27 (PBF_{DXA}); $p < 0.01$ for both comparisons with adjusted BMI. Although levels of DBP were only weakly ($r < 0.10$) associated with any of the anthropometric variables, the associations were stronger for $PBF_{Slaughter}$ and PBF_{DXA} than for adjusted BMI. Among girls, for example, the 3 correlations were $r = -0.01$ (BMI), $r = 0.08$ ($PBF_{Slaughter}$) and $r = 0.05$ (PBF_{DXA}).

There was also relatively little difference in the relation of the 3 body size measures to lipid and

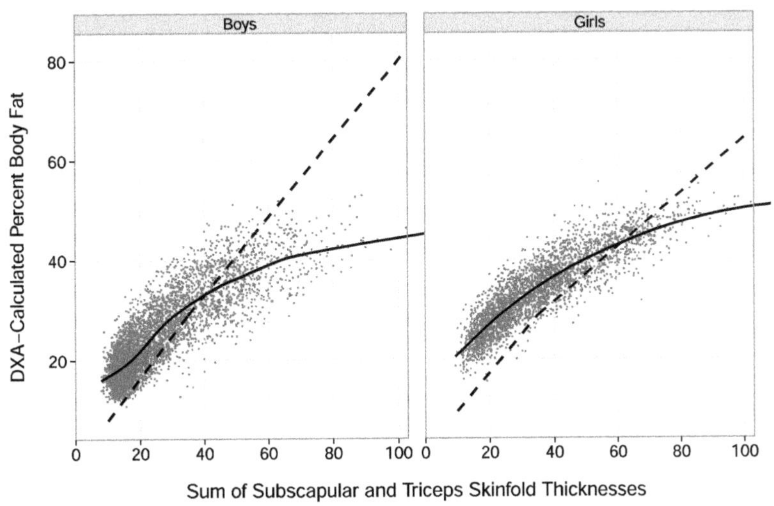

Fig. 2 The relation of the SF sum to levels of PBF_{DXA} for each child (points), along with the predicted relationship of the SF sum to PBF $_{Slaughter}$(dashed line) and PBF $_{DXA}$(solid line, lowess). For boys with a SF sum < 35 mm, the intercept of the SF sum vs. PBF $_{Slaughter}$ line varies by race and sexual maturation in the Slaughter equations,[26] and the illustrated line is for white, pubescent boys. Among pubertal (ages 12 to 13.9 y) boys who have a SF sum ≤ 35 mm, the estimated percent body fat is: -3.4 + 1.21*(SF sum) -0.008*(SF sum)2. For boys with a SF sum >35 mm, the equation is: 1.6 + 0.783*(SF sum) irrespective of pubertal stage

Table 3 Mean levels of obesity, body fatness, and CVD risk factors by categories of sex and percent body fat estimated from the Slaughter Equations

$PBF_{Slaughter}$ Category	N_{TC} [a]	Age (years)	Obese (%)	PBF_{DXA}	Total Cholesterol (mg/dL	Triglycerides (mg/dL)[b]	Non-HDL Cholesterol (mg/L)	LDL Cholesterol (mg/dL)	HDL Cholesterol (mg/dL)	N_{SBP} [a]	SBP (mm Hg)	DBP (mm Hg)
Boys												
<15 %	1703	14 ± 0.1[c]	0 [c]	19 ± 0.1	156 ± 1	69 (66, 72)	103 ± 1	86 ± 1	53 ± 0.6	1825	107 ± 0.4	58 ± 0.5
15 - 24.9 %	1143	14 ± 0.2	4 ± 1	25 ± 0.2	161 ± 1	78 (73, 84)	112 ± 1	94 ± 2	49 ± 0.5	1208	108 ± 0.4	58 ± 0.7
≥ 25 %	1193	14 ± 0.2	58 ± 2*	35 ± 0.3*	172 ± 2*	110 (101,119)*	127 ± 1*	102 ± 2*	44 ± 0.6*	1287	113 ± 0.5*	59 ± 0.6
Girls												
<25 %	1122	13 ± 0.1	0	28 ± 0.2	162 ± 1	72 (67, 77)	107 ± 1	89 ± 2	56 ± 0.5	1255	102 ± 0.4	59 ± 0.5
25 - 34.9 %	960	15 ± 0.2	11 ± 1	35 ± 0.2	165 ± 1	79 (73, 86)	113 ± 1	92 ± 2	52 ± 0.5	1056	106 ± 0.6	60 ± 0.5
≥ 35 %	614	15 ± 0.2	68 ± 4*	43 ± 0.4*	170 ± 2*	84 (76, 92)*	122 ± 2*	99 ± 3*	47 ± 0.6*	679	110 ± 0.5*	62 ± 0.6

[a] Ns in the column heading represent number of children with a non-missing value of that characteristic (total cholesterol or SBP). Ns for levels of TG and LDL-C, which required the child (age, 12–19 y) to be fasting, were about one third of the Ns for total cholesterol. The sample sizes for all risk factors are given in the Methods section

[b] Geometric means are shown for TG levels, which were log-transformed

[c] Values are mean or prevalence ± SE within each SF sum category

* $P < 0.01$ for difference in CVD risk factor level between lowest and highest $PBF_{Slaughter}$ categories based on linear or logistic regression models that controlled for age and 2-year cycle

lipoprotein levels in analyses stratified by race-ethnicity. As seen in Table 5, as compared with $PBF_{Slaughter}$ or PBF_{DXA}, BMI was more strongly associated with levels of HDL cholesterol among white non-Hispanics, and with levels of both total and non-HDL cholesterol among Mexican-Americans. However, among black non-Hispanic children, BMI showed a weaker association with levels of LDL cholesterol than did $PBF_{Slaughter}$.

Discussion

It is sometimes asserted that body fatness is the true outcome of interest in obesity research and that BMI is an inaccurate surrogate. Although BMI is an inaccurate index of body fatness among normal-weight children [3], the results of several studies indicate that BMI is, in general, as strongly associated with adverse levels of various CVD risk factors as are more accurate assessments of body fatness [13–18]. In the current, cross-sectional study of 8- to 19-year-olds in the U.S., $PBF_{Slaughter}$ estimates of body fatness were biased. $PBF_{Slaughter}$ underestimated DXA-calculated percent body fat among relatively thin children, but the extent of underestimation decreased at higher levels of body fatness. Among the heaviest boys, $PBF_{Slaughter}$ overestimated PBF_{DXA} by about 10 percentage points. Despite being less strongly associated with PBF_{DXA} than was $PBF_{Slaughter}$, we found that adjusted levels of BMI were, in general, as strongly associated with levels of lipids and lipoproteins as was either $PBF_{Slaughter}$ or PBF_{DXA}. SBP levels, however, were more strongly associated with BMI, while the weaker associations ($r < 0.10$) with DBP levels were stronger for $PBF_{Slaughter}$ and PBF_{DXA}. These results are similar to our previous findings concerning among children in the Bogalusa Heart Study and the Pediatric Rosetta Body Composition Project [19].

In general, skinfold thicknesses (and estimates derived from them) are more strongly correlated with body fatness than is BMI, but some of the observed differences have been relatively small [3, 43]. Furthermore, the accuracy of skinfold thickness estimates of body fatness likely varies across skinfold sites and equations [21], in part due to differences in the distribution of body fatness

Table 4 Correlations between the CVD risk factors and measures of body size, by sex

Sex	Characteristic	Total cholesterol	Triglycerides	LDL cholesterol	Non-HDL Cholesterol	HDL cholesterol	SBP	DBP
Boys	Adjusted BMI	0.20	0.39	0.24	0.31	−0.34	0.32	−0.01
	$PBF_{Slaughter}$	0.21	0.40	0.25	0.32	−0.34	0.25*	0.02*
	PBF_{DXA}	0.20	0.37	0.25	0.31	−0.33	0.27*	0.03*
Girls	Adjusted BMI	0.07	0.14	0.11	0.19	−0.31	0.32	−0.01
	$PBF_{Slaughter}$	0.10	0.15	0.11	0.21	−0.29	0.21*	0.08*
	PBF_{DXA}	0.11	0.15	0.15	0.22	−0.29	0.21*	0.05*

[a] Levels of triglycerides were log transformed

* P-values assesses whether the correlation between the risk factor and adjusted BMI is equal to the correlation between the risk factor and either $PBF_{Slaughter}$ or PBF_{DXA}. Among boys, for example, levels of SBP were more strongly associated with adjusted BMI ($r = 0.32$) than with PBF_{DXA} ($r = 0.25$). * $p \leq 0.01$, H_0: correlation of risk factor with adjusted BMI is equal to its correlation with $PBF_{Slaughter}$ or PBF_{DXA}

Table 5 Correlations between the CVD risk factors and measures of body size, by race-ethnicity

Race-ethnicity	Characteristic	Total cholesterol	Triglycerides [a]	LDL cholesterol	Non-HDL Cholesterol	HDL cholesterol	SBP	DBP
White non-Hispanics (*N* = 2026)	Adjusted BMI	0.14	0.31	0.17	0.26	−0.35	0.31	−0.03
	$PBF_{Slaughter}$	0.17	0.33	0.17	0.27	−0.30*	0.21*	0.05*
	PBF_{DXA}	0.17	0.25	0.16	0.26	−0.26*	0.22*	0.07*
Black non-Hispanics (*N* = 2433)	Adjusted BMI	0.11	0.32	0.20	0.24	−0.32	0.32	0.03
	$PBF_{Slaughter}$	0.12	0.31	0.24*	0.26	−0.32	0.25*	0.07*
	PBF_{DXA}	0.10	0.24	0.21	0.23	−0.31	0.21*	0.08*
Mexican-Americans (*N* = 2547)	Adjusted BMI	0.19	0.39	0.26	0.30	−0.32	0.35	0.00
	$PBF_{Slaughter}$	0.19	0.37	0.25	0.30	−0.31	0.25*	0.04*
	PBF_{DXA}	0.15*	0.32	0.19	0.25*	−0.30	0.24*	0.06*

[a]Levels of triglycerides were log transformed
**P*-values assesses whether the correlation between the risk factor and adjusted BMI is equal to the correlation between the risk factor and either $PBF_{Slaughter}$ or PBF_{DXA}. Among white non-Hispanics, for example, levels of SBP were more strongly associated with adjusted BMI ($r = 0.31$) than with PBF_{DXA} ($r = 0.22$). * $p \leq 0.01$, H_0: correlation of risk factor with adjusted BMI is equal to its correlation with $PBF_{Slaughter}$ or PBF_{DXA}

[44]. For example, whereas various skinfold thicknesses and equations were stronger predictors of body fatness (determined from a 4-compartment model) than was BMI (R^2s of ~0.85 vs. 0.67) [3], the multiple R^2 for individual skinfolds varied from 0.76 (thigh) to 0.85 (biceps) [45].

It is possible that much of the discrepancy between $PBF_{Slaughter}$ and PBF_{DXA} in the current study results from the relatively thin children and adolescents in the sample ($n = 242$) in which the Slaughter equations were developed [31]. Although BMI levels were not reported in this 1988 paper, these participants weighed less and had much thinner skinfolds than did those in the current analysis. For example, the mean SF sum among the 58 post-pubescent boys in the 1988 study was 18 mm (SD = 7) [31], whereas the mean SF sum among the 2572 14- to 19-year-old boys in the current study was 50 % larger (27 mm). It is unlikely that equations developed among relatively thin children can accurately estimate the body fatness of the much heavier children and adolescents in the current U.S. population.

In agreement with our results among the heaviest children, a previous analysis of data from the Pediatric Rosetta Body Composition Project obtained using Lunar models DPX and DPX-L [19] also found that the Slaughter skinfold thickness equations overestimate DXA-calculated percent body fat among heavy children. As shown in Fig. 2, this overestimation likely results from the functional form of the Slaughter equations. Although the Slaughter equations include a squared term for the SF sum [31], this term has very little influence on the estimated values. Furthermore, at SF sum values > 35 mm, the Slaughter equations are linear, with each 1 mm increase in the SF sum associated with a 0.783 (boys) or 0.546 (girls) increase in the estimate of percent body fat. As shown in Fig. 2, there is a nearly linear relationship between the SF sum and $PBF_{Slaughter}$ throughout the entire range of SF sum values, while the relation of the SF sum to PBF_{DXA} is strongly curvilinear.

In general, the magnitudes of the associations with CVD risk factor levels that we observed agree fairly well with previous reports, including an analysis of NHANES 1999-2004 data that examined the relation of PBF_{DXA} to levels of lipids and lipoproteins [46]. Many investigators have found levels of various risk factors to be related similarly to levels of BMI and to estimates of body fatness calculated from skinfold thicknesses [17, 19], air-displacement plethysmography [13] and DXA [14–16]. This similarity may arise because the associations are largely influenced by risk factor levels among obese children, among whom BMI is a relatively good indicator of fatness [3], or because of the errors in measurement associated with skinfold thicknesses [5]. We did, however, observe some consistent differences in the associations with blood pressure, with BMI showing the strongest ($p < 0.01$) association with SBP but the weakest association with DBP.

There are additional limitations of the current, cross-sectional analyses that should be considered. Although the errors in the measurement of skinfold thicknesses are well known [5]. DXA estimates of the body fatness of an individual can also differ substantially from those obtained with the 4-compartment model and neutron activation [47]. It is also possible that DXA underestimates the body fatness of leaner persons and overestimates the fatness of obese persons [48], but if this occurred in the current study, the $PBF_{Slaughter}$ overestimation of the body fatness of obese children may be even greater than what we observed. Although errors may have also been introduced by our use of age as a surrogate for pubertal maturation, we observed the largest discrepancies between PBF_{DXA} and $PBF_{Slaughter}$ among boys with thick skinfolds; among these boys, $PBF_{Slaughter}$ is based on only the SF sum [31]. It should also be realized that because BMI performs better as an indicator of body fatness among children who have relatively high levels of percent body fat than among thinner children [4, 20, 45], our results may not apply to populations in which the prevalence of obesity is relatively low.

Conclusion

Our results indicate that the Slaughter skinfold thickness equations of percent body fat are biased, with $PBF_{Slaughter}$ overestimating the body fatness of obese children, particularly obese boys. Furthermore, with the exception of very weak associations with DBP levels, adjusted (for sex and age) BMI values are as strongly associated with levels of various CVD risk factors as is $PBF_{Slaughter}$. Our results do not support the possibility that the assessment of CVD risk among children and adolescents could be improved through the measurement of skinfold thicknesses or the use of DXA-calculated percent body fat rather than BMI.

Abbreviations

BMI: Body mass index; CDC: Centers for disease control and prevention; DXA: Dual energy x-ray absorptiometry; NHANES: National health and nutrition examination survey; PBF_{DXA}: Percent body fat estimated by dual energy X-ray absorptiometry; $PBF_{Slaughter}$: Percent body fat estimated by the Slaughter skinfold thickness equations.

Competing interests

The authors declare that they have no competing interests.

Authors' contributions

DF developed the idea for the analyses, performed most of the analyses, and drafted the manuscript. CO and BK critiqued the analyses, performed some of the analyses, helped to draft the manuscript, and made revisions to the text. All authors read and approved the final manuscript.

Acknowledgements

None of the authors received funding for data analysis or for the preparation of the manuscript. We thank the U.S. National Center for Health Statistics for collecting the data used in the current study and for making these data publicly available to researchers (http://wwwn.cdc.gov/Nchs/Nhanes/Search/DataPage.aspx?Component=Examination&CycleBeginYear=2003). Neither scientific editors/writers nor funding bodies had any role in the analysis of data for this paper or in the preparation of the manuscript.
The findings and conclusions in this report are those of the authors and do not necessarily represent the official position of the Centers for Disease Control.

Author details

[1]Division of Nutrition, Physical Activity, and Obesity, Centers for Disease Control and Prevention, Atlanta, GA, USA. [2]National Center for Health Statistics, Centers for Disease Control and Prevention, Hyattsville, MD, USA.

References

1. Reilly JJ, Methven E, McDowell ZC, Hacking B, Alexander D, Stewart L, et al. Health consequences of obesity. Arch Dis Child. 2003;88:748–52.
2. Krebs NF, Himes JH, Jacobson D, Nicklas TA, Guilday P, Styne D. Assessment of child and adolescent overweight and obesity. Pediatrics. 2007;120(Suppl):S193–228.
3. Bray GA, DeLany JP, Volaufova J, Harsha DW, Champagne C. Prediction of body fat in 12-y-old African American and white children: evaluation of methods. Am J Clin Nutr. 2002;76:980–90.
4. Freedman DS, Sherry B. The validity of BMI as an indicator of body fatness and risk among children. Pediatrics. 2009;124(Suppl):S23–34.
5. Ulijaszek SJ, Kerr DA. Anthropometric measurement error and the assessment of nutritional status. Br J Nutr. 1999;82:165–77.
6. Martin AD, Ross WD, Drinkwater DT, Clarys JP. Prediction of body fat by skinfold caliper: assumptions and cadaver evidence. Int J Obes. 1985;9 Suppl 1:31–9.
7. Laurson KR, Eisenmann JC, Welk GJ. Body fat percentile curves for U.S. children and adolescents. Am J Prev Med. 2011;41(4 Suppl 2):S87–92.
8. Going SB, Lohman TG, Cussler EC, Williams DP, Morrison JA, Horn PS. Percent body fat and chronic disease risk factors in U.S. children and youth. Am J Prev Med. 2011;41(4 Suppl 2):S77–86.
9. Goacher PJ, Lambert R, Moffatt PG. Can weight-related health risk be more accurately assessed by BMI, or by gender specific calculations of Percentage Body Fatness? Med Hypotheses. 2012;79:656–62.
10. Sardinha LB, Going SB, Teixeira PJ, Lohman TG. Receiver operating characteristic analysis of body mass index, triceps skinfold thickness, and arm girth for obesity screening in children and adolescents. Am J Clin Nutr. 1999;70:1090–5.
11. Freedman DS, Wang J, Ogden CL, Thornton JC, Mei Z, Pierson RN, et al. The prediction of body fatness by BMI and skinfold thicknesses among children and adolescents. Ann Hum Biol. 2007;34:183–94.
12. Wannamethee SG, Shaper AG, Morris RW, Whincup PH. Measures of adiposity in the identification of metabolic abnormalities in elderly men. Am J Clin Nutr. 2005;81:1313–21.
13. Bosy-Westphal A, Geisler C, Onur S, Korth O, Selberg O, Schrezenmeir J, et al. Value of body fat mass vs anthropometric obesity indices in the assessment of metabolic risk factors. Int J Obes (Lond). 2006;30:475–83.
14. Sun Q, Dam RM, Van Spiegelman D, Heymsfield SB, Willett WC, Hu FB, et al. Comparison of dual-energy x-ray absorptiometric and anthropometric measures of adiposity in relation to adiposity-related biologic factors. Am J Epidemiol. 2010;172:1442–54.
15. Weber DR, Leonard MB, Shults J, Zemel BS. A comparison of fat and lean body mass index to BMI for the identification of metabolic syndrome in children and adolescents. J Clin Endocrinol Metab. 2014;99:3208–16.
16. Hemmingsson E, Uddén J, Neovius M. No apparent progress in bioelectrical impedance accuracy: validation against metabolic risk and DXA. Obesity (Silver Spring). 2009;17:183–7.
17. Freedman DS, Katzmarzyk PT, Dietz WH, Srinivasan SR, Berenson GS. Relation of body mass index and skinfold thicknesses to cardiovascular disease risk factors in children: the Bogalusa Heart Study. Am J Clin Nutr. 2009;90:210–6.
18. Lawlor DA, Benfield L, Logue J, Tilling K, Howe LD, Fraser A, et al. Association between general and central adiposity in childhood, and change in these, with cardiovascular risk factors in adolescence: prospective cohort study. BMJ. 2010;341:c6224.
19. Freedman DS, Horlick M, Berenson GS. A comparison of the Slaughter skinfold-thickness equations and BMI in predicting body fatness and cardiovascular disease risk factor levels in children. Am J Clin Nutr. 2013;98:1417–24.
20. Steinberger J, Jacobs DR, Raatz S, Moran A, Hong CP, Sinaiko AR. Comparison of body fatness measurements by BMI and skinfolds vs dual energy X-ray absorptiometry and their relation to cardiovascular risk factors in adolescents. Int J Obes. 2005;29:1346–52.
21. Lohman TG, Pollock ML, Slaughter MH, Brandon LJ, Boileau RA. Methodological factors and the prediction of body fat in female athletes. Med Sci Sports Exerc. 1984;16:92–6.
22. Ogden CL, Li Y, Freedman DS, Borrud LG, Flegal KM: Smoothed percentage body fat percentiles for U.S. children and adolescents, 1999-2004. Natl Heal Stat Rep 2011:1–7.[http://www.cdc.gov/nchs/products/nhsr.htm.]
23. The 1999-2004 Dual Energy X-ray Absorptiometry (DXA) Multiple Imputation Data Files and Technical Documentation [http://www.cdc.gov/nchs/nhanes/dxx/dxa.htm]
24. National Health and Nutrition Examination Survey: Technical Documentation for the 1999-2004 Dual Energy X-Ray Absorptiometry (DXA) Multiple Imputation Data files [http://www.cdc.gov/nchs/data/nhanes/dxa/dxa_techdoc.pdf]
25. Kuczmarski RJ, Ogden CL, Guo SS, Grummer-Strawn LM, Flegal KM, Mei Z, et al. 2000 CDC Growth charts for the United States: methods and development. Vital Health Stat 11. 2002;11:1–190.
26. Flegal KM, Wei R, Ogden CL, Freedman DS, Johnson CL, Curtin LR. Characterizing extreme values of body mass index-for-age by using the 2000 centers for disease control and prevention growth charts. Am J Clin Nutr. 2009;90:1314–20.

27. Cut-offs to define outliers in the 2000 CDC Growth Charts [http://www.cdc.gov/nccdphp/dnpa/growthcharts/resources/BIV-cutoffs.pdf]
28. Berkey CS, Colditz GA. Adiposity in adolescents: Change in actual BMI works better than change in BMIz score for longitudinal studies. Ann Epidemiol. 2007;17:44–50.
29. AMELIA II: A Program for Missing Data [http://cran.r-project.org/package=Amelia]
30. R: A language and environment for statistical computing. R Foundation for Statistical Computing: Vienna, Austria. [http://www.r-project.org/]
31. Slaughter MH, Lohman TG, Boileau RA, Horswill CA, Stillman RJ, Van Loan MD, et al. Skinfold equations for estimation of body fatness in children and youth. Hum Biol. 1988;60:709–23.
32. NHANES 1999-2000 Data Documentation, Codebook, and Frequencies. Triglycerides and LDL-Cholesterol Data (Lab13am) [http://www.cdc.gov/nchs/nhanes/nhanes1999-2000/Lab13am.htm]
33. NHANES 2003 - 2004: Total Cholesterol and HDL Data Documentation, Codebook, and Frequencies [http://www.cdc.gov/nchs/nhanes/nhanes2003-2004/l13_c.htm]
34. Friedewald WT, Levy RI, Fredrickson DS. Estimation of the concentration of low-density lipoprotein cholesterol in plasma, without use of the preparative ultracentrifuge. Clin Chem. 1972;18:499–502.
35. National High Blood Pressure Education Program Working Group on High Blood Pressure in Children and Adolescents. The fourth report on the diagnosis, evaluation, and treatment of high blood pressure in children and adolescents. Pediatrics. 2004;114(2 Suppl 4th Report):555–76.
36. Lumley T. Analysis of complex survey samples. Hoboken, N.J.: John Wiley & Sons; 2010.
37. Schenker N, Borrud LG, Burt VL, Curtin LR, Flegal KM, Hughes J, et al. Multiple imputation of missing dual-energy X-ray absorptiometry data in the national health and nutrition examination survey. Stat Med. 2010;30:260–76.
38. Little RJA, Rubin DB. Statistical analysis with missing data; second edition. Hoboken, NJ: John Wiley & Sons; 2002.
39. Donders ART, van der Heijden GJMG, Stijnen T, Moons KGM, Donders AR T. Review: a gentle introduction to imputation of missing values. J Clin Epidemiol.2006;59:1087–91.
40. Khare M, Little R, Rubin D, Schafer J: Multiple imputation of NHANES III. Proceedings of the American Statistical Association, Survey Research Methods Section. 1993;297-302.https://scholar.google.com/scholar?hl=en&q=MULTIPLE+IMPUTATION+OF+NHANES+III&btnG=&as_sdt=1%2C11&as_sdtp=]
41. Schafer JL. Multiple imputation: a primer. Stat Methods Med Res. 1999;8:3–15.
42. Bland JM, Altman DG. Statistical methods for assessing agreement between two methods of clinical measurement. Lancet. 1986;1:307–10.
43. Himes JH, Bouchard C. Validity of anthropometry in classifying youths as obese. Int J Obes. 1989;13:183–93.
44. Martin AD, Drinkwater DT. Variability in the measures of body fat. Assumptions or technique? Sports Med. 1991;11:277–88.
45. Bray GA, DeLany JP, Harsha DW, Volaufova J, Champagne CC. Evaluation of body fat in fatter and leaner 10-y-old African american and white children: the baton rouge Children's study. Am J Clin Nutr. 2001;73:687–702.
46. Lamb MM, Ogden CL, Carroll MD, Lacher DA, Flegal KM. Association of body fat percentage with lipid concentrations in children and adolescents: United States, 1999–2004. Am J Clin Nutr. 2011;94:877–83.
47. Toombs RJ, Ducher G, Shepherd JA, De Souza MJ. The impact of recent technological advances on the trueness and precision of DXA to assess body composition. Obesity (Silver Spring). 2012;20:30–9.
48. Van Der Ploeg GE, Withers RT, Laforgia J. Percent body fat via DEXA: comparison with a four-compartment model. J Appl Physiol. 2003;94:499–506.

Permissions

All chapters in this book were first published in PEDIATRICS, by BioMed Central; hereby published with permission under the Creative Commons Attribution License or equivalent. Every chapter published in this book has been scrutinized by our experts. Their significance has been extensively debated. The topics covered herein carry significant findings which will fuel the growth of the discipline. They may even be implemented as practical applications or may be referred to as a beginning point for another development.

The contributors of this book come from diverse backgrounds, making this book a truly international effort. This book will bring forth new frontiers with its revolutionizing research information and detailed analysis of the nascent developments around the world.

We would like to thank all the contributing authors for lending their expertise to make the book truly unique. They have played a crucial role in the development of this book. Without their invaluable contributions this book wouldn't have been possible. They have made vital efforts to compile up to date information on the varied aspects of this subject to make this book a valuable addition to the collection of many professionals and students.

This book was conceptualized with the vision of imparting up-to-date information and advanced data in this field. To ensure the same, a matchless editorial board was set up. Every individual on the board went through rigorous rounds of assessment to prove their worth. After which they invested a large part of their time researching and compiling the most relevant data for our readers.

The editorial board has been involved in producing this book since its inception. They have spent rigorous hours researching and exploring the diverse topics which have resulted in the successful publishing of this book. They have passed on their knowledge of decades through this book. To expedite this challenging task, the publisher supported the team at every step. A small team of assistant editors was also appointed to further simplify the editing procedure and attain best results for the readers.

Apart from the editorial board, the designing team has also invested a significant amount of their time in understanding the subject and creating the most relevant covers. They scrutinized every image to scout for the most suitable representation of the subject and create an appropriate cover for the book.

The publishing team has been an ardent support to the editorial, designing and production team. Their endless efforts to recruit the best for this project, has resulted in the accomplishment of this book. They are a veteran in the field of academics and their pool of knowledge is as vast as their experience in printing. Their expertise and guidance has proved useful at every step. Their uncompromising quality standards have made this book an exceptional effort. Their encouragement from time to time has been an inspiration for everyone.

The publisher and the editorial board hope that this book will prove to be a valuable piece of knowledge for researchers, students, practitioners and scholars across the globe.

List of Contributors

Lewis K Peake, Elizabeth S Draper, Judith LS Budd and David Field
Department of Health Sciences, University of Leicester, Leicester LE1 6TP, UK

Noriko Motoki, Yuji Inaba, Satoshi Matsuzaki, Yohei Akazawa, Takafumi Nishimura, Tetsuhiro Fukuyama and Kenichi Koike
Department of Pediatrics, Shinshu University School of Medicine, Asahi 3-1-1, Matsumoto 390-8621, Japan

Chia-Pei Chou
Department of Family Medicine, Kaohsiung Chang Gung Memorial Hospital and Chang Gung University College of Medicine, No.123, Dapi Rd., Niaosong Dist., Kaohsiung City 833, Taiwan, R.O.C

I-Chun Lin and Kuang-Che Kuo
Department of Pediatrics, Kaohsiung Chang Gung Memorial Hospital and Chang Gung University College of Medicine, No.123, Dapi Rd., Niaosong Dist., Kaohsiung City 833, Taiwan, R.O.C.

Margery A. Connelly, Deborah A. Winegar, Irina Shalaurova, Ray Pourfarzib and James D. Otvos
LipoScience, Laboratory Corporation of America® Holdings, 2500 Sumner Blvd, Raleigh, NC 27616, USA

Chisato Shimizu, John T. Kanegaye, Adriana H. Tremoulet and Jane C. Burns
Department of Pediatrics, University of California, San Diego, CA, USA
Rady Children's Hospital, San Diego, CA, USA

Anthony Batte
Child Health and Development Centre, Makerere University College of Health Sciences, Kampala, Uganda

Peter Lwabi and Sulaiman Lubega
Uganda Heart Institute, Kampala, Uganda

Sarah Kiguli and and Charles Karamagi
Department of Pediatrics and Child Health, Makerere University College of Health Sciences, Kampala, Uganda

Kennedy Otwombe
Perinatal HIV Research Unit, Faculty of Health Sciences, University of the Witwatersrand, Johannesburg, South Africa

Lucy Chimoyi
The Aurum Institute, Johannesburg, South Africa

Violette Nabatte
Nakaseke Hospital, Nakeseke, Uganda

Charles Karamagi
Clinical Epidemiology Unit, Makerere University College of Health Sciences, Kampala, Uganda

Leilei Pei, Yijun Kang, Yaling Zhao and Hong Yan
Department of Epidemiology and Health Statistics, School of Public Health, Xi'an Jiaotong University Health Science Center, Xi'an, Shaanxi 710061, People's Republic of China

Mirthe J. Mebius, Arend F. Bos and Elisabeth M. W. Kooi
University Medical Center Groningen, Beatrix Children's Hospital, Division of Neonatology, University of Groningen, Hanzeplein 1, 9713 GZ Groningen, The Netherlands

Diana W. Wolthuis
University Medical Center Groningen, Beatrix Children's Hospital, Division of Pediatric Intensive Care, University of Groningen, Groningen, The Netherlands

Gideon J. du Marchie Sarvaas and Beatrijs Bartelds
University Medical Center Groningen, Center for Congenital Heart Diseases, Pediatric Cardiology, Beatrix Children's Hospital, University of Groningen, Groningen, The Netherlands

Martin C. J. Kneyber
Critical Care, Anesthesiology, Peri-operative & Emergency medicine (CAPE), the University of Groningen, Groningen, The Netherlands

J . Tony Nengom, S. Sap Ngo Um, D. Chelo, R. Mbono Betoko, J. Boombhi, F. Mouafo Tambo, A. Chiabi, S. Kingue and P. Koki Ndombo
Faculty of Medicine and Biomedical Sciences of Yaounde I University, Yaounde, Cameroon

S. Sap Ngo Um and D. Chelo
Mother and Child Centre of the Chantal Biya Foundation, Yaounde, Cameroon

J. Boombhi, S. Kingue and P. Koki Ndombo
Yaounde General Hospital, Yaounde, Cameroon

Mouafo Tambo and A. Chiabi
Yaounde Gyneco Obstetric and Pediatric Hospital, Yaounde, Cameroon

Xiao-li Wu, Ru Li, Fang Fu, Min Pan, Jin Han, Xin Yang, Yong-ling Zhang, Fa-tao Li and Can Liao
Prenatal Diagnostic Center, Guangzhou Women and Children's Medical Center, Guangzhou Medical University, No. 9 Jinsui Road, Guangdong, China

Enora Laas, Nathalie Lelong, Pierre-Yves Ancel, Thibaut Andrieu, François Goffinet and Babak Khoshnood
Obstetrical, perinatal and pediatric epidemiology research team, Center for biostatistics and epidemiology, INSERM U1153, Maternité de Port-Royal, 6ème étage, 53 av. de l'Observatoire, 75014 Paris, France

Lucile Houyel
Service de chirurgie des cardiopathies congénitales, Hôpital Marie Lannelongue, 133, avenue de la Résistance, 92350 Le Plessis Robinson, France

Damien Bonnet
Centre de référence M3C-Necker, Université Paris Descartes, 140 rue de Sèvres, 75015 Paris, France

Jean-François Magny
Service de pédiatrie et réanimation néonatales CHU Necker Enfants Malades, Paris, France

François Goffinet
Maternité Port Royal, 53 avenue de l'Observatoire, 75014 Paris, France

Ming-Yu Liu, Hsin-Min Liu, Chia-Hui Wu, Chun-An Chen, Shuenn-Nan Chiu, Chun-Wei Lu, Ming-Tai Lin, Luan-Yin Chang, Jou-Kou Wang and Mei-Hwan Wu
Department of Pediatrics, National Taiwan University Hospital and Medical College, National Taiwan University, No. 7, Chung-Shan South Road, Taipei 100, Taiwan

Chin-Hao Chang
Department of Medical Research, National Taiwan University Hospital, Taipei, Taiwan

Guan-Jr Huang
Medical Information Management Office, National Taiwan University Hospital, Taipei, Taiwan

Zhenquan Wang, Fengfeng Weng, Zhangke Tang, Huixian Qiu, Yue'e He, Rongzhou Wu and Maoping Chu
Children's Heart Center, the Second Affiliated Hospital and Yuying Children's Hospital, Institute of cardiovascular development and translational medicine, Wenzhou Medical University, Wenzhou, Zhejiang 325027, China

Chen Li
Children's Hospital, Zhejiang University School of Medicine, Hangzhou, Zhejiang 310051, China

Hongying Shi
Department of Preventive Medicine, School of Environmental Science and Public Health, Wenzhou Medical University, Wenzhou, Zhejiang 325035, China

Christoph E. Schwarz
Department of Neonatology, University Children's Hospital, Calwerstr. 7, 72076 Tuebingen, Germany

Antonio Preusche
Department of Neonatology, University Children's Hospital, Tuebingen, Germany

Martin Wolf
Department of Neonatology, University Hospital Zurich, Zurich, Switzerland

Christian F. Poets
Department of Neonatology, University Children's Hospital, Tuebingen, Germany

Axel R. Franz
Department of Neonatology, University Children's Hospital, Tuebingen, Germany
Center for Pediatric Clinical Studies, University Children's Hospital, Tuebingen, Germany

Lisa Ha Barstad, Pétur B. Júlíusson, Line Kristin Johnson, Jens Kristoffer Hertel, Samira Lekhal and Jøran Hjelmesæth
Morbid Obesity Centre, Vestfold Hospital Trust, 3103 Tønsberg, Norway

Pétur B. Júlíusson
Department of Clinical Science, University of Bergen, 5021 Bergen, Norway

Jøran Hjelmesæth
Department of Endocrinology, Morbid Obesity and Preventive Medicine, Institute of Clinical Medicine, University of Oslo, Oslo, Norway

Julie Korol Wright
Tropical Disease Unit, Division of Infectious Diseases, Department of Medicine, University of Toronto, Toronto, ON, Canada

Kyla Hayford, Vanessa Tran and Kevin C. Kain
Sandra Rotman Centre for Global Health, University Health Network-Toronto General Hospital, Department of Medicine, University of Toronto, Toronto, ON, Canada

Gulam Muhammed Al Kibria
Department of International Health, Bloomberg School of Public Health, Johns Hopkins University, Baltimore, MD, USA

Arif Mahmud, Nazma Begum, Abdullah Baqui and Azadeh Farzin
International Centre for Maternal and Newborn Health, Department of International Health, Bloomberg School of Public Health, Johns Hopkins University, Baltimore, MD, USA

Ali Manajjir
Department of Pediatrics, Sylhet MAG Osmani Medical College Hospital, Sylhet, Bangladesh

Mashuk Siddiquee
Dhaka Shishu (Children's) Hospital, Sher-E-Bangla Nagar, Dhaka, Bangladesh

Azadeh Farzin
Division of Neonatology, Department of Pediatrics, Johns Hopkins University School of Medicine, Baltimore, MD, USA

Elzbieta Pac-Kozuchowska and Paulina Krawiec
Department of Paediatrics and Gastroenterology, Medical University of Lublin, Gebali 6 Street, 20-093 Lublin, Poland

Ewelina Grywalska
Department of Clinical Immunology and Immunotherapy, Medical University of Lublin, Chodzki 4a Street, 20-093 Lublin, Poland

Tadej Petek, Tjaša Hertiš and Nataša Marčun Varda
Faculty of Medicine, University of Maribor, Taborska ulica 8, 2000 Maribor, Slovenia

Nataša Marčun Varda
Department of Paediatrics, University Medical Centre Maribor, Ljubljanska ulica 5, 2000 Maribor, Slovenia

Maria João Fonseca, Milton Severo, Henrique Barros and Ana Cristina Santos
EPIUnit - Instituto de Saúde Pública, Universidade do Porto, Rua das Taipas n° 135, 4050-600 Porto, Portugal

Milton Severo, Henrique Barros and Ana Cristina Santos
Departamento de Ciências da Saúde Pública e Forenses e Educação Médica, Faculdade de Medicina, Universidade do Porto, Porto, Portugal

Debbie A. Lawlor
Medical Research Council Integrative Epidemiology Unit at the University of Bristol, Bristol, UK
School of Social and Community Medicine, University of Bristol, Bristol, UK

Xike Wang, Haitao Wei, Ying Tian and Yue Wu
Department of paediatrics, Guizhou Provincial People's Hospital, Guiyang 550002, China

Lei Luo
Department of science and education, Guizhou Provincial People's Hospital, Guiyang 550002, China

Nicole Ata, David C Hamilton and Stefan Kuhle
Departments of Pediatrics and Obstetrics & Gynaecology, Dalhousie University, Halifax, NS, Canada

Bryan Maguire
Department of Mathematics and Statistics, Dalhousie University, Halifax, NS, Canada

Mariam Noorani and Nuruddin Lakhani
Aga Khan Hospital, Dar es Salaam, Tanzania

Eduardo Macias and Shafkat Anwar
Division of Cardiology, Department of Pediatrics, Washington University School of Medicine in St. Louis, One Children's Place, Campus NWT, St. Louis, MO 63110, USA

Elizabeth Nieman
Division of Dermatology, Department of Medicine, Washington University School of Medicine, St. Louis, MO, USA

Kentaro Yomogida and Kevin Baszis
Division of Rheumatology, Department of Pediatrics, Washington University School of Medicine, St. Louis, MO, USA

Orlando Petrucci
Division of Cardiothoracic Surgery, Department of Surgery, Washington University School of Medicine, St. Louis, MO, USA

Cylen Javidan
Mallinckrodt Institute of Radiology, Washington University School of Medicine, St. Louis, MO, USA

Golaleh Asghari
Department of Clinical Nutrition and Dietetics, Faculty of Nutrition Sciences and Food Technology, National Nutrition and Food Technology Research Institute, Shahid Beheshti University of Medical Sciences, Tehran, Iran

Pooneh Dehghan
Department of Imaging, Research Development Center, Taleghani Hospital, Shahid Beheshti University of Medical Sciences, Tehran, Iran

Parvin Mirmiran
Nutrition and Endocrine Research Center, Research Institute for Endocrine Sciences, Shahid Beheshti University of Medical Sciences, Tehran, Iran

Emad Yuzbashian
Nutrition and Endocrine Research Center, Research Institute for Endocrine Sciences, Shahid Beheshti University of Medical Sciences, Tehran, Iran

Maryam Mahdavi
Obesity Research Center, Research Institute for Endocrine Sciences, Shahid Beheshti University of Medical Sciences, Tehran, Iran

Maryam Tohidi
Prevention of Metabolic Disorders Research Center, Research Institute for Endocrine Sciences, Shahid Beheshti University of Medical Sciences, Tehran, Iran

Tirang R. Neyestani
Laboratory of Nutrition Research, National Nutrition and Food Technology Research Institute, Faculty of Nutrition Sciences and Food Technology, Shahid Beheshti University of Medical Sciences, Tehran, Iran

Farhad Hosseinpanah
Obesity Research Center, Research Institute for Endocrine Sciences, Shahid Beheshti University of Medical Sciences, Tehran, Iran

Fereidoun Azizi
Endocrine Research Center, Research Institute for Endocrine Sciences, Shahid Beheshti University of Medical Sciences, Tehran, Iran

Seo Hee Yoon, Dong Soo Kim and Jong Gyun Ahn
Department of Pediatrics, Severance Children's Hospital, Yonsei University College of Medicine, 50-1 Yonsei-ro, Seodaemun-gu, Seoul 03722, South Korea

Takanori Noto, Hiroki Seto, Junji Fukuhara, Masao Murabayashi, Mamoru Ayusawa and Ichiro Morioka
Department of Pediatrics, Numazu City Hospital, 550, Harunoki, Higashi-Shiroji, Numazu 4100302, Japan

Takanori Noto, Hiroki Seto, Junji Fukuhara, Masao Murabayashi, Mamoru Ayusawa and Ichiro Morioka
Department of Pediatrics and Child Health, Nihon University School of Medicine, 30-1, Oyaguchi, Kami-cho, Itabashi-ku, Tokyo 173-8610, Japan

Akihiro Yachie
Department of Pediatrics, School of Medicine, Institute of Medical, Pharmaceutical and Health Sciences, Kanazawa University, 13-1, Takaramachi, Kanazawa 9208641, Japan

Tonje Bårdsen, Mari Hoven Sørbye, Gottfried Greve and Ansgar Berg
Department of Clinical Science, University of Bergen, Bergen, Norway

Håvard Trønnes
Department of Global Public Health and Primary Care, University of Bergen, Bergen, Norway

Håvard Trønnes and Ansgar Berg
Department of Paediatrics, Haukeland University Hospital, Bergen, Norway

Gottfried Greve
Department of Heart Disease, Haukeland University Hospital, Bergen, Norway

Michael Khoury, Cedric Manlhiot, Nita Chahal and Brian W. McCrindle
Labatt Family Heart Centre, Department of Pediatrics, The Hospital for Sick Children, University of Toronto, 555 University Avenue, Toronto, ON M5G 1X8, Canada

Don Gibson, Karen Stearne and Stafford Dobbin
Heart Niagara Inc., Niagara Falls, ON, Canada

Christoph E. Schwarz, Antonio Preusche, Christian F. Poets and Axel R. Franz
Department of Neonatology, University Children's Hospital of Tuebingen, University of Tuebingen, Calwerstr. 7, 72076 Tuebingen, Germany

Winfried Baden
Department of Pediatric Cardiology, University Children's Hospital of Tuebingen, University of Tuebingen, Tuebingen, Germany

Axel R. Franz
Center for Pediatric Clinical Studies, University Children's Hospital of Tuebingen, University of Tuebingen, Tuebingen, German

David S. Freedman
Division of Nutrition, Physical Activity, and Obesity, Centers for Disease Control and Prevention, Atlanta, GA, USA

Cynthia L. Ogden and Brian K. Kit
National Center for Health Statistics, Centers for Disease Control and Prevention, Hyattsville, MD, USA

Index

CPSIA information can be obtained
at www.ICGtesting.com
Printed in the USA
LVHW060900030122
707669LV00002B/266

9 781639 274239